Posture, Balance, and Gait: Assessment Techniques and Rehabilitation Strategies

Posture, Balance, and Gait: Assessment Techniques and Rehabilitation Strategies

Guest Editors

Vasiliki Sakellari
George Gioftsos

MDPI

Basel • Beijing • Wuhan • Barcelona • Belgrade • Novi Sad • Cluj • Manchester

Guest Editors
Vasiliki Sakellari
Department of Physiotherapy
University of West Attica
(UniWA)
Athens
Greece

George Gioftsos
Department of Physiotherapy
University of West Attica
(UniWA)
Athens
Greece

Editorial Office
MDPI AG
Grosspeteranlage 5
4052 Basel, Switzerland

This is a reprint of the Special Issue, published open access by the journal *Journal of Functional Morphology and Kinesiology* (ISSN 2411-5142), freely accessible at: https://www.mdpi.com/journal/jfmk/special_issues/76CZ2L40OD.

For citation purposes, cite each article independently as indicated on the article page online and as indicated below:

Lastname, A.A.; Lastname, B.B. Article Title. *Journal Name* **Year**, *Volume Number*, Page Range.

ISBN 978-3-7258-6414-0 (Hbk)
ISBN 978-3-7258-6415-7 (PDF)
https://doi.org/10.3390/books978-3-7258-6415-7

Cover image courtesy of Vasiliki Sakellari

Contents

About the Editors

Vasiliki Sakellari

Vasiliki Sakellari is a Professor in the Department of Physiotherapy at the University of West Attica (UniWA), Athens, Greece, and serves as Director of the Postgraduate Programme "New Methods of Physiotherapy". She is a qualified physiotherapist and an Executive Committee Member of the International Federation of Physiotherapy in Occupational Health and Ergonomics (IFPOHE), an ENPHE representative for UniWA, and an active member of the Panhellenic Physiotherapists' Association. She holds an MSc in Ergonomics from University College London and a PhD from the University of London, Institute of Neurology. Her previous academic and administrative roles include Director of the School of Health and Welfare Professions of the TEI of Lamia, Institutional Coordinator of the SOCRATES–Erasmus Program, full member of the General Assembly of the Hellenic Foundation for Research and Innovation (ELIDEK), and Director of the Center for Technological Research of Central Greece. She has extensive experience in coordinating and participating in European-funded research and educational projects, including COST Action CA21122, FP7, and ESPA programs. Her teaching and research interests focus on ergonomics and consulting in physiotherapy, geriatric physiotherapy, evidence-based practice, and clinical education in neurological physiotherapy. She has authored numerous peer-reviewed publications and supervises postgraduate and doctoral research in these fields. ORCID: 0000-0002-9481-996X.

George Gioftsos

George Gioftsos is a Professor of Physiotherapy and Head of the Department of Physiotherapy at the University of West Attica (UniWA), Athens, Greece. He holds a Diploma in Physiotherapy from the Athens Institute of Technology, an MSc in Biomedical Engineering from the University of Surrey, United Kingdom, and a PhD in Biomechanics from the Royal Free Hospital School of Medicine, University of London, where his doctoral research focused on human movement classification using artificial neural networks. He has extensive clinical experience in physiotherapy practice. Prior to joining UniWA, he held senior academic and administrative positions at the Lamia Institute of Technology, including Rector, Vice- Rector, and Director of the School of Health and Welfare Professions. He has supervised doctoral research in collaboration with international institutions, including the University of Manchester, and has participated in major European-funded research projects such as ProFouND and Archimedes, with a focus on fall prevention, movement analysis, and rehabilitation science. His research interests include biomechanics, human movement measurement, musculoskeletal and neurological rehabilitation, fall prevention in older adults, and the evaluation of physiotherapy education. He has received distinctions from the Hellenic Scientific Physiotherapy Society and the Greek State Scholarships Foundation and has served as President of the Scientific Council of the Panhellenic Physiotherapists' Association.

Preface

This Reprint brings together peer reviewed contributions from the Special Issue entitled "Posture, Balance, and Gait: Assessment Techniques and Rehabilitation Strategies", published in the *Journal of Functional Morphology and Kinesiology*. The subject matter of the Reprint lies at the intersection of human movement science, clinical assessment, and rehabilitation practice, with a focus on posture control, balance regulation, and gait performance across the lifespan and across health conditions.

The scope of the Reprint encompasses foundational biomechanical and sensorimotor mechanisms, objective and technology assisted assessment methods, and contemporary rehabilitation interventions applied in diverse populations, including older adults, individuals with neurological or musculoskeletal disorders, and pediatric patients. Collectively, the included studies reflect the current state of knowledge while highlighting emerging methodological and therapeutic directions within physiotherapy and rehabilitation sciences.

The primary aim of this Reprint is to provide clinicians, researchers, educators, and postgraduate students with a coherent and accessible collection of evidence that supports evidence based decision making in the assessment and rehabilitation of posture, balance, and gait. By assembling experimental studies, systematic analyses, and applied clinical research in a single volume, the Reprint facilitates effective knowledge translation from research to practice.

The motivation for preparing this Reprint arises from the growing clinical relevance of movement impairments and fall related risks, alongside rapid advances in wearable technologies, sensor based analysis, and individualized rehabilitation strategies. These developments create both opportunities and challenges for health professionals, reinforcing the need for integrated scientific resources that bridge theory, measurement, and intervention.

This Reprint is addressed to professionals and scholars in physiotherapy, physical medicine and rehabilitation, ergonomics, orthopedics, neurology, geriatrics, and allied health disciplines, as well as to researchers with an interest in human movement, biomechanics, and functional performance. It is our hope that this Reprint will serve as a useful reference, stimulate interdisciplinary dialogue, and support continued innovation in rehabilitation research and clinical practice.

Vasiliki Sakellari and George Gioftsos
Guest Editors

Journal of
Functional Morphology and Kinesiology

MDPI

Editorial

Special Issue "Posture, Balance, and Gait: Assessment Techniques and Rehabilitation Strategies"

Vasiliki Sakellari * and George Gioftsos

Physiotherapy Department, Faculty of Health and Care Sciences, University of West Attica, Agiou Spidonos 28, Egaleo, 12243 Athens, Greece; gioftsos@uniwa.gr
* Correspondence: vsakellari@uniwa.gr

1. Editorial Introduction

Posture, balance, and gait are central determinants of human movement, independence, and quality of life. Their integrity depends on the coordinated interaction of musculoskeletal, sensory, and neural systems. Impairments—whether due to aging, neurological or musculoskeletal conditions, or environmental constraints—can substantially increase the risk of falls, disability, and reduced autonomy.

This Special Issue, "Posture, Balance, and Gait: Assessment Techniques and Rehabilitation Strategies", https://www.mdpi.com/journal/jfmk/special_issues/76CZ2L40OD (accessed on 13 November 2025), presents a curated collection of studies spanning foundational science, methodological innovations, therapeutic strategies, and applied population research. Together, these contributions represent a continuum from theory to clinical application, enhancing our understanding of human movement and guiding evidence-based rehabilitation practice.

Foundational research continues to refine our knowledge of the physiological, biomechanical, and sensory–motor mechanisms that underpin posture, balance, and musculoskeletal function. Spatial attention, for instance, operates through both goal-directed and stimulus-driven processes within the fronto-parietal cortex, enhancing multisensory processing at attended locations regardless of modality [1]. Exercise-based interventions have been shown to improve postural alignment and physical capacities, though their long-term benefits often require continuous training [2]. Conversely, sagittal spinal curves have not demonstrated strong associations with health outcomes such as spinal pain [3]. Somatosensory inputs play a pivotal role in postural control by triggering and scaling automatic postural responses [4], while the cerebellar nuclei integrate diverse sensorimotor signals to support the execution and adaptation of dexterous limb movements—processes disrupted in cerebellar dysfunction [5].

Epidemiological data emphasize the importance of accurate and objective assessment methods: in 2018, more than one in four older adults reported at least one fall, and over 10% sustained a fall-related injury [6]. These findings underline the need for precise tools that move beyond subjective observation. Wearable technologies, such as accelerometers, activity monitors, and pressure sensors, now provide noninvasive, real-time evaluations of gait parameters including cadence, stride length, gait cycle duration, and symmetry [7]. Sensor-based and motion analysis systems further enhance the precision of clinical assessment, supporting data-driven and individualized rehabilitation planning.

Progress in assessment has been matched by advances in therapeutic interventions. Wearable sensors enable clinicians to monitor gait abnormalities over time- and design-personalized rehabilitation strategies [7]. Augmented feedback derived from sensor-based

 https://doi.org/10.3390/jfmk10040457

gait reports offers a valuable complement to traditional assessments, improving treatment planning and outcomes in stroke rehabilitation [8].

Population-focused research provides additional clinical relevance. Osteoarthritis, for example, is strongly associated with limitations in activities of daily living among older adults. Hip or knee osteoarthritis significantly affects mobility, self-care, and domestic activities, with some evidence suggesting stronger effects in men for specific mobility-related tasks [9]. As global mobility limitations rise, such insights underscore the need for targeted, population-specific rehabilitation approaches.

The contributions in this Special Issue can be conceptually grouped into four thematic areas that reflect the translational pathway of rehabilitation research:

1. Foundational and Conceptual Frameworks—studies elucidating the physiological, biomechanical, and sensory–motor bases of posture, balance, and movement.
2. Clinical Assessment Methods—research developing and validating objective measurement tools and predictive models for postural control and gait performance.
3. Rehabilitation Strategies and Interventions—evidence-based approaches ranging from sensory stimulation and exercise to robotic and sensor-assisted therapies.
4. Population-Specific and Applied Research—investigations focusing on distinct cohorts such as athletes, older adults, or patients undergoing surgery.

Collectively, the studies presented in this Special Issue advance both scientific knowledge and clinical practice, offering innovative perspectives on how posture, balance, and gait can be preserved, improved, and optimized across the lifespan.

2. Highlights of Contributions

2.1. Foundational and Conceptual Frameworks (Contribution 1 and 2)

Two contributions, Lerida-Ponce et al. (Contribution 1) and Akao et al. (Contribution 2), provide fundamental insights into the physiological, biomechanical, and sensory–motor mechanisms underlying posture, balance, and musculoskeletal function. Lerida-Ponce et al. focus on the interplay between visual demands and cervical muscle activation, revealing how ocular input integrates with motor control and proprioception. Akao et al. demonstrate how spinal–pelvic alignment and intersegmental interactions shape muscle length and postural control. Together, they establish a conceptual framework that informs both research and clinical approaches to assessment and rehabilitation.

Lerida-Ponce et al. (2025, Contribution 1) conducted a systematic review investigating the links between visual accommodation, cervical muscle activity, and related symptomatology, analyzing seven experimental studies with 308 participants. The findings indicated that accommodative stress consistently increased trapezius electromyographic activity, suggesting a direct connection between ocular effort and cervical muscle activation. This work highlights a functional and anatomical coupling between the visual and cervical systems, expanding the conceptual framework of posture by integrating visual demands with proprioceptive and motor mechanisms. Clinically, it supports interdisciplinary interventions, including optometric training, ergonomic adjustments, and postural re-education to mitigate cervical strain associated with visual fatigue.

Complementing this perspective, Akao et al. (2025, Contribution 2) examined spinal–pelvic alignment and its relationship to muscle shortening in 41 healthy young men, using Shapley Additive Explanation (SHAP) analysis to assess individual and interactive effects of thoracic kyphosis, lumbar lordosis, and anterior pelvic tilt on six key muscles. Results showed that hip-related muscles—iliopsoas, rectus femoris, gluteus maximus, and hamstrings—were strongly influenced by both individual alignments and intersegmental interactions, particularly the thoracic–lumbar interplay. In contrast, back extensors and abdominals were minimally affected. These findings emphasize the need to consider segmental spinal interactions in postural assessment and muscle flexibility interventions.

2.2. Clinical Assessment Methods (Contribution 3, 4, 5, 6 and 7)

A second group of contributions in this Special Issue (Contribution 3, 4, 5, 6 and 7) addresses the evaluation of postural control, gait, and musculoskeletal function, emphasizing objective measurement, psychometric validation, and clinically meaningful interpretation.

Mirando et al. (2025, Contribution 3) investigated the distribution of plantar pressures during quiet stance and gait in 60 healthy adults using a baropodometric platform. The study assessed pressures across ten regions of the foot, revealing that although gait increased overall plantar pressures, the spatial distribution patterns closely resembled those observed during quiet stance. Significant positive correlations between static and dynamic measurements suggested that plantar pressure during gait could, to some extent, be estimated from quiet stance data. Clinically, this provides a practical approach for assessing foot loading, guiding orthotic prescription, and informing postural and gait rehabilitation. By integrating static and dynamic assessments, clinicians can efficiently evaluate foot biomechanics even in settings with limited sensorized equipment, supporting interventions that reduce injury risk and optimize functional performance.

Polo-Ferrero et al. (2025, Contribution 4) focused on fall risk assessment in older adults by evaluating the predictive capacity of the 3-Meter Backward Walk Test (3m-BWT) in 483 community-dwelling participants aged 60–96 years, including 101 individuals with a prior history of falls. Results indicated that slower 3m-BWT performance was significantly associated with previous falls and moderately correlated with established functional assessments, including the Short Physical Performance Battery, Five-Repetition Sit-to-Stand, gait speed, Timed Up-and-Go, and Four-Square Step Test. Optimal cut-off points were proposed to stratify risk, balancing sensitivity and specificity. Although no single test can fully capture the multifactorial nature of falls, the 3m-BWT offers a rapid, easily administered, and sensitive tool to complement comprehensive geriatric evaluations, supporting early identification of individuals at risk and informing targeted preventive interventions.

Gianzina et al. (2025, Contribution 5) extended the application of objective clinical assessment to a clinical population, examining gait impairments in individuals awaiting total knee arthroplasty compared with healthy age-matched controls using wearable inertial sensors. The study assessed 17 gait parameters, including stride duration, cadence, symmetry indices, pelvic tilt, rotation, and obliquity, and propulsion indices for both legs. Patients awaiting TKA demonstrated significantly longer gait cycles, reduced cadence, lower symmetry indices, and decreased propulsion compared with controls, highlighting compensatory gait strategies adopted to reduce knee joint load. The findings emphasize the potential of wearable sensors to provide objective, high-resolution biomechanical data for prehabilitation, functional monitoring, and tailored rehabilitation programs aimed at improving gait performance prior to surgery. This approach also underscores the importance of assessing multiple gait dimensions rather than relying solely on global measures, enhancing sensitivity to subtle functional impairments.

Matsuda et al. (2025, Contribution 6) used two small motion sensors placed on the shank and lower back to estimate knee loading during walking at different step rates. The method showed strong agreement with standard 3D motion analysis, particularly at normal or faster walking speeds, suggesting a simple and practical way to assess knee biomechanics in clinical settings.

Coetzee et al. (2025, Contribution 7) employed a preoperative clinical phenotyping approach in patients with end-stage knee osteoarthritis awaiting total knee replacement in

South Africa. Using exploratory factor analysis on a combination of demographic, functional, physical, and patient-reported variables, three distinct phenotypes were identified: (1) gait and weight—characterized by poor gait mechanics, obesity, and low self-efficacy; (2) central pain—encompassing central sensitization, depressive symptoms, and reduced functional performance; and (3) functional factors—reflecting muscular weakness and sedentary behavior. These phenotypes illustrate the heterogeneity of clinical presentations in end-stage knee osteoarthritis and highlight the need for tailored, multidisciplinary preoperative interventions addressing gait, strength, pain management, psychosocial support, and behavioral change strategies. By stratifying patients according to phenotypic characteristics, clinicians can optimize rehabilitation and enhance post-surgical outcomes.

2.3. Rehabilitation Strategies and Interventions (Contributions 8, 9, and 10)

This group of contributions is classified under "Rehabilitation Strategies and Interventions". Each test structured therapeutic approaches designed to improve balance, gait, and motor recovery in diverse populations. These works evaluate the efficacy of active interventions—ranging from sensory stimulation protocols to treadmill-based and robotic therapies—that aim to enhance postural control, functional mobility, and independence. Taken together, these three contributions reflect the breadth and innovation of contemporary rehabilitation strategies. They highlight the shift toward multimodal, evidence-based rehabilitation strategies that are tailored to both populations needs and technological possibilities. As a group, Contributions 8, 9, and 10 demonstrate how physiotherapy research is increasingly positioned at the intersection of sensory science, motor learning, and technological innovation, paving the way for more precise, effective, and accessible rehabilitation solutions.

Tanaka et al. (2025, Contribution 8) investigated the effects of a novel sensory stimulation protocol targeting the trunk and plantar surfaces in older adults. Using a randomized design, the authors demonstrated that repeated tactile stimulation significantly improved dynamic balance, as measured by center-of-pressure displacement and stability indices. These findings suggest that augmenting sensory input from key postural regions can compensate for age-related declines in proprioception and somatosensation. By activating sensory–motor integration pathways, this low-cost and non-invasive intervention offers a promising avenue for fall prevention and functional mobility support in geriatric populations.

Lepoura et al. (2025, Contribution 9) extended the focus to pediatric neurorehabilitation, evaluating Functional Partial Body Weight Support Treadmill Training (FPBWSTT) in children with ataxia. The study found that structured treadmill-based training improved gait symmetry, walking speed, and dynamic balance, while also reducing ataxic movement patterns. Importantly, the intervention was well tolerated by children, underscoring its clinical feasibility and potential as a complementary therapy in managing balance and mobility deficits associated with pediatric ataxia. By integrating partial weight support with functional, repetitive locomotor practice, FPBWSTT highlights the therapeutic value of task-specific, intensive training paradigms for children with neurological disorders.

Bonanno et al. (2025, Contribution 10) explored the application of robotic-assisted gait training compared with conventional physiotherapy in individuals with chronic stroke. Their randomized controlled trial demonstrated that robotic training resulted in superior improvements in gait parameters, balance control, and lower-limb motor function. The findings underline the ability of robotic systems to deliver high-intensity, repetitive, and precisely controlled locomotor practice, which may surpass the dosage and consistency achievable in standard therapy. By harnessing advanced technology, robotic gait training exemplifies a forward-looking approach that complements therapist-led rehabilitation while expanding therapeutic possibilities for individuals with persistent motor impairments.

2.4. Population-Specific and Applied Research (Contribution 11)

Classified under "Population-Specific and Applied Research", this study shows how examining surfers yields insights not captured in broader populations. By addressing the unique demands of aquatic sports, it demonstrates that targeted activity enhances postural stability and flexibility. Beyond sport performance, these results have translational value for rehabilitation and fall-prevention, illustrating how population-centered research can inform applied health and performance practices.

De Castro-Maqueda et al. (2025, Contribution 11) investigated balance, flexibility, and self-esteem in surfers compared to non-surfers and physically active controls, employing established clinical measures such as the SEBT, Flamenco Test, Sit-and-Reach, and Rosenberg Scale. The study found that surfers demonstrated superior static and dynamic balance, suggesting sport-specific adaptations that surpass the benefits of general physical activity, while no differences emerged in self-esteem.

3. Translational Significance

The collective contributions of this Special Issue underscore the relevance of posture, balance, and gait research for clinical translation. For example, Lerida-Ponce et al. (2025, Contribution 1) identified physiological links between visual accommodation and cervical muscle activity, suggesting that visual demand may influence musculoskeletal tone and pain pathways, with implications for patient management in cervical disorders. Similarly, Mirando et al. (2025, Contribution 3) demonstrated that plantar pressure distribution during gait can be reliably estimated from quiet stance in healthy adults, a finding that may streamline clinical screening protocols and broaden assessment strategies beyond laboratory contexts. Translational value is also evident in the applied studies: Tanaka et al. (2025, Contribution 8) showed that vibratory sensory stimulation of the trunk and sole significantly improves balance and reduces fall risk in older adults, while Lepoura et al. (2025, Contribution 9) provided robust evidence that functional partial bodyweight support treadmill training enhances motor performance and daily mobility in children with ataxia. Complementary to these approaches, Polo-Ferrero et al. (2025, Contribution 4) validated the 3-Meter Backward Walk Test as a promising, though not stand-alone, predictor of fall risk in older adults, underscoring the need for multidimensional screening. Together, these findings illustrate how biomechanical insights, population-specific adaptations, and innovative rehabilitation techniques can be translated into practical strategies for prevention, assessment, and intervention.

4. Future Directions

While the studies in this Special Issue advance both theoretical understanding and clinical application, they also identify key knowledge gaps that outline a forward-looking research agenda. Akao et al. (2025, Contribution 2) underscored the importance of analyzing the interactive effects of thoracic, lumbar, and pelvic alignment on muscle shortening, calling for future investigations that incorporate strength measures and frontal-plane parameters into comprehensive, multidimensional models. Likewise, Gianzina et al. (2025, Contribution 5) reported notable gait impairments among individuals awaiting total knee arthroplasty and emphasized the need for prehabilitation research—particularly interventions integrating strengthening and wearable-sensor feedback—to enhance surgical outcomes. Bonanno et al. (2025, Contribution 10) demonstrated that end-effector robotic gait training may improve motor coordination even in chronic stroke, yet they highlighted the necessity for long-term and cost-effectiveness studies to establish sustainability and clinical value. De Castro-Maqueda et al. (2025, Contribution 11) introduced an innovative perspective by showing that surfing can enhance postural stability, suggesting potential therapeutic applications for balance disorders if validated within controlled rehabilitation settings. Finally, Coetzee et al. (2025, Contribution 7) advanced clinical phenotyping in end-stage knee osteoarthritis, identifying patient subgroups based on gait characteristics, body weight, central sensitization, and functional impairment—thereby supporting the development of phenotype-specific rehabilitation strategies.

Taken together, these directions trace a translational pathway that integrates biomechanical, sensory, technological, and population-focused perspectives, moving toward more personalized and effective rehabilitation paradigms.

5. Conclusions

Taken together, the contributions in this Special Issue illustrate how conceptual advances, methodological innovations, targeted interventions, and applied research collectively shape a coherent framework for translating posture, balance, and gait science into effective clinical and real-world applications. Progress in this field clearly depends on bridging foundational neurophysiological and biomechanical mechanisms with validated assessment tools, developing and testing innovative rehabilitation strategies, and addressing population-specific needs.

This growing body of work reflects a clear shift toward individualized, evidence-based care—emphasizing both prevention and functional recovery across diverse populations. Building on the success of this first edition, we are pleased to announce the launch of the second edition of the Special Issue, "Posture, Balance, and Gait: Assessment Techniques and Rehabilitation Strategies—2nd Edition" https://www.mdpi.com/journal/jfmk/special_issues/C731740M3W (accesssed on 13 November 2025). We warmly invite researchers and clinicians to contribute new insights, technologies, and interdisciplinary approaches that will continue to advance this dynamic and clinically meaningful area of rehabilitation science.

Conflicts of Interest: The authors declare no conflicts of interest.

List of Contributions

1. Lérida-Ponce, M.A.; Lérida-Ortega, M.A.; Sedeño-Vidal, A.; Ibáñez-Vera, A.J. Associations Between Visual Accommodation and Cervical Muscle Activity and Symptomatology: A Systematic Review. *J. Funct. Morphol. Kinesiol.* **2025**, *10*, 252. https://doi.org/10.3390/jfmk10030252.
2. Akao, M.; Ishikura, Y.; Isshiki, T.; Tsukada, S.; Shigetoh, H.; Miyazaki, J. Comprehensive Associations Between Spinal–Pelvic Alignment and Muscle Shortening in Healthy Young Men: An Analysis of Individual and Interactive Effects in the Sagittal Plane Using SHapley Additive exPlanation. *J. Funct. Morphol. Kinesiol.* **2025**, *10*, 259. https://doi.org/10.3390/jfmk10030259.
3. Mirando, M.; Pavese, C.; Pingue, V.; Sozzi, S.; Nardone, A. Can Plantar Pressure Distribution During Gait Be Estimated from Quiet Stance in Healthy Individuals? *J. Funct. Morphol. Kinesiol.* **2025**, *10*, 301. https://doi.org/10.3390/jfmk10030301.
4. Polo-Ferrero, L.; Torres-Alonso, J.; Sánchez-Sánchez, M.C.; Puente-González, A.S.; Barbero-Iglesias, F.J.; Méndez-Sánchez, R. The Predictive Capacity of the 3-Meter Backward Walk Test for Falls in Older Adults: A Case–Control Analysis. *J. Funct. Morphol. Kinesiol.* **2025**, *10*, 154. https://doi.org/10.3390/jfmk10020154.
5. Gianzina, E.; Yiannakopoulos, C.K.; Armenis, E.; Chronopoulos, E. Wearable Sensor Assessment of Gait Characteristics in Individuals Awaiting Total Knee Arthroplasty: A Cross-Sectional, Observational Study. *J. Funct. Morphol. Kinesiol.* **2025**, *10*, 288. https://doi.org/10.3390/jfmk10030288.

6. Matsuda, T.; Watanabe, J.; Sotokawa, T.; Shishime, T.; Katoh, H. Estimation of the External Knee Adduction Moment Using Inertial Measurement Unit Sensors on the Shank and Lower Back: A Pilot Study. *J. Funct. Morphol. Kinesiol.* **2025**, *10*, 356. https://doi.org/10.3390/jfmk10030356.
7. Coetzee, M.; Clifford, A.M.; Bedada, D.T.; Bergh, O.; Louw, Q.A. Preoperative Clinical Phenotyping for Individualised Rehabilitation in End-Stage Knee Osteoarthritis. *J. Funct. Morphol. Kinesiol.* **2025**, *10*, 360. https://doi.org/10.3390/jfmk10030360.
8. Tanaka, T.; Maeda, Y.; Miura, T. Effects of Tactile Sensory Stimulation Training of the Trunk and Sole on Standing Balance Ability in Older Adults: A Randomized Controlled Trial. *J. Funct. Morphol. Kinesiol.* **2025**, *10*, 96. https://doi.org/10.3390/jfmk10010096.
9. Lepoura, A.; Lampropoulou, S.; Galanos, A.; Papadopoulou, M.; Gkrimas, G.; Tziomaki, M.; Sakellari, V. Effects of Functional Partial Body Weight Support Treadmill Training on Mobility in Children with Ataxia: A Randomized Controlled Trial. *J. Funct. Morphol. Kinesiol.* **2025**, *10*, 123. https://doi.org/10.3390/jfmk10020123.
10. Bonanno, M.; De Pasquale, P.; Lombardo Facciale, A.; Dauccio, B.; De Luca, R.; Quartarone, A.; Calabrò, R.S. May Patients with Chronic Stroke Benefit from Robotic Gait Training with an End-Effector? A Case-Control Study. *J. Funct. Morphol. Kinesiol.* **2025**, *10*, 161. https://doi.org/10.3390/jfmk10020161.
11. De Castro-Maqueda, G.; Rosety-Rodríguez, M.A.; Rivero-Vila, M.; Del Rosario Fernández-Santos, J.; Abiko, T. Surf's Up for Postural Stability: A Descriptive Study of Physical Activity, Balance, Flexibility, and Self-Esteem in Healthy Adults. *J. Funct. Morphol. Kinesiol.* **2025**, *10*, 290. https://doi.org/10.3390/jfmk10030290.

References

1. Macaluso, E. Orienting of spatial attention and the interplay between the senses. *Cortex* **2010**, *46*, 282–297. [CrossRef] [PubMed]
2. Porto, A.B.; Nascimento Guimarães, A.; Alves Okazaki, V.H. The effect of exercise on postural alignment: A systematic review. *J. Bodyw. Mov. Ther.* **2024**, *40*, 99–108. [CrossRef] [PubMed]
3. Christensen, S.T.; Hartvigsen, J. Spinal curves and health: A systematic critical review of the epidemiological literature dealing with associations between sagittal spinal curves and health. *J. Manip. Physiol. Ther.* **2008**, *31*, 690–714. [CrossRef] [PubMed]
4. Chiba, R.; Takakusaki, K.; Ota, J.; Yozu, A.; Haga, N. Human upright posture control models based on multisensory inputs; in fast and slow dynamics. *Neurosci. Res.* **2016**, *104*, 96–104. [CrossRef] [PubMed]
5. Thanawalla, A.R.; Chen, A.I.; Azim, E. The cerebellar nuclei and dexterous limb movements. *Neuroscience* **2020**, *450*, 168–183. [CrossRef] [PubMed]
6. Moreland, B.; Kakara, R.; Henry, A. Trends in nonfatal falls and fall-related injuries among adults aged ≥65 years—United States, 2012–2018. *MMWR Morb. Mortal. Wkly. Rep.* **2020**, *69*, 875–881. [CrossRef] [PubMed]
7. Peters, D.; O'Brien, E.; Kamrud, K.; Roberts, S.; Rooney, T.; Thibodeau, K.; Balakrishnan, S.; Gell, N.; Mohapatra, S. Utilization of wearable technology to assess gait and mobility post-stroke: A systematic review. *J. NeuroEng. Rehabil.* **2021**, *18*, 84. [CrossRef] [PubMed]
8. Johansson, G.M.; Öhberg, F. Augmented feedback in post-stroke gait rehabilitation derived from sensor-based gait reports—A longitudinal case series. *Sensors* **2025**, *25*, 3109. [CrossRef] [PubMed]
9. Clynes, M.A.; Jameson, K.A.; Edwards, M.H.; Cooper, C. Impact of osteoarthritis on activities of daily living: Does joint site matter? *Aging Clin. Exp. Res.* **2019**, *31*, 1049–1056. [CrossRef] [PubMed]

Journal of
Functional Morphology and Kinesiology

MDPI

Review

Associations Between Visual Accommodation and Cervical Muscle Activity and Symptomatology: A Systematic Review

Miguel Ángel Lérida-Ponce [1], Miguel Ángel Lérida-Ortega [1,2], Ana Sedeño-Vidal [1,*] and Alfonso Javier Ibáñez-Vera [1]

1 Department of Health Sciences, University of Jaen, 23071 Jaén, Spain
2 Área de Gestión Sanitaria Norte de Jaén, Servicio Andaluz de Salud, 23700 Jaén, Spain
* Correspondence: asedeno@ujaen.es

Abstract

Objectives: The aim of this study was to investigate the potential anatomical and physiological interconnections between the visual system and the cervical muscular system, as well as to examine the role of the visual system in the etiology and manifestation of cervical musculoskeletal pain or discomfort. **Methods**: A systematic review was conducted following the PRISMA guidelines, using databases such as PubMed, Scopus, Web of Science, CINAHL, and PEDro. The protocol was registered in PROSPERO. The included study designs comprised experimental studies, randomized controlled trials (RCTs), and pilot RCTs. **Results**: The literature search was conducted between January and May 2025 and yielded 51 studies across all databases. Seven experimental studies were finally included, all of which met the inclusion criteria and presented a mean methodological quality score of 5 on the PEDro methodological quality scale. The studies included data from a total of 308 participants (n = 261; 84.74% females). Subjects in the intervention group reported cervical pain or visual fatigue. **Conclusions**: Our results indicated a relationship between visual accommodation and increased electromyographic activity of the trapezius muscle, suggesting that accommodative stress may induce cervical muscle fatigue and pain.

Keywords: visual accommodation; visual function; neck pain; cervical pain

1. Introduction

Alterations in the visual system and musculoskeletal disorders are significant public health issues that affect a large portion of the general population. Near visual tasks, reading, and screen use require precise coordination between the head-stabilizing muscles and the visual system. Head orientation in space and posture rely on the visual, vestibular, and proprioceptive systems [1].

During near visual work, the eyes are subjected to continuous accommodative and convergence effort, which leads to reduced use of distance vision and less frequent far-to-near-far focus shifts. This prolonged visual demand results in sustained activation of the extrinsic and intrinsic eye muscles, causing distortion and imbalance in visual behavior, which can lead to accommodative dysfunctions [2].

Accommodative anomalies and non-strabismic binocular dysfunctions are visual disorders that affect the binocular system and the patient's visual performance. These visual disorders are associated with musculoskeletal discomfort in the cervical and shoulder regions, as well as headaches, often leading to the adoption of sustained non-ergonomic postures such as forward head position or asymmetric postures [3].

Uncorrected alterations in the visual system and the need for corrective lenses primarily increase the strain on the visual system and the head-stabilizing muscles, leading to visual fatigue, headaches, and cervicodorsal pain, as well as difficulty concentrating and poor coordination [1].

The visual effort based on the continued contraction of the ciliary muscles not only causes ocular discomfort but may also increase musculoskeletal tension, especially in the cervical and scapular regions, associated with increased activation of the trapezius muscle and the suboccipital musculature [4,5], thereby linking a visual disorder with a postural adaptation intended to maintain binocular function and visual comfort.

These discomforts may be physiologically connected or may result from postural adjustments unconsciously adopted as a response to visual fatigue or the use of inadequate optical correction. In this context, the cervical spine serves as a primary source for neuromuscular control [5]. Fatigue of the ocular muscles could lead to secondary changes in nerve activation, for example, linking a dysfunction in the sympathetic innervation of the eye in patients with whiplash injury to alterations in accommodation [6]. Therefore, this opens the possibility of a cross-dysfunction between the two systems.

The main objective of this systematic review is to determine the potential anatomical and physiological relationships between the ocular system and the cervical musculoskeletal system. The specific objectives are to justify the relationship between visual accommodation and the cervical muscular system, as well as its influence on musculoskeletal pain or discomfort related to the cervical region.

2. Materials and Methods

2.1. Clinical Literature Review

This systematic review and meta-analysis was conducted in accordance with the recommendations of the Preferred Reporting Items for Systematic Reviews and Meta-Analyses (PRISMA) [7] statement and the Cochrane Handbook for Systematic Reviews of Interventions [8]. The review was registered in PROSPERO (CRD420251053840).

2.2. Search Strategy

A literature search was carried out independently by two authors (MALP, ASV) from January to May 2025, across various health science databases, including PubMed (Medline), SCOPUS, Web of Science (WOS), CINAHL Complete, and the Physiotherapy Evidence Database (PEDro). To formulate the research question, the PICOS method proposed by the Cochrane Collaboration was used, as follows: P—population (patients with neck pain), I—intervention (visual tasks), C—comparison (pre-intervention and post-intervention results), and O—outcome (accommodation/vergence response, electromyographic muscle activity). For the search strategy, free-text terms such as "neck pain " and "lens accommodation" were combined with MeSH terms and their synonyms indexed in PubMed MEDLINE. The search strategy incorporated MeSH terms and Boolean operators as follows: "((neck pain) OR (trapezius muscle activity)) AND ((ocular accommodation) OR (lens accommodation))". No filters were applied for language or publication date. This phase was overseen by a third author with expertise in search strategies (AJIV). Table 1 shows the search strategy used.

Table 1. Search Strategy.

Database	Search Strategy
PubMed Medline	((cervical pain) OR (cervicalgia) OR (neckache) OR (neck pain) OR (neck muscles) OR (trapezius muscle activity)) AND ((ocular accommodation) OR (lens accommodation))

Table 1. *Cont.*

Database	Search Strategy
Cinahl	AB (cervical pain or neck pain or cervicalgia or neckache or neck muscles or trapezius muscle activity) AND AB (ocular accommodation or lens accommodation)
Web Of Science	TOPIC (cervical pain or neck pain or cervicalgia or neckache or neck muscles or trapezius muscle activity) TOPIC (ocular accommodation or lens accommodation)
PEDro	Cervical pain and Ocular accommodation
Scopus	TITLE-ABS-KEY "cervical pain" OR "cervicalgia" OR "neckache" OR "neck pain" OR "neck muscles" OR "trapezius muscle activity" AND "ocular accommodation" OR "lens accommodation"

2.3. Eligibility Criteria

Two authors (MALP, ASV) independently and carefully reviewed all records retrieved in the literature search by title and abstract. When a study was identified as potentially eligible in the review, the full text was read and examined by the two authors. Disagreements and uncertainties were resolved by a third author (AJIV).

The inclusion criteria were as follows: (1) experimental studies, randomized controlled trials (RCTs), or pilot RCTs; (2) patients with neck pan, upper limb pain, or visual dysfunctions based on the accommodative capacity of the lens; (3) studies that assessed the variability in visual accommodation and the perception of ocular and cervical fatigue and pain; (4) studies with a control group that received another type of intervention or no intervention; and (5) studies that evaluated outcome related to subjective symptoms of neck pain, visual accommodation, and cervical muscle activity.

The exclusion criteria were as follows: (1) a sample that was not entirely composed of patients with neck pain or studies where the visual accommodation was not alterations; (2) patients with concomitant conditions affecting cranio-cervical function and postural alterations; and (3) subjects who had ocular motility defects, strabismus, nystagmus, amblyopia, or any ocular or systemic disease that could affect the results.

2.4. Data Extraction

Data from the selected studies were extracted and coded into a data sheet standardized Microsoft® Excel file, created for this review by two authors (M.A.L.P., A.S.V.). Any discrepancies were resolved by consulting a third author (A.J.I.V.).

After joint data comparison and review, a consensus on result interpretation was sought, ensuring validity and objectivity. From each study, the following data were extracted: (1) general features (authorship, publication date, country and funding); (2) patient characteristics (total sample size, number of participants in each group, age, and sex); (3) characteristics of the experimental and control groups (type of intervention, number of sessions); and (4) data related to variables (evaluated variable, test used, and time point of assessment).

2.5. Outcomes

The variables assessed in this systematic review were the following: the accommodative/vergence response (measured using an infrared refractometer); heart rate variability (measured through electrocardiography and electromyography); trapezius muscle activity (measured using electromyography); and ocular and cervical fatigue (evaluated using the Borg CR-10 Scale).

2.6. Risk of Bias and Quality of Evidence Assessments

The evaluation of the risk of bias in each included study and the quality of the evidence of the main findings was carried out by 2 authors independently (M.A.L.P. and A.S.V.). The methodological quality and the risk of bias of the included studies were assessed using the PEDro scale [9]. It consists of 11 items that assess the internal validity and the interpretability of trial results. The scale evaluates essential methodological aspects including randomization, blinding, and follow-up, with a score range from 0 to 10 (since one item is not scored). The total score indicates excellent (10–9 points), good (8–6 points), moderate (5–4 points), or poor (<3 points) methodological quality. Any discrepancies between researchers were resolved by a third investigator (A.J.I.V.).

3. Results

3.1. Study Selection

After removing duplicates, twenty-two references were excluded. Thirty studies were excluded based on the title/abstract, and fourteen studies were excluded based on the selection criteria. A total of twenty-one distinct articles were obtained, which were assessed for eligibility based on the inclusion criteria: three were excluded due to study design, five for not analyzing the variables of interest, four for involving healthy populations, and one for not linking cervical pain with ocular dysfunctions. Additionally, one potential article was not included as it did not have a digital version (published in 1985 and in Norwegian) [10]. A total of seven studies [11–17] met the eligibility criteria and were included in this systematic review. The PRISMA flow chart (Figure 1) shows the study selection process.

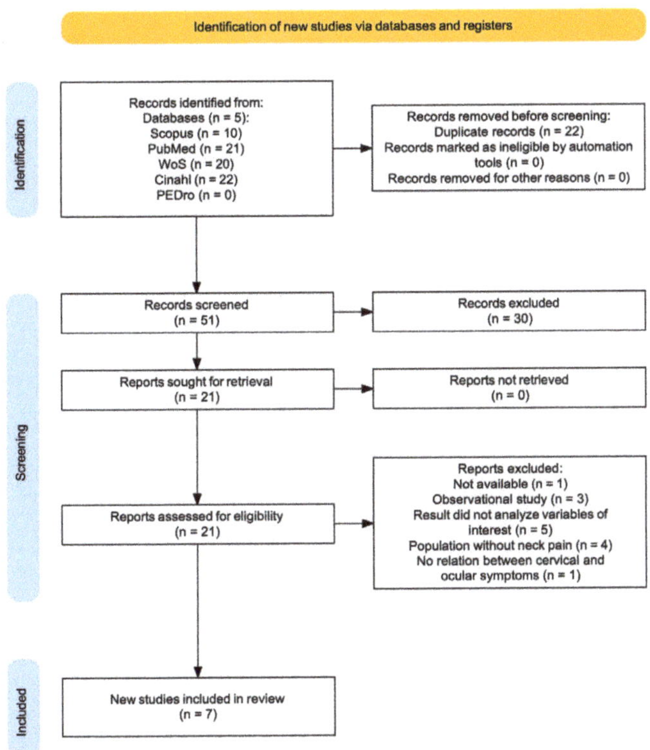

Figure 1. PRISMA flow diagram.

3.2. Characteristics of the Studies Included in the Review

The studies included [11–17] were conducted between 2010 and 2017. A total of 308 participants were provided by the included studies (150 in the control group; 158 in the experimental group) with a mean age of 18 ± 47 years (75.64% female). All the studies reported data on the immediate effects of demanding visual tasks, which varied in duration, distance, and visual condition. The sessions lasted between 10 and 30 min. Regarding the variables, the accommodative/vergence response was assessed using infrared technology, neck/shoulder discomfort and muscle fatigue were assessed using Borg's CR-10 scale [17], muscle activity was measured with electromyography [11–16], and heart rate variability was measured using electrocardiography [12,15,16] to reduce disturbances from heart signals on raw electromyography and as an indicator of autonomic reactivity during the experiments. No external funding was reported in any of the studies. Table 2 shows the main characteristics of the included studies.

Table 2. The main characteristics of the included studies in the review.

Study	N (F/M)	D	Experimental Group			Control Group			Outcomes/Measured
			Sample	Intervention		Sample	Intervention		
			Ne (Age)	Tt	Ses	Ne (Age)	Tt	Ses	
Richter et al., 2010 (Sweden) [14] FN: Yes	28 (18/10)	Ne: chronic neck pain and/or professional oculomotor problems (asthenopia) Nc: healthy symptom	13 (32 ± 7)	Four near-to-far vision tasks under different visual conditions	1 ses of 5 min	15 (27 ± 8)	Four near-to-far vision tasks	1 ses of 5 min	Accommodative/vergence response (refractor) Heart rate variability (electrocardiography; electromyography) Trapezius muscle activity (electromyography)
Richter et al., 2011 (Sweden) [15] FN: Yes	28 (18/10)	Ne: chronic neck pain and/or professional oculomotor problems (asthenopia) Nc: healthy symptom	13 (32 ± 7)	Two near-to-far vision tasks under different visual conditions	1 ses of 5 min	15 (27 ± 8)	Two near-to-far vision tasks	1 ses of 5 min	Accommodative/vergence response (refractor) Heart rate variability (electrocardiography; electromyography) Trapezius muscle activity (electromyography)
Forsman et al., 2012 (Sweden) [13] FN: No	28 (18/10)	Ne: chronic neck pain and/or professional oculomotor problems (asthenopia) Nc: healthy symptom	13 (32 ± 7)	Near-to-far vision tasks under different visual conditions	1 ses Near 15 times and at Far 15 times	15 (27 ± 8)	Near-to-far vision tasks under different visual conditions	1 ses Near 15 times and at Far 15 times	Accommodative/vergence response (refractor) Heart rate variability (electrocardiography; electromyography) Trapezius muscle activity (electromyography)
Zetterberg et al., 2013 (Sweden) [12] FN: Yes	66 (54/12)	Ne: neck/shoulder pain in the last 12 weeks Nc: healthy symptom	33 (median age 39 [range 20–47])	Visually demanding near work at a computer screen under different visual conditions	1 ses 4 series of 7 min	33 (median age 39 [range 20–47])	Visually demanding near work at a computer screen under different visual conditions	1 ses 4 series of 7 min	Accommodative/vergence response (refractor) Heart rate variability (electrocardiography; electromyography) Trapezius muscle activity (electromyography)
Richter et al., 2015 (Sweden) [16] FN: Yes	66 (54/12)	Ne: chronic neck pain Nc: healthy symptom	33 (median age 39 [range 20–47])	Four near-to-far vision tasks under different visual conditions	1 ses 4 series of 7 min	33 (median age 39 [range 20–47])	Four near-to-far vision tasks under different visual conditions	1 ses 4 series of 7 min	Accommodative/vergence response (refractor) Heart rate variability (electrocardiography; electromyography) Trapezius muscle activity (electromyography)
Zetterberg et al., 2015 (Sweden) [11] FN: Yes	26 (17/9)	Ne: chronic neck pain and/or professional oculomotor problems (asthenopia) Nc: healthy symptom	12 (26 ± 8) 26 ± 8	Near-to-far vision tasks under different visual conditions	1 ses of 2.5 min	14 (32 ± 7)	Near-to-far vision tasks under different visual conditions	1 ses of 2.5 min	Accommodative/vergence response (refractor) Heart rate variability (electrocardiography; electromyography) Trapezius muscle activity (electromyography)

Table 2. *Cont.*

Study	N (F/M)	D	Experimental Group			Control Group			Outcomes/Measured
			Sample	Intervention		Sample	Intervention		
			Ne (Age)	Tt	Ses	Ne (Age)	Tt	Ses	
Zetterberg et al., 2017 (Sweden) [17] FN: Yes	66 (54/12)	Ne: chronic neck pain Nc: healthy symptom	33 (median age 39 [range 20–47])	Four near-to-far vision tasks under different visual conditions	1 ses of 7 min	33 (median age 39 [range 20–47])	Four near-to-far vision tasks under different visual conditions	1 ses of 7 min	Accommodative/vergence response (refractor) Heart rate variability (electrocardiography; electromyography) Ocular and cervical fatigue (Borg CR-10 scale)

FN: funding N: total sample size; D: diagnostic; F/M: female/male; Ne: experimental group sample size; Tt: Treatment; Ses: session; Nc: control group sample size; min: minutes.

3.3. Assessment of Methodological Quality and Main Biases Identified

Table 3 reports the PEDro score for each study included in the review. The studies showed moderate methodological quality and a medium risk of bias (PEDro score of 5 points). None of the studies blinded the participants, evaluators, or therapists, nor was there any concealed allocation or masking, which increased the risk of performance biases.

Table 3. PEDro methodological quality scale.

Author	C1	C2	C3	C4	C5	C6	C7	C8	C9	C10	C11	Total Score
Richter et al., 2010 [14]	✓	✓	✗	✓	✗	✗	✗	✓	✗	✓	✓	5
Richter et al., 2011 [15]	✓	✓	✗	✓	✗	✗	✗	✓	✗	✓	✓	5
Forsman et al., 2012 [13]	✓	✓	✗	✓	✗	✗	✗	✓	✗	✓	✓	5
Zetterberg et al., 2013 [12]	✓	✓	✗	✓	✗	✗	✗	✓	✗	✓	✓	5
Zetterberg et al., 2015 [11]	✓	✓	✗	✓	✗	✗	✗	✓	✗	✓	✓	5
Richter et al., 2015 [16]	✓	✓	✗	✓	✗	✗	✗	✓	✗	✓	✓	5
Zetterberg et al., 2017 [17]	✓	✓	✗	✗	✗	✗	✗	✓	✓	✓	✓	5

C: criteria; ✓: yes; ✗: no.

3.4. Main Findings in Systematic Review

3.4.1. Effects of Visual Work on the Accommodation Response

In six of the seven selected studies [11,12,14–17], a greater accommodative response was observed with negative lenses compared to neutral lenses. The study by Richter et al., 2015 [16] showed an insufficient response, as the accommodation of the lens did not need to compensate for the accommodative load under both binocular and monocular negative conditions. The study by Richter et al., 2010 [14], used Prism-Out lenses (which induce an external deviation of the eyes), showing an appropriate visual accommodation response. Only in the study by Richter et al., 2011 [15] was an inconsistency observed between accommodation and convergence with positive lenses. No significant differences were found between the symptomatic group and the control group in the selected studies, except for the study by Zetterberg et al., 2015 [11], where the accommodative response was greater in the control group ($p = 0.049$) compared to the group with cervical symptoms. Table 4 presents the primary outcomes with statistical data from the selected studies.

Table 4. Summary of primary outcomes from the selected studies.

Reference	Variable/Condition	Main Results (Experimental Group)
Richter et al., 2010 [14]	Accommodative error (D)/EMG (% RVE)	Binocular with −3.5 D: r^2 =0.38; $p = 0.0012$ Binocular with 0.0 D: $r^2 = 0.003$; $p = 0.79$ Binocular with 1–2 Prism D: $r^2 = 0.07$; $p = 0.203$ Binocular with +3.5 D: $r^2 = 0.316$; $p = 0.0022$

Table 4. *Cont.*

Reference	Variable/Condition	Main Results (Experimental Group)
Richter et al., 2011 [15]	Response diopters (D)/EMG (% RVE)	Binocular with −3.5 D: r^2 = 0.25; p = 0.013 Binocular with 0.0 D: r^2 = 0.016; p = 0.563
	Accommodative error (D)/EMG (% RVE)	Binocular with −3.5 D: r^2 = 0.3686 p = 0.001 Binocular with 0.0 D: r^2 = 0.0018; p = 0.845
Forsman et al., 2012 [13]	EMG/refraction signals	R(tau) = 0.019; p = 0.001
Zetterberg et al., 2013 [12]	Accommodation response (D)/EMG (%RVE)	Binocular with −3.5: r = 0.377; p = 0.017 Monocular with −3.5: r = 0.147; p = 0.326 Monocular neutral with 0.0 D: r = −0.018; p = 0.897 Monocular with +3.5: r = 0.088; p = 0.524
Zetterberg et al., 2015 [11]	Trapezius muscle activity (in %RVE)	Neutral lenses: 1.82 [0.79, 2.86]; p = 0.034 Negative −3.5 D lenses: 2.36 [0.72, 3.99]; p > 0.1 Positive +3.5 D lenses: 1.74 [0.28, 3.21]; p = p > 0.1
Richter et al., 2015 [16]	Trapezius muscle activity (% RVE) during the visual tasks	Binocular −3.5 D: p = 0.007 Monocular −3.5 D: p = 0.048 Monocular 0 D: p = 0.043 Monocular +3.5 D: p > 0.5
Zetterberg et al., 2017 [17]	Accommodation response	Binocular −3.5 D: 3.39 (2.09) Monocular −3.5 D: 3.68 (2.00) Monocular 0 D: 1.51 (0.74) Monocular +3.5 D: 0.97 (0.99)
	BOR's scale internal eye discomfort	Binocular −3.5 D: 3.0 (0 ± 9.0) * Monocular −3.5 D: 2.0 (0 ± 7.0) Monocular 0 D: 2.0 (0 ± 7.0) Monocular +3.5 D: 3.0 (0 ± 9.0)
	BOR's scale external eye discomfort	Binocular −3.5 D: 3.0 (0 ± 7.0) Monocular −3.5 D: 2.5 (0.3 ± 7.0) Monocular 0 D: 2.0 (0 ± 7.0) Monocular +3.5 D: 2.5 (0 ± 7.0)
	BOR's scale neck/shoulder discomfort	Binocular −3.5 D: 3.0 (1.0 ± 9.0) Monocular −3.5 D: 3.0 (0.5 ± 10.0) Monocular 0 D: 3.0 (1.0 ± 10.0) Monocular +3.5 D: 3.0 (0.5 ± 9.0)

D: diopters; EMG: electromyography; RVE: reference voluntary electrical activity; r-value: Pearson correlation coefficient; *: values presented are medians with the range in brackets.

3.4.2. Effects of Visual Work on Cervical Muscle Tone

Six of the seven selected studies [11–16] analyzed the effects of visual work on trapezius muscle activity. Three of the studies [13–15] showed that accommodative stress induced by the use of lenses with positive or negative load increased trapezius muscle tone (p = 0.001). Two studies [12,16] identified a significant correlation between accommodative stress and an increase in trapezius muscle tone, but only under binocular vision conditions (p = 0.009) according to Zetterberg et al., 2013 [12] and (p = 0.007) Richter et al., 2015 [16]. Under other visual conditions, trapezius activity remained low with no statistically significant differences, while one of the included studies found no significant differences in muscle tone across the different visual tasks (p = 0.1) [11]. In the six studies [11–16], muscle tone was quantified by recording electromyographic activity (Table 4).

3.4.3. Effects of Visual Work on Heart Rate

In three of the selected studies [11,13,14] electrocardiography was not a primary variable but a technical tool to optimize the electromyographic recording. Conversely, in another three studies [12,15,16], electrocardiography, in addition to being used to optimize the electromyographic recording, was used to measure heart rate variability, thereby assessing the influence of the autonomic nervous system. Across these latter studies, the autonomic nervous system was not altered at any point during the experiment with any of the proposed visual tasks. Only in the study by Richter et al., 2015 [16] was a statistically significant decrease observed in the binocular vision condition with negative lenses ($p = 0.024$).

3.4.4. Effects of Visual Work on the Perception of Fatigue and Pain

Only one of the included studies [17] analyzed the perception of fatigue and pain in the eyes, cervical region, and glenohumeral area. This study observed that, after accommodative stress induced by negative lenses, there was a significant increase in fatigue and pain in the eyes, cervical area, and glenohumeral region ($p = 0.001$). This variable also increased with positive lenses, although in this case, the differences were not significant ($p = 0.3$). In this study [17], the Borg CR-10 Scale, a numerical scale with verbal expressions used to quantify pain intensity, was employed to assess the perception of fatigue [18].

4. Discussion

All studies [11–17] have demonstrated a relationship between the visual system and the cervical musculoskeletal system. On the one hand, the authors have established a relationship between ocular accommodation and the cervical region [11–16]. These studies induced visual accommodation changes through the use of positive, negative, and neutral lenses. However, most of the reviewed literature did not directly ascertain whether ocular accommodation affects cervical conditions. The various authors described variations in trapezius electromyographic activity induced by changes in lens accommodation. However, the findings were inconsistent across studies. These findings suggest the possibility of increased cervical muscle tone as a mechanism to stabilize gaze in response to a mismatch in visual accommodation.

Previous studies observed a relationship between binocular vision and the neck system. Sánchez-González et al. [3] evaluated binocular vision status and confirmed a relationship between nonstrabismic binocular dysfunctions and musculoskeletal neck disorders. Giffard et al. [19] demonstrated a relationship between convergence insufficiency and cervical pain, demonstrating reduced ocular convergence in patients with cervical pain compared to asymptomatic subjects. Matheron et al. [20] reported head rotation in an attempt to compensate for the vertical deviation produced by a prism placed in front of the eye.

Other studies, such as that by Domkin et al. (2019) [21], observed that visually demanding tasks lead to increased trapezius muscle activity. Moreover, Richter et al. (2012) [22] emphasized that the patient's accommodative effort is more closely related to trapezius EMG activity than the actual inability to focus.

Several authors have reported accommodative and vergence disorders in whiplash patients. Roca et al. [23] and Burke et al. [24] found that convergence and accommodation are reduced in whiplash patients. Ischebeck et al. [25] suggested that these patients exhibit altered eye reflexes and smooth pursuit movements, which may impair the coordination of the head and eyes. Stiebel-Kalish et al. [26] stated that whiplash patients exhibited convergence insufficiency and accommodative disorder symptoms. Ischebeck et al. [27] noted that severely impaired chronic neck pain patients have an elevated cervico-ocular reflex (COR) compared to healthy controls. These results are similar to those obtained in our study, supporting the hypothesis that there is an adaptive postural modification of the cervical spine related to vision.

Physiological processes that connect accommodative stress with activation of the trapezius muscle, such as the coordination between sensory and motor systems and mechanisms for postural control, can lead to postural changes including tilting or turning the head, lifting the chin, lowering it, or a mix of these, depending on the underlying cause [28]. According to Nucci et al., tension in the neck muscles may occur as a secondary effect when the head tilts to compensate for a vertical misalignment caused by dysfunction in the superior oblique muscle [29]. This head position can reduce the strain on the affected ocular muscles through reflexive responses. Although such an adjustment may support better visual function, over time, it may also result in musculoskeletal issues in the cervical region. From this perspective, discomfort or pain in the neck may arise as a consequence of the body's effort to optimize visual performance. In this context, cervical disorders may develop due to sustained postural compensation aimed at maintaining visual comfort, highlighting the clinical implications of integrating optometric and postural interventions [30].

On the other hand, one of the selected studies [17] focused on cervical musculoskeletal symptoms and ocular symptoms. The Borg CR-10 Scale was measured before and after performing the visually demanding task, and it was concluded that a change in accommodative load led to an increase in ocular and cervical discomfort. This suggests that cervical pain may be caused by accommodative stress. In this regard, we found studies such as the one published by Lodin et al. (2012) [4], which concluded that a demanding visual exercise can lead to the onset of cervical and ocular symptoms. The study published by Sánchez-González et al. (2018) [2] determined a significant association between accommodative dysfunctions and the presence of pain in the cervical region, measured using the Neck Disability Index, the Visual Analogue Scale, cervical range of motion, deep flexor muscle activation score, and performance index.

While the findings of this work offer clinical relevance, further clarification is needed regarding the percentage of change in EMG trapezius activity during vision tasks. Future studies should address the median and standard deviation values of each group over time and the group interaction. It is also important to consider some limitations: the inclusion of a limited number of studies, the relatively small sample sizes in some of these studies, the local recruitment (all studies performed in Sweden), and the predominance of female participants may reduce the robustness and generalizability of our findings. Another limitation is the potential for publication bias to influence several of our results. Nonetheless, several studies seem to have used the same sample, and the quality of evidence reported was moderated. None of the studies presented random selection or blinding of participants, assessors, or therapists. Additionally, it is important to note that the possibility of patient follow-up could not be considered for the studies included due to limitations in their design. Future studies with larger sample sizes are necessary to elucidate the impact of the relationship between visual accommodation and trapezius tone.

5. Conclusions

Given the descriptive nature of the data and the lack of statistical synthesis, the findings of this systematic review suggest that there is an anatomical and physiological relationship between the ocular system and the cervical musculoskeletal system, indicating a possible influence on trapezius muscle tone due to visual demand. The limited differences between the control and symptomatic groups reflect that cervical pain does not worsen visual accommodation. However, insufficient accommodative capacity could potentially induce a painful muscular process in the cervical region. Further studies are required to enhance the generalizability, evidence base, and robustness of these findings.

Author Contributions: Conceptualization, A.J.I.-V. and A.S.-V.; methodology A.J.I.-V. and A.S.-V.; validation, M.Á.L.-O. and A.S.-V.; investigation, M.Á.L.-P. and A.J.I.-V.; resources, M.Á.L.-O. and A.S.-V.; data curation, M.Á.L.-P. and A.J.I.-V.; writing—original draft preparation, M.Á.L.-P. and A.S.-V.; writing—review and editing, A.J.I.-V.; supervision, M.Á.L.-O. All authors have read and agreed to the published version of the manuscript.

Funding: No funding was received for this study.

Data Availability Statement: The data of this review are available upon request to the corresponding author.

Conflicts of Interest: The authors declare no conflicts of interest.

References

1. Espí López, G.V.; Sentandreu Mañó, T.; Colorado Lluch, M.I.; Dueñas Moscardó, L. Efectos de Un Programa de Ejercicios Oculocervicales En Adultos En La Movilidad Cervical. *Fisioterapia* **2011**, *33*, 41–49. [CrossRef]
2. Sánchez-González, M.C.; Pérez-Cabezas, V.; López-Izquierdo, I.; Gutiérrez-Sánchez, E.; Ruiz-Molinero, C.; Rebollo-Salas, M.; Jiménez-Rejano, J.J. Is It Possible to Relate Accommodative Visual Dysfunctions to Neck Pain? *Ann. N. Y. Acad. Sci.* **2018**, *1421*, 62–72. [CrossRef]
3. Sánchez-González, M.C.; Gutiérrez-Sánchez, E.; Sánchez-González, J.M.; Rebollo-Salas, M.; Ruiz-Molinero, C.; Jiménez-Rejano, J.J.; Pérez-Cabezas, V. Visual System Disorders and Musculoskeletal Neck Complaints: A Systematic Review and Meta-Analysis. *Ann. N. Y. Acad. Sci.* **2019**, *1457*, 26–40. [CrossRef]
4. Lodin, C.; Forsman, M.; Richter, H. Eye- and Neck/Shoulder-Discomfort during Visually Demanding Experimental near Work. *Work* **2012**, *41* (Suppl. S1), 3388–3392. [CrossRef]
5. Domkin, D.; Forsman, M.; Richter, H.O. Ciliary Muscle Contraction Force and Trapezius Muscle Activity during Manual Tracking of a Moving Visual Target. *J. Electromyogr. Kinesiol.* **2016**, *28*, 193–198. [CrossRef] [PubMed]
6. Enix, D.E.; Scali, F.; Pontell, M.E. The Cervical Myodural Bridge, a Review of Literature and Clinical Implications. *J. Can. Chiropr. Assoc.* **2014**, *58*, 184. [PubMed]
7. Moher, D.; Liberati, A.; Tetzlaff, J.; Altman, D.G.; Antes, G.; Atkins, D.; Barbour, V.; Barrowman, N.; Berlin, J.A.; Clark, J.; et al. Preferred Reporting Items for Systematic Reviews and Meta-Analyses: The PRISMA Statement. *PLoS Med.* **2009**, *6*, e1000097. [CrossRef]
8. Cochrane Handbook for Systematic Reviews of Interventions | Cochrane Training. Available online: https://training.cochrane.org/handbook (accessed on 23 April 2025).
9. Mather, C.G.; Sherrington, C.; Herbert, R.D.; Moseley, A.M.; Elkins, M. Reliability of the PEDro Scale for Rating Quality of Randomized Controlled Trials. *Phys. Ther.* **2003**, *83*, 713–721. [CrossRef] [PubMed]
10. Lie, I.; Watten, R. [Visually Induced Muscle Stress]. *Tidsskr. Nor. Laegeforening* **1985**, *105*, 1714–1718.
11. Zetterberg, C.; Richter, H.O.; Forsman, M. Temporal Co-Variation between Eye Lens Accommodation and Trapezius Muscle Activity during a Dynamic near-Far Visual Task. *PLoS ONE* **2015**, *10*, e0126578. [CrossRef]
12. Zetterberg, C.; Forsman, M.; Richter, H.O. Effects of Visually Demanding near Work on Trapezius Muscle Activity. *J. Electromyogr. Kinesiol.* **2013**, *23*, 1190–1198. [CrossRef]
13. Forsman, M.; Lodin, C.; Richter, H. Co-Variation in Time between near-Far Accommodation of the Lens and Trapezius Muscle Activity. *Work* **2012**, *41*, 3393–3397. [CrossRef] [PubMed]
14. Richter, H.O.; Bänziger, T.; Abdi, S.; Forsman, M. Stabilization of Gaze: A Relationship between Ciliary Muscle Contraction and Trapezius Muscle Activity. *Vis. Res.* **2010**, *50*, 2559–2569. [CrossRef]
15. Richter, H.O.; Bänziger, T.; Forsman, M. Eye-Lens Accommodation Load and Static Trapezius Muscle Activity. *Eur. J. Appl. Physiol.* **2011**, *111*, 29–36. [CrossRef] [PubMed]
16. Richter, H.O.; Zetterberg, C.; Forsman, M. Trapezius Muscle Activity Increases during near Work Activity Regardless of Accommodation/Vergence Demand Level. *Eur. J. Appl. Physiol.* **2015**, *115*, 1501–1512. [CrossRef]
17. Zetterberg, C.; Forsman, M.; Richter, H.O. Neck/Shoulder Discomfort Due to Visually Demanding Experimental near Work Is Influenced by Previous Neck Pain, Task Duration, Astigmatism, Internal Eye Discomfort and Accommodation. *PLoS ONE* **2017**, *12*, e0182439. [CrossRef]
18. Zamunér, A.R.; Moreno, M.A.; Camargo, T.M.; Graetz, J.P.; Rebelo, A.C.; Tamburús, N.Y.; Da Silva, E. Evaluación Del Esfuerzo Percibido Subjetivo En El Umbral Anaeróbico Con La Escala de Borg CR-10. *J. Sports Sci. Med.* **2010**, *2010*, 130–136.
19. Giffard, P.; Daly, L.; Treleaven, J. Influence of Neck Torsion on near Point Convergence in Subjects with Idiopathic Neck Pain. *Musculoskelet. Sci. Pract.* **2017**, *32*, 51–56. [CrossRef]
20. Matheron, E.; Zandi, A.; Wang, D.; Kapoula, Z. A 1-Diopter Vertical Prism Induces a Decrease of Head Rotation: A Pilot Investigation. *Front Neurol.* **2016**, *7*, 62. [CrossRef] [PubMed] [PubMed Central]
21. Domkin, D.; Forsman, M.; Richter, H.O. Effect of Ciliary-Muscle Contraction Force on Trapezius Muscle Activity during Computer Mouse Work. *Eur. J. Appl. Physiol.* **2019**, *119*, 389–397. [CrossRef]
22. Richter, H.O.; Camilla, L.; Forsman, M. Temporal Aspects of Increases in Eye-Neck Activation Levels during Visually Deficient near Work. *Work* **2012**, *41*, 3379–3384. [CrossRef] [PubMed]
23. Roca, P.D. Ocular Manifestations of Whiplash Injuries. *Ann. Ophthalmol.* **1972**, *4*, 63–73. [PubMed]

24. Burke, J.P.; Orton, H.P.; West, J.; Strachan, I.M.; Hockey, M.S.; Ferguson, D.G. Whiplash and Its Effect on the Visual System. *Graefes Arch. Clin. Exp. Ophthalmol.* **1992**, *230*, 335–339. [CrossRef]
25. Ischebeck, B.K.; De Vries, J.; Van Der Geest, J.N.; Janssen, M.; Van Wingerden, J.P.; Kleinrensink, G.J.; Frens, M.A. Eye Movements in Patients with Whiplash Associated Disorders: A Systematic Review. *BMC Musculoskelet. Disord.* **2016**, *17*, 441. [CrossRef]
26. Stiebel-Kalish, H.; Amitai, A.; Mimouni, M.; Bach, M.; Saban, T.; Cahn, M.; Gantz, L. The Discrepancy between Subjective and Objective Measures of Convergence Insufficiency in Whiplash-Associated Disorder versus Control Participants. *Ophthalmology* **2018**, *125*, 924–928. [CrossRef]
27. Ischebeck, B.K.; de Vries, J.; Janssen, M.; van Wingerden, J.P.; Kleinrensink, G.J.; van der Geest, J.N.; Frens, M.A. Eye Stabilization Reflexes in Traumatic and Non-Traumatic Chronic Neck Pain Patients. *Musculoskelet. Sci. Pract.* **2017**, *29*, 72–77. [CrossRef]
28. Zhang, D.; Zhang, W.H.; Dai, S.Z.; Peng, H.Y.; Wang, L.Y. Binocular Vision and Abnormal Head Posture in Children When Watching Television. *Int. J. Ophthalmol.* **2016**, *9*, 746–749. [CrossRef] [PubMed]
29. Nucci, P.; Kushner, B.J.; Serafino, M.; Orzalesi, N. A Multi-Disciplinary Study of the Ocular, Orthopedic, and Neurologic Causes of Abnormal Head Postures in Children. *Am. J. Ophthalmol.* **2005**, *140*, e1–e65. [CrossRef]
30. Richter, H.O. Neck Pain Brought into Focus. *Work* **2014**, *47*, 413–418. [CrossRef]

Journal of
Functional Morphology and Kinesiology

MDPI

Article

Comprehensive Associations Between Spinal–Pelvic Alignment and Muscle Shortening in Healthy Young Men: An Analysis of Individual and Interactive Effects in the Sagittal Plane Using SHapley Additive exPlanation

Minami Akao †, Yuna Ishikura †, Takuma Isshiki, Shinnosuke Tsukada, Hayato Shigetoh * and Junya Miyazaki

Department of Physical Therapy, Faculty of Health Science, Kyoto Tachibana University, 34 Yamada-cho, Oyake, Yamashina-ku, Kyoto 607-8175, Japan; a903022004@st.tachibana-u.ac.jp (M.A.); a903022028@st.tachibana-u.ac.jp (Y.I.); a903022032@st.tachibana-u.ac.jp (T.I.); a903022164@st.tachibana-u.ac.jp (S.T.); j-miyazaki@tachibana-u.ac.jp (J.M.)

* Correspondence: shigeto@tachibana-u.ac.jp; Tel.: +81-75-574-4313

† These authors contributed equally to this work.

Abstract

Objectives: To comprehensively examine the association between spinopelvic alignment and muscle shortening in healthy young men, focusing on the individual and interactive effects of thoracic kyphosis, lumbar lordosis, and anterior pelvic tilt using SHapley Additive exPlanation (SHAP) analysis. **Methods**: Forty-one healthy young adult men participated in this cross-sectional study. Thoracic kyphosis, lumbar lordosis, and anterior pelvic tilt were measured using a flexible curve ruler and inclinometer. Muscle length indices for six muscles (iliopsoas, rectus femoris, gluteus maximus, hamstrings, back extensors, and abdominals) were assessed via standardized physical examinations and image analysis. A machine learning model was developed, and SHAP analysis applied to determine individual and interactive contributions of spinopelvic angles to each muscle length index. **Results**: SHAP analysis showed that hip-related muscle shortening (iliopsoas, rectus femoris, hamstrings, gluteus maximus) was influenced by both individual alignments and interactions, especially between thoracic kyphosis and lumbar lordosis. Lumbar lordosis was most associated with iliopsoas shortening (SHAP = −0.09), while anterior pelvic tilt was linked to hamstring shortening (SHAP = −0.30). Thoracic kyphosis was the key factor for rectus femoris shortening (SHAP = −0.05). Interactive effects exceeded individual contributions for the rectus femoris, gluteus maximus, and hamstrings. In contrast, spinal alignment had minimal influence on the back extensors and abdominals. **Conclusions**: Both individual and intersegmental spinal alignments are associated with muscle shortening, particularly in hip-related muscles. The interaction between thoracic kyphosis and lumbar lordosis plays a pivotal role. These findings underscore the importance of evaluating segmental spinal interactions when assessing muscle flexibility and posture.

Keywords: sagittal spinal alignment; pelvic tilt; muscle shortening; SHAP (SHapley Additive exPlanation); posture analysis; machine learning

1. Introduction

Postural alignment in humans is one of the critical elements influencing the activities of daily living and physical function. Standing posture is the state wherein the center of the body mass is maintained within the base of support and the body is aligned vertically [1]. In particular, the sagittal-plane standing posture is affected by the spinal alignment curvature, including thoracic kyphosis and lumbar lordosis, and is associated with displacement of the center of mass. One of the representative classifications based on the sagittal spinal curvature is the Kendall classification, which categorizes posture into four types based on the characteristics of the spinal curvature: ideal posture, kyphotic–lordotic, flat back, and sway back [2]. Abnormal sagittal spinal curvature is reportedly associated with deviations in postural alignment and adverse health outcomes, including pain, reduced mobility, impaired physical function, and increased mortality [3]. The spinal sagittal curvature is not limited to isolated regions such as the thoracic or lumbar spine. However, it is regulated by the spinal–pelvic complex, which reflects its interrelationships with other body regions. Therefore, to understand normative alignment in the sagittal plane, it is essential not only to evaluate spinal curvature alone but also to analyze each postural alignment type by considering the positional relationship of the spinal-pelvic complex in relation to other body regions [4].

Muscle shortening is one factor associated with the spinal alignment. The shortening or overactivity of specific muscle groups may be related to trunk inclination [3]. Janda classified muscles into two groups: tonic muscles, which contain a higher proportion of red fibers and are responsible for sustained postural contractions; and phasic muscles, which have a higher proportion of white fibers and are involved in rapid, dynamic joint movements [5,6]. Tonic muscles are prone to tightness or shortening, whereas phasic muscles are more susceptible to weakness. Postural alignment during standing is thought to be associated with muscle length. For example, the shortening of the hip flexors is associated with anterior pelvic tilt, whereas the shortening of the hip extensors is associated with posterior pelvic tilt [2]. When the lumbar erector spinae are shortened and the abdominal muscles are relatively lengthened, the pelvic tilt and lumbar lordosis tend to increase beyond the normal ranges. This suggests that pelvic tilt is related to lumbar curvature in normal standing posture and that both are influenced by the performance and length of the trunk muscles [7]. Thus, muscle shortening is likely associated with the alignment of the pelvis and lumbar spine. However, conflicting findings have been reported, with some studies indicating that hamstring muscle length is not associated with pelvic tilt angle [8]. Walker et al. suggested that abdominal muscle length may also be associated with lumbar lordosis and pelvic tilt [9]. However, a combination of complex factors can influence this relationship. Therefore, postural alignment may not be determined solely by muscle shortening. In summary, while some studies report associations between spinal alignment and muscle shortening, others report no such relationship; the association remains inconclusive.

Although previous studies have suggested a potential relationship between individual spinal alignment and muscle shortening, spinal alignment is inherently interrelated across different spinal regions. Therefore, interactions between spinal regions may also contribute to muscle shortening. However, the relationship between individual spinal alignments and interregional interactions related to muscle length has not been sufficiently explored. Recent studies have begun to apply machine learning approaches to elucidate complex biomechanical interactions within the spinal–pelvic region. For example, Pasha et al. demonstrated the utility of machine learning analysis in interpreting spinal alignment features from spinal imaging data, highlighting the potential of explainable AI in musculoskeletal research contexts [10]. However, few studies have extended such approaches to analyze the contribution of spinal alignment patterns to muscle length indices, particularly in a standing posture. Clarifying the relationship between spinal alignment and muscle length could enhance clinical decision-making for assessment and treatment. These insights may support the development of individualized interventions to improve postural alignment, flexibility, and overall physical performance. Accordingly, the present study aimed to investigate the association among muscle length, individual contributions, and interregional interactions of spinal alignment, focusing specifically on the thoracic, lumbar, and pelvic regions.

2. Materials and Methods

2.1. Participants

The participants were 41 healthy young adult men (mean age: 20.7 ± 0.6 years; height: 170.5 ± 6.0 cm; weight: 61.9 ± 9.8 kg; BMI: 21.2 ± 2.7). The exclusion criteria included a history of spinal fractures or other spinal disorders, known neurological conditions, and spinal asymmetry. Specifically, participants with a known diagnosis of scoliosis made by a medical professional were excluded, as radiographic assessment (e.g., Cobb angle) was not performed in this study. This study was approved by the ethics committee of Kyoto Tachibana University (approval no. 24-74). All participants received a verbal explanation of the study and provided written informed consent before participation.

2.2. Study Protocol

All participants underwent the following measurements: muscle length indices, spinal curvature angles, and pelvic tilt angles. All measurements were conducted under standardized conditions, with the participants wearing swimwear for the lower body and no clothing for the upper body.

2.3. Measurement of Spinal Curvature Angles

Spinal curvature angles were measured in a static standing posture using a flexible curve ruler (Shinwa Rules Co., Ltd., Niigata, Japan). The participants stood barefoot with their feet shoulder-width apart and maintained a static standing posture while flexing their shoulder and elbow joints to 90° [11] (Figure 1). Anatomical landmarks were identified, and markers were placed on the spinous processes of the seventh cervical vertebra (C7) and the first lumbar vertebra (L1), as well as on the left and right posterior superior iliac spines (PSIS). The flexible curved ruler was molded along the contour of the spine by gently pressing it with the fingers to ensure that it conformed closely to the spinal shape. The ruler was then carefully transferred to the paper without deformation and traced [12]. This procedure was repeated twice, and the mean value was used for the analysis. Following the method described in previous studies [12], the thoracic kyphosis angle was calculated using a straight line (L) drawn between C7 and L1 and a perpendicular line (H) from the apex of the curve to the L.

$$\text{Thoracic kyphosis angle} = 4 \times \text{arctangent}\ (2H/L)$$

Similarly, the lumbar lordosis angle was calculated using a straight line (L') drawn between L1 and the midpoint of the left and right PSIS and a perpendicular line (H') from the apex of the curve to L' (Figure 1).

$$\text{Lumbar lordosis angle} = 4 \times \text{arctangent}\ (2H'/L')$$

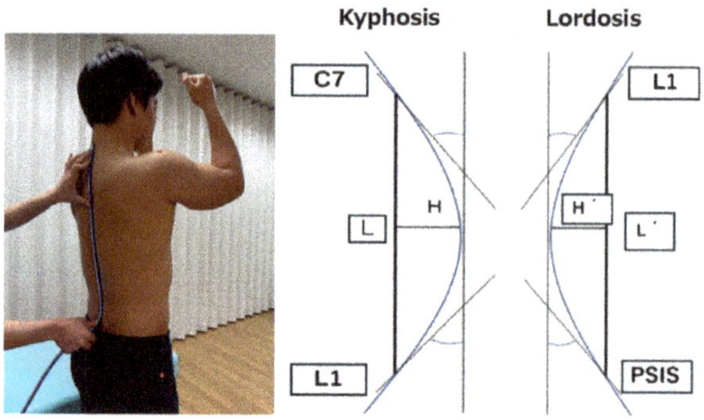

Figure 1. The evaluation of spinal alignment using a flexible curve ruler and method for calculating spinal curvature angles.

2.4. Measurement of Sagittal Pelvic Alignment

Sagittal pelvic alignment was measured using an inclinometer (BWT61 Gyroscope Sensor; WitMotion Co., Ltd., Shenzhen, China). The measurement posture was identical to that of the spinal curvature assessment: participants stood barefoot with feet shoulder-width apart, maintaining a static standing posture with both the shoulder and elbow joints flexed to 90°. The inclinometer was placed at the midpoint between the left and right posterior superior iliac spines (PSIS), and the angle relative to the vertical axis was measured. The anterior tilt angle of the sacrum, which is related to the pelvic tilt, was used to indicate the anterior pelvic inclination [13].

2.5. Measurement of Muscle Length Indices

To comprehensively assess the flexibility of the primary hip flexor and extensor muscle groups as well as the trunk muscles, muscle length indices were measured for six specific muscles: the iliopsoas, rectus femoris, gluteus maximus, hamstrings, abdominal muscles, and back extensor muscles. Lateral images of the participants were captured using the rear camera of a 7th-generation iPad (Apple Inc., Cupertino, CA, USA) running iPadOS 16.3.1. The device was positioned approximately 3 m from the participant at the level of the greater trochanter to ensure full-body visibility in the frame. Images were taken using the default camera application, and the resolution was 1920 × 1080 pixels, consistent with the standard output of the device. Angle measurements were performed using ImageJ image analysis software (NIH, Bethesda, MD, USA; available from https://imagej.net/ij/download.html; accessed on 13 May 2025), with anatomical landmarks marked at the acromion, greater trochanter, lateral femoral epicondyle, and lateral malleolus.

For the rectus femoris and iliopsoas, a modified Thomas test was used to calculate the hip and knee joint angles [14]. The participants lay in a supine position with both legs hanging off the edge of the examination table. The non-measured leg was brought as close to the chest as possible while maintaining contact between the lumbar spine and table. The leg to be measured remained relaxed and hanging below the table. The reference axis for the rectus femoris was defined as the femoral shaft (the line between the greater trochanter and lateral femoral epicondyle), and the movement axis was defined as the lower leg shaft (the line between the fibular head and lateral malleolus) (Figure 2A). For the iliopsoas, the reference axis was the line between the acromion and greater trochanter, and the movement axis was the femoral shaft (Figure 2B).

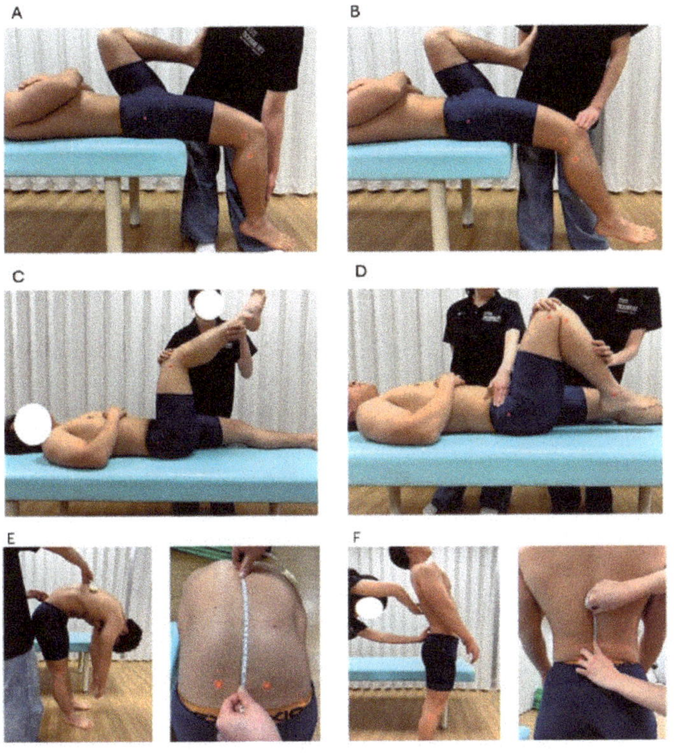

Figure 2. Measurement methods for each muscle length index. (**A**): rectus femoris; (**B**): iliopsoas; (**C**): hamstrings; (**D**): gluteus maximus; (**E**): back extensor muscles; (**F**): abdominal muscles.

The participants lay supine with their hip and knee joints flexed to 90° to evaluate the hamstrings. The knee was extended as much as possible from this position, and the knee joint angle was measured at full extension [14]. The reference axis was the femoral shaft and the movement axis was the shaft of the lower leg (Figure 2C).

For the gluteus maximus, with the anterior superior iliac spine (ASIS) stabilized, the hip joint was passively flexed while keeping the knee flexed. The hip flexion angle was measured when the ASIS began to move [15] (Figure 2D). The reference axis was the line from the acromion to the greater trochanter and the movement axis was the femoral shaft.

A line connecting the left and right PSIS was drawn to assess the back and abdominal muscles, and a point 15 cm above the intersection with the spine was used as a landmark. The participants flexed and extended their trunks while keeping their arms relaxed. The distance between the two landmarks during flexion and extension was measured using a tape measure, and the change in distance was used as the muscle length index [16] (Figure 2E,F). An increase in the distance during flexion and a decrease during extension indicate greater lumbar mobility.

The rectus femoris, iliopsoas, hamstrings, and gluteus maximus were measured on both sides, and the side showing the most significant muscle shortening was used for the analysis. All measurements were performed twice, and the minimum value was used for analysis.

2.6. Data Analysis

To investigate the individual and interactive effects of thoracic, lumbar, and pelvic alignment on muscle length, we first constructed random forest regression models for each muscle. The dataset comprised 41 participants, and each model used 17 spinopelvic alignment parameters as input variables to predict a single muscle length index. The models were built using scikit-learn with 100 estimators (n_estimators = 100) and a fixed random state (random_state = 42) for reproducibility. All other hyperparameters were set to default. Given the limited sample size, we did not use cross-validation but instead assessed model performance using mean absolute error (MAE) to quantify prediction accuracy. No normalization (e.g., z-score standardization or min–max scaling) was applied to the muscle length indices, as the values were already expressed in interpretable physical units (degrees or centimeters), making further transformation unnecessary. Subsequently, we employed SHAP analysis, a model interpretation method based on machine learning. SHAP is a game-theoretic approach that quantifies the contribution of each independent variable to the predicted value of the dependent variable [17]. The SHAP values indicate the magnitude and direction of each variable's contribution to the prediction, not causality. A positive SHAP value implies that the variable increases the predicted outcome, whereas a negative value indicates a contribution that decreases the prediction.

In this study, the dependent variables were the muscle length indices, and the independent variables were the thoracic kyphosis, lumbar lordosis, and anterior pelvic tilt angles. A negative SHAP value for the muscle length index was interpreted as a tendency toward muscle shortening, except for the abdominal muscles, for which a positive SHAP value indicates shortening. To evaluate the individual effects of spinal alignment, SHAP summary plots and mean SHAP values were used to visualize and quantify the relative contribution of each angle to muscle length indices. The summary plot shows the contribution of each independent variable (SHAP value) to the prediction, providing a comprehensive view of the variables that influence muscle-shortening tendencies. Additionally, to assess the interactions between spinal regions, we calculated the mean interaction SHAP values to examine their combined influence on the muscle length indices. The interaction SHAP quantifies the contribution of the interaction between two variables to the predicted outcome. We also visualized the relationship between the SHAP values and spinal curvature angles using dependence plots, focusing on the spinal alignment variable with the most substantial contribution (individually or through interaction). In the dependence plot, the x axis represents the feature value, the y axis represents the SHAP value, and each point represents an individual participant. This allows for a visual interpretation of how feature values relate to the prediction contributions. Moreover, dependence plots can visualize the interaction effects using color-coding points based on the value of a second variable. When interaction effects are present, noticeable shifts in the color patterns are observed, indicating the presence and nature of the interaction.

3. Results

3.1. Characteristics of Participant Measures

The characteristics of the spinal alignment and muscle length indices of the study participants are presented in Table 1.

Table 1. Characteristics of spinal alignment and muscle length indices in study participants.

Measurement Index	Value (Mean ± SD) (n = 40)
Thoracic kyphosis angle (°)	25.9 ± 8.7
Lumbar lordosis angle (°)	26.7 ± 7.2
Anterior pelvic tilt angle (°)	12.6 ± 5.1
Iliopsoas (°)	−9.8 ± 5.2
Rectus femoris (°)	70.8 ± 14.1
Hamstrings (°)	140.4 ± 10.0
Gluteus maximus (°)	69.0 ± 10.8
Back extensor muscles (cm)	21.2 ± 1.1
Abdominal muscles (cm)	12.3 ± 0.7

3.2. Effects of Spinal Alignment on Muscle Length Indices

The mean absolute error (MAE) for each model was as follows: iliopsoas, 3.2°; rectus femoris, 8.1°; gluteus maximus, 8.6°; hamstrings, 7.1°; back extensor muscles, 0.9 cm; and abdominal muscles, 0.6 cm. These values indicate that the models reasonably approximated each muscle length index based on spinopelvic alignment parameters. Figure 3 shows the SHAP summary plots for each muscle length index derived from the random forest model. The features are ranked in descending order based on their mean absolute SHAP values, indicating their relative contributions to the model's prediction. Table 2 displays the mean SHAP values for the individual and interaction effects of spinal alignment on each muscle length index.

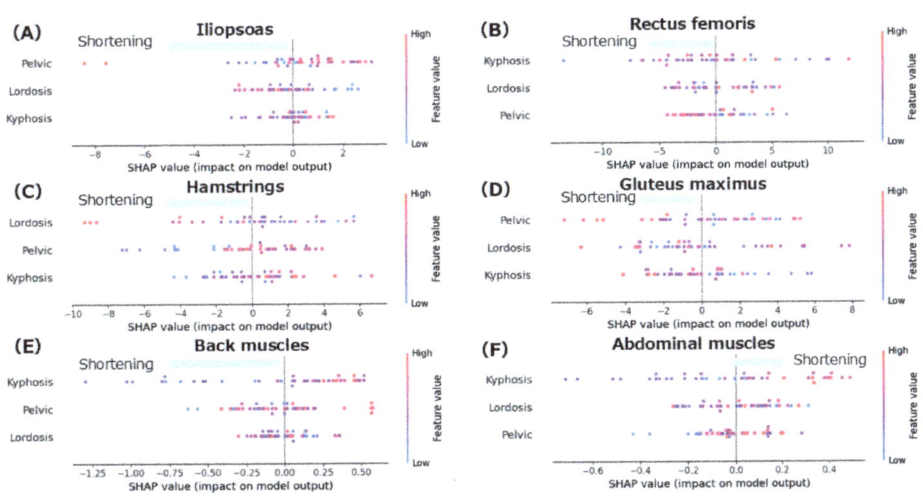

Figure 3. SHAP summary plots for each muscle length index. (**A**): iliopsoas; (**B**): rectus femoris; (**C**): hamstrings; (**D**): gluteus maximus; (**E**): back extensor muscles; (**F**): abdominal muscles. Color coding in the SHAP summary plots indicates the magnitude of each spinal alignment parameter: red represents higher values of the corresponding feature (e.g., greater kyphosis, lordosis, or pelvic tilt), while blue indicates lower values.

Table 2. Mean SHAP values for individual and interaction effects of spinal alignment on each muscle length index.

	RF	IP	HAM	GM	BA	AB
Kyphosis	−0.05	0.00	0.29	0.05	−0.02	−0.01
Lordosis	0.16	−0.09	0.16	−0.08	0.00	0.02
Pelvic	0.02	0.07	−0.30	0.27	−0.02	−0.01
Kyphosis × Lordosis	−0.08	0.00	−0.27	−0.16	0.00	0.00
Kyphosis × Pelvic	−0.05	0.01	−0.03	−0.04	0.00	0.00
Lordosis × Pelvic	0.00	0.04	0.06	0.19	−0.01	−0.01
Kyphosis	−0.05	0.00	0.29	0.05	−0.02	−0.01

RF: rectus femoris, IP: iliopsoas, HAM: hamstrings, GM: gluteus maximus, BA: back muscles, AB: abdominal muscles.

3.2.1. Iliopsoas

The summary plot for the iliopsoas (Figure 3A) shows that greater anterior pelvic tilt angles were associated with negative SHAP values, indicating a contribution to iliopsoas muscle shortening. Notably, even in patients with smaller anterior pelvic tilt angles, negative SHAP values were observed, indicating a shortening tendency. Similarly, increased lumbar lordosis angles were associated with negative SHAP values, suggesting a contribution to the shortening of the iliopsoas. In contrast, the thoracic kyphosis angles showed a mixed distribution of positive and negative SHAP values with no consistent trend. According to the mean SHAP values in Table 2, lumbar lordosis had the strongest individual contribution to iliopsoas muscle shortening (mean SHAP = −0.09). Given that lumbar lordosis was the most influential factor, a dependence plot of the lordosis angle was generated (Figure 4A). This plot revealed that lumbar lordosis angles between 20° and 35° were associated with negative SHAP values, indicating a contribution to iliopsoas shortening.

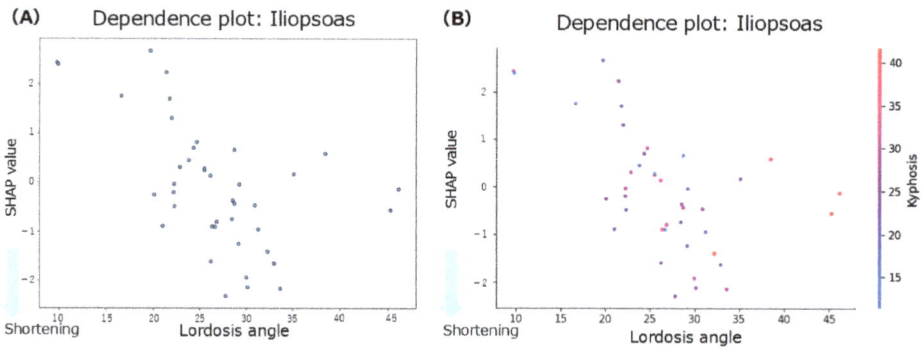

Figure 4. Dependence plots for the iliopsoas muscle. (**A**): dependence plot for the lumbar lordosis angle; (**B**): dependence plot for the interaction between the thoracic kyphosis and lumbar lordosis angles.

Focusing on interregional spinal interactions, the mean interaction SHAP values (Table 2) were positive across all spinal region combinations, suggesting that interaction effects did not contribute to iliopsoas shortening. However, a dependence plot of the interaction between lumbar lordosis and thoracic kyphosis (Figure 4B) showed that lumbar lordosis angles between 20° and 40° and thoracic kyphosis angles between 20° and 50° were associated with negative SHAP values, indicating a potential interaction-related contribution to the shortening of the iliopsoas within this specific range.

3.2.2. Rectus Femoris

The summary plot for the rectus femoris (Figure 3B) shows that the SHAP values for thoracic kyphosis were positively and negatively distributed with no clear trend observed. However, when the lumbar lordosis angles were high, the SHAP values tended to be negative, indicating a contribution to rectus femoris shortening. Similarly, greater anterior pelvic tilt angles were associated with negative SHAP values, suggesting a tendency towards shortening. According to the mean SHAP values in Table 2, thoracic kyphosis showed the strongest individual contribution to rectus femoris shortening (mean SHAP = −0.05). The dependence plot for thoracic kyphosis (Figure 5A) revealed that the SHAP values were negative within the 10–35° range, indicating a contribution to rectus femoris shortening in this angle range.

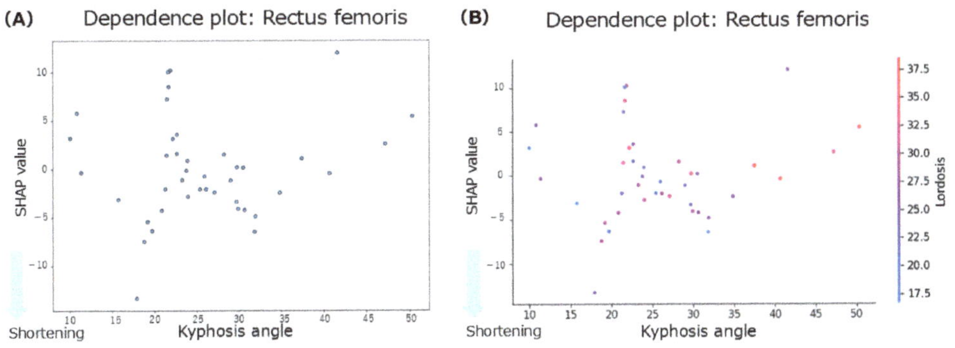

Figure 5. Dependence plots for the rectus femoris muscle. (**A**): dependence plot for the thoracic kyphosis angle. (**B**): dependence plot for the interaction between the thoracic kyphosis and lumbar lordosis angles.

Focusing on the interactions between spinal regions, the interaction of SHAP values (Table 2) indicated that the interaction between thoracic kyphosis and lumbar lordosis contributed to rectus femoris shortening (interaction mean SHAP = −0.08). The dependence plot for this interaction (Figure 5B) showed that the SHAP values were negative when the thoracic kyphosis and lumbar lordosis angles were within the 10–35° range, indicating a shortening-related contribution from their interaction.

3.2.3. Hamstrings

The summary plot for the hamstrings (Figure 3C) shows that greater lumbar lordosis angles were associated with negative SHAP values, indicating a contribution to hamstring shortening. Similarly, smaller anterior pelvic tilt angles were associated with negative SHAP values, suggesting a tendency toward muscle shortening. In contrast, the SHAP values for thoracic kyphosis were positively and negatively distributed with no consistent trend observed. According to the Mean SHAP values in Table 2, pelvic tilt showed the strongest individual contribution to hamstring shortening (Mean SHAP = −0.30). The dependence plot for anterior pelvic tilt (Figure 6A) indicated that the SHAP values were negative in the 0–10° range, suggesting a contribution to hamstring shortening in this angle range.

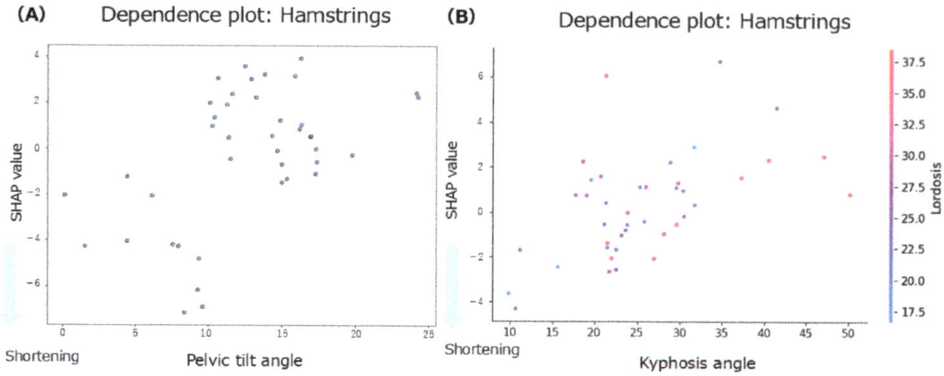

Figure 6. Dependence plots for the hamstrings. (**A**): dependence plot for the anterior pelvic tilt angle; (**B**): dependence plot for the interaction between the thoracic kyphosis and lumbar lordosis angles.

Focusing on inter-regional spinal interactions, the interaction mean SHAP values (Table 2) showed that both the thoracic–lumbar interaction (interaction mean SHAP = −0.27) and the thoracic–pelvic interaction (interaction mean SHAP = −0.03) contributed to hamstring shortening. The dependence plot for the interaction between thoracic kyphosis and lumbar lordosis (Figure 6B) demonstrated that when thoracic kyphosis was between 10° and 30° and lumbar lordosis was between 18° and 35°, the SHAP values were negative, indicating a contribution to hamstring shortening in this range.

3.2.4. Gluteus Maximus

The summary plot for the gluteus maximus (Figure 3D) showed that the SHAP values for anterior pelvic tilt were positively and negatively distributed, indicating no consistent trend. When the lumbar lordosis angles were small, the SHAP values tended to be negative, suggesting a contribution to shortening of the GM. In contrast, at higher lumbar lordosis angles, the SHAP values were mixed, with no clear directional patterns. High thoracic kyphosis angles were associated with negative SHAP values, indicating their contribution to gluteus maximus shortening. According to the mean SHAP values in Table 2, lumbar lordosis had the strongest individual contribution to gluteus maximus shortening (mean SHAP = −0.08). The dependence plot for lumbar lordosis (Figure 7A) revealed that the SHAP values were negative in the 10–45° range, suggesting a shortening tendency in this range.

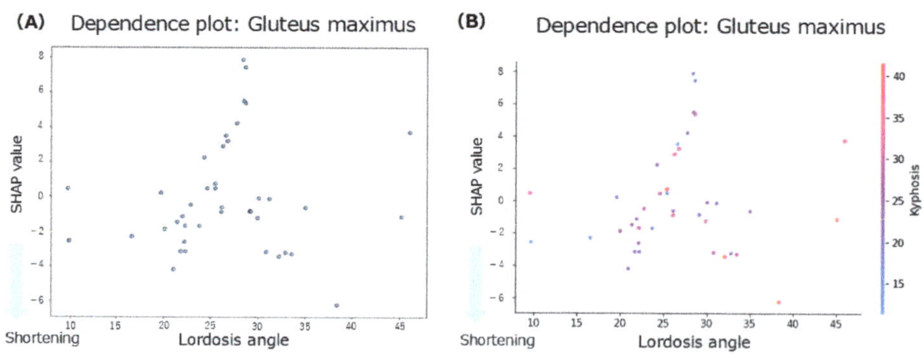

Figure 7. Dependence plots for the gluteus maximus concerning lumbar lordosis. (**A**): Dependence plot for the lumbar lordosis angle. (**B**): Dependence plot for the interaction between the lumbar lordosis and thoracic kyphosis angles.

Regarding inter-regional spinal interactions, the mean interaction SHAP values (Table 2) showed that the interaction between thoracic kyphosis and lumbar lordosis contributed to gluteus maximus shortening (interaction mean SHAP = −0.16). The dependence plot for this interaction (Figure 7B) indicated that when thoracic kyphosis was between 10° and 40° and lumbar lordosis was between 10° and 45°, the SHAP values were negative, suggesting a contribution to gluteus maximus shortening in this range.

3.2.5. Back Muscles

The summary plot for the back extensor muscles (Figure 3E) showed a tendency toward negative SHAP values when the thoracic kyphosis angles were small, indicating a contribution to muscle shortening. In contrast, the SHAP values for pelvic tilt were positively and negatively distributed, showing no clear trends. When the thoracic kyphosis angles were high, the SHAP values tended to be negative, suggesting a shortening effect. According to the mean SHAP values in Table 2, both thoracic kyphosis (mean SHAP = −0.02) and pelvic tilt (mean SHAP = −0.02) contributed to back extensor shortening. The dependence plot for thoracic kyphosis (Figure 8) showed that the SHAP values were negative in the 10–23° range, indicating an association with muscle shortening in that angular range.

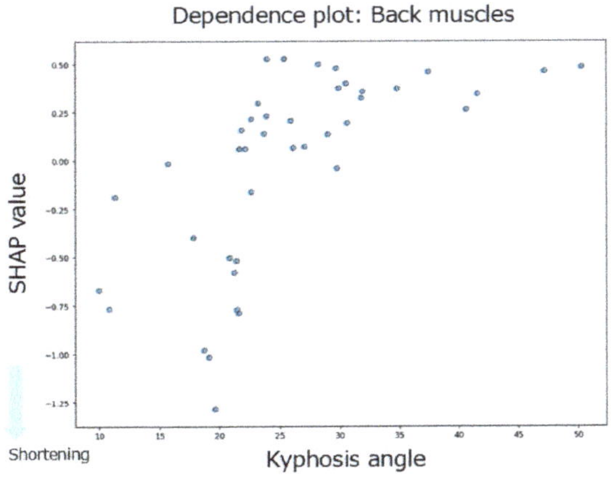

Figure 8. A dependence plot for the back extensor muscles about the thoracic kyphosis angle.

Regarding inter-regional spinal interactions, the interaction of SHAP values (Table 2) did not contribute to the shortening of the back extensor muscles. Additionally, the absolute SHAP values for the back extensor muscles were lower than those observed for the hip-related muscles, indicating that both the individual and interaction effects of spinal alignment contributed minimally to the variation in back extensor muscle length.

3.2.6. Abdominal Muscles

The summary plot for the abdominal muscles (Figure 3F) shows that greater thoracic kyphosis angles tended to be associated with positive SHAP values, indicating a contribution to abdominal muscle shortening. Similarly, smaller lumbar lordosis angles also tended to produce positive SHAP values, which contributed to shortening. In contrast, overall, the SHAP values for lumbar lordosis were distributed positively and negatively, showing no consistent trend. According to the mean SHAP values shown in Table 2, lumbar lordosis had the strongest individual contribution to abdominal muscle shortening (mean SHAP = 0.02). The dependence plot for lumbar lordosis (Figure 9) revealed that the

SHAP values were positive in the 10–35° range, indicating a shortening-related effect in this region.

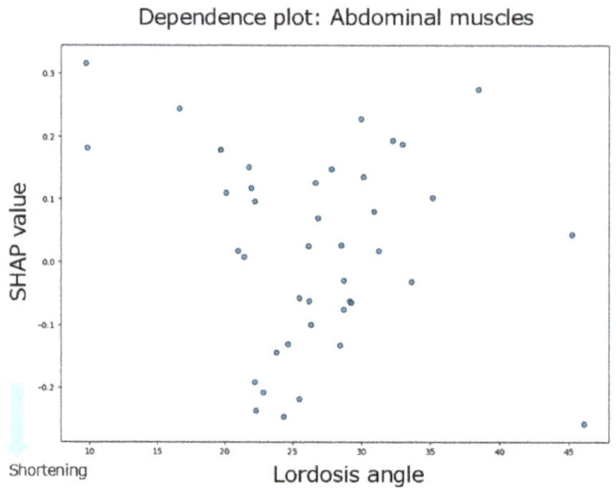

Figure 9. Dependence plot for the abdominal muscles about lumbar lordosis.

Regarding inter-regional spinal interactions, none of the interaction SHAP values between the spinal regions contributed to abdominal muscle shortening (Table 2). Moreover, the absolute SHAP values for the abdominal muscles were lower than those for the hip-related muscles, suggesting that both the individual and interaction effects of spinal alignment had a limited influence on abdominal muscle length.

4. Discussion

This study investigated the associations between the individual and interactive effects of thoracic, lumbar, and pelvic alignment and trunk and hip-related muscle lengths. The SHAP summary plots derived from the random forest model revealed that the degree of the spinal alignment's contribution to muscle shortening varied across different muscles. For the rectus femoris, thoracic alignment contributed the most to muscle shortening, with the interaction between the thoracic and lumbar regions showing the most substantial contribution among the interaction effects. The lumbar alignment had the greatest influence on the iliopsoas; however, no significant interaction effect was observed. Hamstring shortening was associated with pelvic alignment alone and with the interaction between the thoracic and lumbar regions. In the gluteus maximus, the lumbar alignment and thoracolumbar interactions contribute to muscle shortening. In contrast, the contributions from both the individual and interaction effects were minimal for the back extensor and abdominal muscles. These findings suggest that muscle shortening, particularly in the muscles surrounding the hip joint, may be associated with both the individual influence of spinal alignment and interactions between spinal regions.

Regarding the effect of individual spinal alignment on muscle shortening, thoracic kyphosis contributed to the shortening of the rectus femoris, with a mean SHAP value of −0.05. Although the summary plot indicated that thoracic kyphosis had the most significant impact on the rectus femoris, SHAP values exhibited bidirectional contributions (both positive and negative), suggesting no consistent trend. However, the dependence plot revealed that the SHAP values were predominantly negative within the thoracic kyphosis angle range of 10–35°, indicating an association with rectus femoris shortening. According to previous studies, the average thoracic kyphosis angle in healthy young men is 31.2 ± 5.32° [18], and an excessive thoracic kyphosis is defined as an angle of 42° or greater [19]. In the present study, the participants had an average thoracic kyphosis angle of 25.9 ± 8.7°, suggesting a tendency toward smaller than average thoracic curvature. Furthermore, the dependence plot showed a concentration of negative SHAP values, particularly within the 20–30° range, indicating that individuals with reduced thoracic curvature tended to shorten the rectus femoris. Although the rectus femoris originates from the anterior inferior iliac spine and does not attach to the thoracic spine, it is directly connected to the pelvis. Therefore, anterior pelvic tilt places the rectus femoris in a shortened position. This suggests that changes in pelvic alignment may indirectly influence other regions, such as the thoracic kyphosis, through kinetic chains and compensatory mechanisms. Additionally, previous reports have indicated that shortening of the rectus femoris may promote anterior pelvic tilt and increase lumbar lordosis as a compensatory response [20]. This is consistent with the summary plot of the present study, which showed a tendency for rectus femoris shortening with a more significant anterior pelvic tilt, aligning with the anatomical and biomechanical functions of the muscle. These findings suggest that rectus femoris shortening may be associated with changes in pelvic alignment and indirectly with thoracic kyphosis, potentially serving as a compensatory mechanism for maintaining the overall spinal alignment. Moreover, a previous study reported a significant negative correlation between thoracic kyphosis and rectus femoris length, indicating that more significant thoracic kyphosis is associated with rectus femoris shortening [21]. This suggests that, as the thoracic spine becomes more kyphotic and the center of gravity shifts, changes in the rectus femoris length may occur, stabilizing the center of mass over the lumbar spine and pelvis. In summary, the contribution of thoracic kyphosis to the rectus femoris shortening may be interpreted as a compensatory adjustment in the spinal curvature among individuals with average or below-average thoracic kyphosis in response to changes in pelvic and lumbar alignment, although thoracic kyphosis itself does not directly influence the rectus femoris through movement.

Concerning lumbar lordosis, the most significant contributions to muscle shortening were observed for the iliopsoas (mean SHAP = −0.09) and the gluteus maximus (mean SHAP = −0.08). In the summary plot for the iliopsoas, the anterior pelvic tilt showed the highest contribution; however, the SHAP values were widely dispersed, indicating a lack of consistency. In contrast, lumbar lordosis angles within the 20–35° range were associated with negative SHAP values, suggesting a contribution to iliopsoas shortening. Previous research has reported an average lumbar lordosis angle of 30.2 ± 5.21° in healthy young men [18]. In contrast, the average value in the present study was 26.7 ± 7.2°, indicating a tendency toward reduced lumbar curvature in the current sample. The dependence plot further supported this finding, showing a predominance of negative SHAP values in the 25–35° range, indicating an overall trend of iliopsoas shortening. Among the iliopsoas components, the psoas major is directly attached to the lumbar spine and facilitates lumbar lordosis. A previous study reported that shortening of the iliopsoas muscle was associated with increased lumbar lordosis [4]. For the gluteus maximus, the mean SHAP value was −0.08, indicating a contribution to muscle shortening. Although anterior pelvic tilt showed the highest contribution in the summary plot, the SHAP values for this variable were distributed across both positive and negative directions, with no clear trend. The dependence plot revealed negative SHAP values in individuals with lordosis angles > 30° and reduced angles of <30°. Notably, negative SHAP values in participants with reduced lumbar lordosis support previous findings, suggesting that a smaller lumbar lordosis angle contributes to gluteus maximus shortening [22]. The gluteus maximus attaches to the posterior aspect of the pelvis and plays a role in posterior pelvic tilt. In a posture in which the posterior pelvic tilt reduces lumbar lordosis, gluteus maximus shortening may occur. A previous study reported that individuals with gluteus maximus contracture demonstrated decreased lumbar lordosis compared with healthy individuals [23]. This has been interpreted as a compensatory mechanism for maintaining the global spinopelvic balance through pelvic morphological changes. Although some variability exists in the lumbar lordosis angle at which gluteus maximus shortening occurs, the finding that reduced lumbar lordosis is associated with gluteus maximus shortening is consistent with those of previous studies [4]. These results suggest that specific ranges of lumbar lordosis angles contribute to the shortening of the iliopsoas and gluteus maximus. This may be explained by a combination of direct anatomical effects and indirect compensatory mechanisms involving other body segments, highlighting the multifactorial relationship between lumbar alignment and muscle length.

Regarding anterior pelvic tilt, the hamstrings showed the most substantial contribution to muscle shortening, with a mean SHAP value of -0.30. The summary plot also indicated that smaller anterior pelvic tilt angles were associated with hamstring shortening, suggesting a tendency towards muscle shortening in the presence of a posterior pelvic tilt. The dependence plot further confirmed this relationship, with many participants exhibiting negative SHAP values when the anterior pelvic tilt was $\leq 10°$, indicating a contribution to muscle shortening. In this study, the average anterior pelvic tilt angle was $12.6 \pm 5.1°$, which is consistent with previous reports indicating an average of $12.6 \pm 5.8°$ in healthy young men [13]. According to a previous study [13], the primary role of the hamstrings in standing posture is to induce posterior pelvic tilt. As hip extensors, the hamstrings pull the posterior pelvis downward, counteracting an excessive anterior tilt. Similarly, a previous study reported that the hamstrings promote posterior pelvic tilt [4]. Moreover, a previous study noted that hamstring shortening is generally associated with a significant increase in posterior pelvic tilt, suggesting a relationship between reduced hamstring flexibility and increased pelvic retroversion [24]. However, in the present study, some participants who did not show a posterior pelvic tilt still exhibited SHAP values, indicating hamstring shortening. A previous study reported that hamstring length is not always associated with anterior pelvic tilt during standing [25]. They suggested that when multiple muscle groups are simultaneously shortened, their effects may cancel each other out, resulting in no observable alignment changes. Nevertheless, in our study, the contribution of hamstring shortening was relatively small in participants without a posterior pelvic tilt, whereas it was substantially greater in those with a posterior pelvic tilt. These findings suggest that, when a posterior pelvic tilt is present, the hamstrings, which attach directly to the pelvis, may have direct anatomical and biomechanical roles in muscle shortening.

This study examined whether interactions between spinal regions enhance muscle shortening. Using interaction SHAP analysis, we found that all hip-related muscles contributed the most to muscle shortening through the interaction between thoracic kyphosis and lumbar lordosis. In contrast, for the back extensors and abdominal muscles, the contributions from both individual and interaction effects were minimal. When comparing the contributions of individual versus interactive effects, thoracic kyphosis alone contributed to rectus femoris shortening; however, the thoracolumbar interaction showed an even more significant contribution. Similarly, thoracolumbar interaction influenced gluteus maximus shortening more strongly than lumbar lordosis alone. For the hamstrings, pelvic alignment showed the strongest individual contribution, but interaction SHAP analysis revealed that the thoracolumbar interaction was the dominant factor. In contrast, lumbar lordosis showed the strongest individual contribution to the iliopsoas; however, the interaction effects were weaker. Based on these findings, we further explored the dependence plots for the rectus femoris, gluteus maximus, and hamstrings, which showed increased contributions under interaction effects, to identify the characteristic angle ranges. For the rectus femoris, participants with thoracic kyphosis angles of 20–30° and lumbar lordosis angles of 20–35° exhibited concentrated negative SHAP values, indicating a contribution to muscle shortening. For the gluteus maximus, a similar concentration of negative SHAP values was observed in the ranges of thoracic kyphosis 20–30° and lumbar lordosis 15–30°. Similarly, for the hamstrings, negative SHAP values were concentrated in the range of thoracic kyphosis 10–30° and lumbar lordosis 18–35°. Despite their different anatomical locations and functions (i.e., anterior versus posterior hip musculature), these muscles share similar thoracolumbar interaction ranges associated with shortening. A previous study suggested that although the rectus femoris does not anatomically attach to the thoracic spine, thoracic kyphosis may still indirectly influence its function via compensatory adjustments of the spine and pelvis to maintain postural balance [21]. Similarly, a previous study reported that individuals with gluteus maximus contracture showed reduced lumbar lordosis and increased thoracic kyphosis, indicating that compensatory mechanisms in spinopelvic alignment may preserve the overall sagittal balance even in symptomatic populations [23]. For the hamstrings, increased tension has been reported to influence spinal curvature [26], and associations between lumbar lordosis and anterior pelvic tilt in the standing position have also been established [27], suggesting that spinal and pelvic alignments jointly contribute to postural regulation. Physiological spinal curvatures, such as lordosis and kyphosis, help efficiently absorb and distribute mechanical loads. These curvatures also influence the position of the center of gravity, thereby contributing to balance and postural stability. Curvature levels, angles, and combinations of spinal and pelvic alignments vary widely and can be classified into multiple alignment types [10]. Taken together, these findings suggest that the spine and pelvis function as a coordinated complex, the spinopelvic unit, which adjusts posture in response to changes in the center of gravity and load distribution. Therefore, changes in thoracic kyphosis and lumbar lordosis may influence pelvic alignment through kinetic chains, and the interaction between these regions may play a key role in contributing to the shortening of the hip-related muscles.

The novelty and strength of this study lie in its investigation of how individual spinal alignments and inter-regional spinal interactions are associated with muscle length, using a machine learning-based analytical method that enables interpretability. The analysis revealed that among the hip-related muscles, individual spinal regions tended to contribute to muscle shortening. Furthermore, in the rectus femoris, hamstring, and gluteus maximus, the combined effects of lumbar lordosis and thoracic kyphosis were associated with a more substantial contribution to muscle shortening. These findings suggest that the direct anatomical effects of muscles attached to the spine and indirect effects, such as spinal curvature-induced shifts in the center of gravity and compensatory adjustments due to muscle length imbalance, play a role in whole-body postural balance. The results of this study enhance the interpretation of the relationship between standing postural alignment and muscle shortening, offering the potential for more integrated and precise interpretations of combined postural and muscle assessments. Moreover, if muscle-shortening tendencies in spinal alignment can be understood, it is possible to prioritize intervention strategies targeting specific muscles based on their relevance to postural alignment. Consequently, the interpretative framework established in this study regarding the relationship between spinal alignment and muscle length may contribute to improved clinical assessments and more effective treatment decision-making.

The present study has several limitations. This study focused on the individual associations between spinal alignment and the lengths of specific muscles. As such, it did not account for the interactive influence of the agonist and antagonist muscle groups. Given the variability in muscle development and usage patterns influenced by individual motor experiences and neuromuscular adaptations, antagonistic muscle activity may influence spinal alignment and muscle lengths. The study sample consisted exclusively of young adult males, which limits the generalizability of the findings to other populations, including females and older adults. This restriction intentionally excludes the confounding effects of sex and spinal pathology. Future studies should examine whether the relationships identified in this study differ by sex or age, as muscle characteristics and spinal alignment may vary accordingly. The analysis in this study was limited to the sagittal plane alignment. Frontal plane factors such as scoliosis were not assessed, and the precise vertical level of the spinal curvatures (e.g., curvature apex) was not examined in detail. Previous research has indicated that spinal alignment varies significantly depending on the combination of thoracic, lumbar, and pelvic configurations [10]. Future studies should include frontal plane alignment and curvature apex positioning to examine detailed and characteristic relationships between spinal posture and muscle shortening. While this study focused on muscle length, it is important to recognize that muscle strength influences spinal alignment. The muscle strength data were not collected in this study. While we focused on muscle length indices estimated from postural data, the potential influence of muscle strength on postural alignment and compensatory mechanisms remains unexplored. Future research should incorporate strength measurements to more comprehensively understand the interaction between spinal alignment, muscle function, and flexibility. Therefore, the results cannot be interpreted as a comprehensive analysis of all the spinal alignment factors. Future investigations should incorporate a broader range of variables, including strength and connective tissue properties, to further clarify the contribution of muscle length to spinal alignment within a multidimensional framework. These findings may have clinical implications in rehabilitation strategies; for instance, targeted flexibility exercises for the rectus femoris could potentially reduce compensatory increases in thoracic kyphosis, thereby improving sagittal balance in individuals with anterior pelvic tilt. Future research directions may also be highlighted.

5. Conclusions

This study investigated how the individual effects and interregional interactions of thoracic, lumbar, and pelvic alignments are associated with muscle length. These findings suggest that individual spinal alignment and the interaction between multiple spinal regions contribute to muscle shortening, particularly in the hip-related musculature. Among these, the interaction between thoracic kyphosis and lumbar lordosis showed the strongest association with muscle shortening, indicating that the combined influence of thoracic and lumbar alignments may play a key role in shortening hip-related muscles.

Author Contributions: These authors contributed equally: M.A. and Y.I. conceptualization, M.A., Y.I. and H.S.; methodology, M.A., Y.I. and H.S.; software, H.S.; validation, M.A., Y.I. and H.S.; formal analysis, M.A., Y.I. and H.S.; investigation, M.A., Y.I., and H.S.; resources, H.S. and J.M.; data curation, M.A. and Y.I.; writing—original draft preparation, M.A. and Y.I.; writing—review and editing, T.I., S.T., H.S. and J.M.; visualization, M.A., Y.I. and H.S.; supervision, H.S. and J.M.; project administration, H.S. and J.M.; funding acquisition, H.S. and J.M. All authors have read and agreed to the published version of the manuscript.

Funding: This research was funded by a grant from JSPS KAKENHI (grant number 23K165580).

Institutional Review Board Statement: The study was conducted in accordance with the Declaration of Helsinki and approved by the Ethics Committee of Kyoto Tachibana University (approval no. 24-74, 13 February 2025).

Informed Consent Statement: Informed consent was obtained from all participants involved in the study. Written informed consent was obtained from all patients to publish this paper.

Data Availability Statement: The original contributions presented in this study are included in the article. Further inquiries can be directed to the corresponding authors.

Acknowledgments: We would like to thank all the study participants for their time and willingness to respond and complete the study protocol.

Conflicts of Interest: The authors declare no conflicts of interest.

References

1. Nashner, L.M.; McCollum, G. The organization of human postural movements: A formal basis and experimental synthesis. *Behav. Brain Sci.* **1985**, *8*, 135–150. [CrossRef]
2. Conroy, V.M.; Murray, B.N., Jr.; Alexopulos, Q.T.; McCreary, J. *Kendall's Muscles: Testing and Function with Posture and Pain*; Lippincott Williams & Wilkins: Philadelphia, PA, USA, 2022.
3. Dolphens, M.; Cagnie, B.; Coorevits, P.; Vleeming, A.; Danneels, L. Classification system of the normal variation in sagittal standing plane alignment: A study among young adolescent boys. *Spine* **2013**, *38*, E1003–E1012. [CrossRef]
4. Dolphens, M.; Vleeming, A.; Castelein, R.; Vanderstraeten, G.; Schlösser, T.; Plasschaert, F.; Danneels, L. Coronal plane trunk asymmetry is associated with whole-body sagittal alignment in healthy young adolescents before pubertal peak growth. *Eur. Spine J.* **2018**, *27*, 448–457. [CrossRef]
5. Janda, V.; Frank, C.; Liebenson, C. Evaluation of muscular imbalance. In *Rehabilitation of the Spine: A Practitioner's Manual*; Liebenson, C., Ed.; Lippincott Williams & Wilkins: Philadelphia, PA, USA, 2006; pp. 203–225.
6. Janda, V. On the concept of postural muscles and posture. *Aust. J. Physiother.* **1983**, *29*, S83–S84. [CrossRef] [PubMed]
7. Youdas, J.W.; Garrett, T.R.; Harmsen, S.; Suman, V.J.; Carey, J.R. Lumbar lordosis and pelvic inclination of asymptomatic adults. *Phys. Ther.* **1996**, *76*, 1066–1081. [CrossRef]
8. Fasuyi, F.O.; Fabunmi, A.A.; Adegoke, B.O.A. Hamstring muscle length and pelvic tilt range among individuals with and without low back pain. *J. Bodyw. Mov. Ther.* **2017**, *21*, 246–250. [CrossRef]
9. Walker, M.L.; Rothstein, J.M.; Finucane, S.D.; Lamb, R.L. Relationships between lumbar lordosis, pelvic tilt, and abdominal muscle performance. *Phys. Ther.* **1987**, *67*, 512–516. [CrossRef]
10. Pasha, S.; Shah, S.; Newton, P. Machine learning predicts the 3D outcomes of adolescent idiopathic scoliosis surgery using patient-surgeon specific parameters. *Spine* **2021**, *46*, 579–587. [CrossRef] [PubMed]
11. Hannink, E.; Dawes, H.; Shannon, T.M.L.; Barker, K.L. Validity of sagittal thoracolumbar curvature measurement using a non-radiographic surface topography method. *Spine Deform.* **2022**, *10*, 1299–1306. [CrossRef]
12. Youdas, J.W.; Suman, V.J.; Garrett, T.R. Reliability of measurements of lumbar spine sagittal mobility obtained with the flexible curve. *J. Orthop. Sports Phys. Ther.* **1995**, *21*, 13–20. [CrossRef]
13. Ludwig, O.; Wilhelm, L.; Fröhlich, M. Correlation between the sacral tilt measured with an inclinometer and the pelvic tilt as a tool for assessing the pelvic position. *J. Phys. Ther. Sci.* **2024**, *36*, 186–189. [CrossRef]
14. Corkery, M.; Briscoe, H.; Ciccone, N.; Foglia, G.; Johnson, P.; Kinsman, S.; Legere, L.; Lum, B.; Canavan, P.K. Establishing normal values for lower extremity muscle length in college-age students. *Phys. Ther. Sport* **2007**, *8*, 66–74. [CrossRef]
15. Magee, D.J.; Mancke, R.C. *Orthopedic Physical Assessment*, 7th ed.; Elsevier: Amsterdam, The Netherlands, 2020; pp. 813–817.
16. Chatchawan, U.; Jupamatangb, U.; Chanchitc, S.; Puntumetakul, R.; Donpunha, W.; Yamauchi, J. Immediate effects of dynamic sitting exercise on the lower back mobility of sedentary young adults. *J. Phys. Ther. Sci.* **2015**, *27*, 3359–3363. [CrossRef] [PubMed]
17. Martini, M.L.; Neifert, S.N.; Gal, J.S.; Oermann, E.K.; Gilligan, J.T.; Caridi, J.M. Drivers of prolonged hospitalization following spine surgery: A game-theory-based approach to explaining machine learning models. *J. Bone Jt. Surg.* **2021**, *103*, 64–73. [CrossRef] [PubMed]
18. Farokhmanesh, K.; Shirzadian, T.; Mahboubi, M.; Shahri, M.N. Effect of foot hyperpronation on lumbar lordosis and thoracic kyphosis in standing position using 3-dimensional ultrasound-based motion analysis system. *Glob. J. Health Sci.* **2014**, *6*, 254–260. [CrossRef]
19. Seidi, F.; Rajabi, R.; Ebrahimi, I.; Alizadeh, M.H.; Minoonejad, H. The efficiency of corrective exercise interventions on thoracic hyper-kyphosis angle. *J. Back Musculoskelet. Rehabil.* **2014**, *27*, 7–16. [CrossRef]
20. Evangelista, J.K. Influence of muscular imbalances on pelvic position and lumbar lordosis: A theoretical basis. *J. Nurs. Soc. Stud. Public Health Rehabil.* **2013**, *4*, 25–36.
21. Chow, S.B.; Moffat, M. Relationship of thoracic kyphosis to functional reach and lower-extremity joint range of motion and muscle length in women with osteoporosis or osteopenia. *Top. Geriatr. Rehabil.* **2004**, *20*, 297–306. [CrossRef]
22. Jeon, I.; Jang, J. Comparison of prone hip extension exercise and prone hip extension exercise after iliopsoas stretching on lumbopelvic control and gluteus maximus activity in subjects with short iliopsoas. *J. Musculoskelet. Sci. Technol.* **2017**, *1*, 19–25. [CrossRef]
23. Liu, J.; Huang, P.; Jiang, G.; Gao, L.; Zhang, M.; Dong, X.; Zhang, W.; Zhang, X. Spinal-pelvic sagittal parameters in patients with gluteal muscle contracture: An imaging study. *PeerJ* **2022**, *10*, e13093. [CrossRef]

24. Herrington, L. The effect of pelvic position on popliteal angle achieved during 90:90 hamstring-length test. *J. Sport Rehabil.* **2013**, *22*, 254–256. [CrossRef] [PubMed]
25. Gajdosik, R.L.; Albert, C.R.; Mitman, J.J. Influence of hamstring length on the standing position and flexion range of motion of the pelvic angle, lumbar angle, and thoracic angle. *J. Orthop. Sports Phys. Ther.* **1994**, *20*, 213–219. [CrossRef] [PubMed]
26. López-Miñarro, P.A.; Alacid, F. Influence of hamstring muscle extensibility on spinal curvatures in young athletes. *Sci. Sports* **2010**, *25*, 188–193. [CrossRef]
27. Day, J.W.; Smidt, G.L.; Lehmann, T. Effect of pelvic tilt on standing posture. *Phys. Ther.* **1984**, *64*, 510–516. [CrossRef]

Journal of
Functional Morphology and Kinesiology

MDPI

Article

Can Plantar Pressure Distribution During Gait Be Estimated from Quiet Stance in Healthy Individuals?

Marta Mirando [1], Chiara Pavese [1,2], Valeria Pingue [1,2], Stefania Sozzi [3] and Antonio Nardone [1,2,*]

1 Department of Clinical-Surgical, Diagnostic and Pediatric Sciences, University of Pavia, 27100 Pavia, Italy; marta.mirando01@universitadipavia.it (M.M.); chiara.pavese@unipv.it (C.P.)
2 Istituti Clinici Scientifici Maugeri IRCCS, Centro Studi Attività Motorie (CSAM) and Neurorehabilitation and Spinal Units of Pavia Institute, 27100 Pavia, Italy
3 Department of Electrical, Computer and Biomedical Engineering, University of Pavia, 27100 Pavia, Italy; stefania.sozzi@unipv.it
* Correspondence: antonio.nardone@unipv.it

Abstract

Objectives: We assessed the difference between quiet stance and gait in the spatial distribution and intensity of foot plantar pressures and whether it is possible to estimate the distribution during gait from data obtained during stance. **Methods**: A total of 60 healthy subjects with a mean age of 31.0 ± 9.4 years performed two trials for quiet stance and four trials for gait on a baropodometric walkway with their eyes open. Foot plantar pressures were recorded from 10 areas of the foot sole. **Results**: During quiet stance, the highest plantar pressure occurred at metatarsal heads (M2 to M4) and the medial (MH) and lateral halves of the heel (LH). During gait, the profile of plantar pressure values was like that during stance, but significantly higher. The differences concentrated at the big toe (T1), M2 to M4, MH, and LH, whilst toes (T2,3,4,5) and midfoot (MF) showed the smallest difference. A significant positive correlation was found between the corresponding areas of foot pressure during gait and stance. **Conclusions**: During quiet stance and gait, the overall profile of plantar pressure distribution was similar. During quiet stance, the subjects loaded more on the heels, in keeping with the known position of the center of pressure just in front of the ankles. During gait, higher pressures on the metatarsal areas are related to the forward propulsion of the center of mass. The correlation between the corresponding areas of foot pressure during gait and stance suggests that the pressure distribution during gait can partly be estimated from that during stance. This finding might be useful in most clinical settings when a single sensorized platform rather than a complete walkway is available.

Keywords: plantar pressures; quiet stance; gait; baropodometry; stabilometry; healthy subjects; rehabilitation

1. Introduction

In assessing human gait and posture, foot pressures play a role in accessing the information hidden beneath the foot's interaction with the surface in contact [1]. During quiet stance and gait, the spatial distribution of foot plantar pressures over time determines the average position of the center of pressure (CoP) as the centroid of the total number of active sensors [2,3]. During quiet stance, the CoP sways in both anteroposterior and mediolateral directions due to the forces exerted on the ground through the feet to control the center of mass (CoM) to maintain stability [4]. The sway of the CoP in both the AP and ML directions is a manifestation of the dynamic interplay between the gravitational forces acting on the CoM and the neuromuscular responses required to counteract these forces [5]. On the other hand, during the stance phase of gait, the progression of the CoP consists of a path formed by a series of coordinates passing from the hindfoot to the midfoot and finally to the forefoot, again as a product of the spatial and temporal distribution of the foot plantar pressures [2].

Analyzing plantar pressures during gait is essential for understanding foot function, biomechanics, and their implications for various activities of daily living and clinical conditions. By evaluating plantar pressure distribution, clinicians can identify asymmetries, abnormal loading patterns, and areas of excessive pressure, which may indicate underlying musculoskeletal or neurological impairments [6]. Initially, the analysis of foot pressures was used mostly for clinical foot deformities or foot illness diagnosis [7], such as those of patients affected by diabetes mellitus [8,9], calcaneal [10,11], or ankle fractures (see Mirando et al. [12] for a review) and pes cavus [13,14]. In these conditions, plantar pressures allow for the estimation of the severity of the pathology and assess the possible risk of complications [15].

Although plantar pressures during gait have been thoroughly studied in both healthy subjects and patients, little consideration has been given to plantar pressures during quiet stance [16]. For example, at variance with the latter condition, when the plantar pressures are constantly acting at the interface between the foot sole and the ground, during the stance phase of gait, the plantar pressures progress during three distinct phases (loading response, mid-stance, and terminal stance) [17,18]. In addition, the plantar pressures are affected by gait speed in a non-uniform way but with some differences in the various areas of the foot sole [19]. Finally, both leg and intrinsic foot muscles are active during double leg support [20,21] as much as during quiet stance, but they are active to a larger extent during the single leg stance phase of gait [20], thus affecting the intensity and pattern of distribution of foot plantar pressures [22].

To our knowledge, few data have been published directly comparing plantar pressures across different areas of the foot sole during balance and gait in the same healthy subjects. Dragulinescu et al. [22] reviewed the pattern of contact areas of the foot sole during different types of standing and gait tasks using different wearable devices. In turn, Cleland et al. [2] focused on the relationship between the contact area of the foot sole and the position of the CoP. They found that the location of CoP is a consequence of different contact regions spread across the foot sole and that, during standing, a great part of the foot sole is in contact with the ground at any time. On the contrary, during gait, only a small part of the foot sole is in contact with the ground. However, neither study focused on the differences in distribution and height of plantar pressures within the various areas of the foot sole between quiet stance and gait. Only Merry et al. [23] addressed this issue. They investigated which regions of the foot can differentiate walking, standing, and sitting in a small sample of young healthy subjects. They aimed to identify the foot sole areas most affected during each activity in a typical working environment to find a connection between work exposure and plantar heel pain.

Although quantitative differences exist in the distribution of plantar pressures between quiet standing and walking, it is not clear to what extent it is possible to estimate plantar pressure distribution during gait from data obtained during quiet stance. This finding might be of some interest since, in most clinical settings, a single sensorized platform rather than a complete walkway is available, thus allowing for recording plantar pressures during quiet stance but not during gait. In addition, we wondered whether any difference in foot plantar pressures between stance and gait was only related to the absolute values being higher during gait [23] or whether there were also spatial differences in plantar pressure distribution between the two tasks. These spatial differences could be the consequence of the biomechanical events characterizing quiet stance and gait and the larger activation of the intrinsic and extrinsic foot muscles under the latter condition [20]. Preliminary results have been presented in abstract form [24].

2. Materials and Methods

2.1. Subjects

This study was approved (#2461CE, 06 October 2020) by the local Ethics Committee of the Istituti Clinici Scientifici Maugeri of Pavia, Italy. Written informed consent was obtained from each subject before the experiment in accordance with the Declaration of Helsinki. The sample size of 60 was an estimate based on what is usual in the field [25] and considering the aim of measuring a diverse age group of healthy volunteers.

The inclusion criteria were the following: (1) age between 18 and 65 years old; (2) no cardiac, pulmonary, or neurological diseases; (3) no previous major trauma or surgical intervention on the musculoskeletal system; and (4) ability to understand and sign the informed consent form. The anthropometric measures collected in our sample were weight, height, and lower limb length (from the greater trochanter to the ground). The subjects were tested at the Centre for the Study of Motor Activities (CSAM) of the Istituti Clinici Scientifici Maugeri in Pavia.

2.2. Assessment Protocol

Plantar pressure was recorded using a baropodometric walkway (P-walk, BTS Bioengineering, Garbagnate Milanese, Italy). The multiple pressure platform system consists of four modules for a total of 9216 resistive load cells (2304 for each platform), with a total length of 2 m and a sampling frequency of 50 Hz. The walkway was calibrated using the manufacturer's proprietary software. Calibration followed standard procedures, applying known weights and verifying sensor response. Prior validation studies regarding the above walkway support excellent accuracy (Pearson's r = 0.99) and low intra-session variability (CV < 5%) during static loading tests [26,27].

Each subject performed two trials barefoot in the quiet stance condition with their eyes open (EO). The participants remained upright with the arms extended alongside the trunk, with the feet forming an open angle of 30° and the malleoli spaced 5 cm apart, following the international standardization criteria for baropodometric tests [28]. To ensure uniformity of position between the subjects, a foot template was placed on the first module of the platform, the one used for static measurements. The path length and surface of the 95% confidence ellipse of the center of pressure (CoP) were recorded for 30 s. The recording did not start immediately, but we waited about ten seconds to avoid recording any initial adaptation of the subjects. The mean of the two trials was calculated for the subsequent analyses.

Four gait trials with EO were performed, asking subjects to start when they felt ready at least two meters before the beginning of the platform, to walk at their usual speed, and to stop two meters after the end of the sensorized platform. We recorded walking speed and single and double support time from the mean of the four trials.

2.3. Plantar Pressure Evaluation

Under both static and walking condition, the software of the sensorized platform divided the foot into the following ten anatomical areas (Figure 1): T1, big toe; T2,3,4,5, toes 2 to 5; M1, metatarsal 1; M2, metatarsal 2; M3, metatarsal 3; M4, metatarsal 4; M5, metatarsal 5; MF, midfoot; MH, medial half of heel; and LH, lateral half of heel. For each area, peak plantar pressure (kPa) was calculated during both quiet stance and gait. The mean peak plantar pressure of the ten-foot areas was calculated separately from the trials under the static condition and the trials under the walking condition for each subject. In such a way, we further analyzed the average value of the areas of the right and the left footprints, which was carried out separately for the static and dynamic conditions.

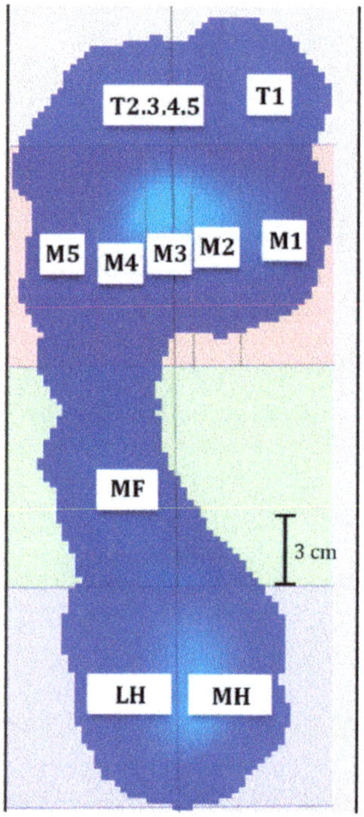

Figure 1. Graphical representation of foot areas in the left foot. The foot is divided into ten areas: T1, big toe; T2,3,4,5, toes 2 to 5; M1, metatarsal 1; M2, metatarsal 2; M3, metatarsal 3; M4, metatarsal 4; M5, metatarsal 5; MF, midfoot; MH, medial half of heel; and LH, lateral half of heel.

In the case of gait trials, given the 2 m length of the walkway, one of the authors (M.M.) selected one step of the right foot and one of the left foot for each trial. Those footprints partially contained by the walkway or with unclearly delineated foot shape were excluded from further analysis. In the latter case, the trial was repeated to obtain four steps for each foot.

2.4. Statistical Analysis

The distribution of the data was assessed for skewness, kurtosis, and equality of variance (Levene's test). As the assumption of normality was met for each variable, data were then expressed as the mean ± standard deviation (SD). For both the right and left foot, we first calculated the average of the peak plantar pressure of the ten-foot areas and tested whether the average value differed between the right and left foot (paired Student's *t*-test). This was performed separately for quiet stance and gait. As we found no difference between the right and left foot mean pressure values during either quiet stance [26] or gait [29], for each condition, we considered the mean pressure of each corresponding area averaged over the two feet for further analysis.

We then assessed the difference in the ten plantar pressure areas and task (stance or gait) using a 2-way repeated measure analysis of variance (ANOVA) with quiet stance and gait and the ten areas as repeated measures. On the other hand, the differences in plantar pressure at each single-foot area calculated between gait and stance were analyzed using a one-way ANOVA. When the assumption of sphericity was violated, the Greenhouse–Geisser correction was applied. Partial eta squared (η^2_p) was reported as a measure of effect size, with 0.01, 0.06, and 0.14 considered as small, medium, and large effect sizes, respectively. Multiple comparison of the mean differences was performed using Tukey's adjustment. The Cohen's d effect size (with 0.2, 0.5, and 0.8 considered as small, medium, and large effect sizes, respectively) was also reported. p values < 0.05 were considered statistically significant.

The relationships between plantar pressures during gait and age, weight, height, body mass index (BMI), and plantar pressures during stance were investigated using regression analyses. All statistical tests were performed using SPSS version 21 for Windows (IBM Corporation, Armonk, NY, USA).

3. Results

3.1. Subject Characteristics

We enrolled 60 healthy subjects, including 29 men (48.3%) and 31 women (51.7%), with a mean age of 31.0 ± 9.4 years (standard deviation, SD), weight of 67.0 ± 13.7 kg, height of 172.0 ± 8.9 cm, body mass index of 22.5 ± 3.1 kg/m^2, and lower limb length of 90.2 ± 5.9 cm and 90.2 ± 5.8 cm for the right and left limbs, respectively.

3.2. CoP Sway and Total Plantar Pressure Distribution During Quiet Stance

During quiet stance, the surface of the 95% confidence ellipse of the CoP and its path were 36.8 ± 12.9 mm^2 and 128.3 ± 29.8 mm, respectively. The average peak pressure between the ten areas of the right and left foot was 30.0 ± 6.6 kPa and 32.5 ± 6.9 kPa (paired *t*-test, p = 0.10, d = 1.05), respectively. As no differences were found between the right and left foot, the mean pressure of each corresponding area from both feet was considered for further analysis.

3.3. Spatial-Temporal Variables of Gait and Total Plantar Pressure Distribution

During gait, the mean speed was 1.20 ± 0.16 m/s. The mean time of single support was 0.46 ± 0.05 s for the right foot and 0.44 ± 0.08 s for the left foot. The mean time of double support was 0.10 ± 0.03 s for the right foot and 0.11 ± 0.03 s for the left foot. We did not find any difference in the support times between the two feet (paired *t*-test for the time of single and double support, respectively; p = 0.20, d = 0.17 and p = 0.55, d = 0.08).

The mean peak plantar pressure of the ten areas of the right and left foot was 132.0 ± 12.5 kPa and 129.1 ± 11.2 kPa, respectively. As in the quiet stance condition, also during gait, the peak plantar pressure averaged over the ten plantar areas did not show a significant (paired *t*-test, p = 0.11, d = 1.17) difference between the right and left foot. Therefore, also in this case, the mean peak plantar pressure of each corresponding area from both feet was considered for further analysis.

The strong similarity between corresponding areas of the right and left foot is apparent in Figure 2, showing that both in the case of quiet stance and gait a significant (p < 0.0001) positive relationship (stance, y = 1.03x + 1.54, R^2 = 0.99; gait, y = 0.97x + 0.47, R^2 = 0.99) existed between mean peak plantar pressures averaged over each of the ten-foot areas of right and left foot.

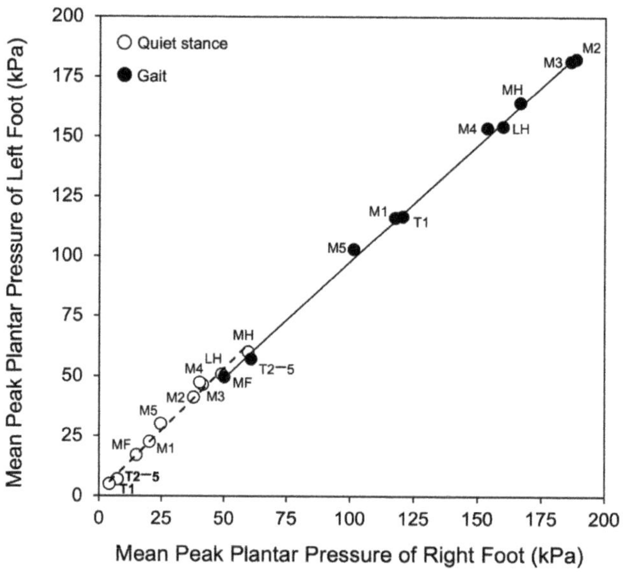

Figure 2. Relationship between the mean peak plantar pressure of each anatomical area of the foot sole during quiet stance and gait in the right and left foot. Each symbol represents the mean peak plantar pressure of the corresponding area of both feet of all subjects.

3.4. Peak Pressures of the Foot Areas During Quiet Stance and Gait

As shown in Figure 3, there was a significant difference between quiet stance and gait condition (F (1,59) = 2345.93, $p < 0.001$, $\eta^2_p = 0.98$). There was a significant difference between foot areas (F (4.35,256.99) = 500.51, $p < 0.001$, $\eta^2_p = 0.89$) and a significant interaction between quiet stance and gait condition and foot areas (F (3.98,234.71) = 207.58, $p < 0.001$, $\eta^2_p = 0.78$). As shown in Figure 3 and Table 1, during quiet stance (open bars), the highest mean peak pressures were recorded at the metatarsal heads (from M2 to M4) and the heel (MH and LH). These areas showed significantly ($p < 0.001$ and d > 0.6 for all comparisons) higher pressure than the others. In turn, the pressure at the metatarsal areas M2 and M3 was significantly ($p < 0.05$ and d > 0.33 for all comparisons) lower than at the heel (MH and LH). The lowest pressures occurred at the toes (T1 and T2–T5) and at the midfoot (MF) ($p < 0.001$ and d > 0.5 for all comparisons).

During gait (Figure 3 and Table 1), overall, the profile of the plantar pressure distribution was superimposable to that during quiet stance. Plantar pressures were significantly ($p < 0.001$) higher in all areas of the foot sole than the corresponding ones during quiet stance. As in the latter case, the highest pressures were found at the metatarsal heads (from M2 to M4) and at the heel (both MH and LH) compared with other areas ($p < 0.001$ and d > 3.04 for all comparisons). At variance with a quiet stance, the pressure at the metatarsal areas M2 and M3 was significantly ($p < 0.001$ and d > 1.04 for all comparisons) higher than at the heel (MH and LH). On the contrary, the lowest pressure occurred at the toes (T2–T5, $p < 0.001$ and d > 2.4 for all comparisons), except for the big toe (T1), which showed a great increase in pressure with respect to T2–T5 ($p < 0.001$, d = 6.37), and at the midfoot (MF, $p < 0.001$, d > 2.5 for all comparisons). There was no difference in the pressure value between T2–T5 and MF area ($p = 0.07$, d = 0.52).

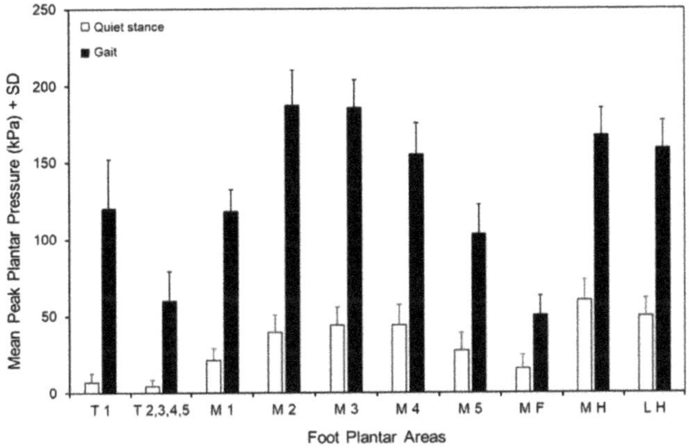

Figure 3. Mean + standard deviation (SD) of peak plantar pressure distribution over the ten anatomical areas of the foot sole during quiet stance (open bars) and gait (filled bars). T1, big toe; T2,3,4,5, toes 2 to 5; M1, metatarsal 1; M2, metatarsal 2; M3, metatarsal 3; M4, metatarsal 4; M5, metatarsal 5; MF, midfoot; MH, medial half of heel; LH, lateral half of heel.

Table 1. Mean ± standard deviation of peak plantar pressure distribution values over the ten anatomical areas of the foot sole averaged from both feet during quiet stance and gait.

Foot Areas	Peak Pressure (kPa) During Quiet Stance	Peak Pressure (kPa) During Gait
T1	7.1 ± 5.8	118.6 ± 34.2
T2–5	4.5 ± 4.0	59.0 ± 20.2
M1	21.3 ± 7.7	116.8 ± 17.6
M2	39.3 ± 11.3	185.4 ± 26.6
M3	43.8 ± 11.8	183.9 ± 22.4
M4	43.7 ± 13.2	153.6 ± 23.1
M5	27.4 ± 11.3	102.2 ± 21.0
MF	15.9 ± 8.5	49.7 ± 13.5
MH	59.9 ± 13.5	165.3 ± 23.2
LH	49.8 ± 11.4	157.0 ± 23.3

3.5. Differences in Peak Pressures of the Foot Areas Between Gait and Quiet Stance

To put into evidence the changes in plantar pressure distribution between quiet stance and gait, we calculated the difference in pressure at each relevant foot area (Figure 4). As already observed, there was a significant difference between the ten-foot area ($F(3.86,227.97) = 219.03$, $p < 0.001$, $\eta^2_p = 0.79$). It appeared that the difference in pressure between gait and stance was not evenly distributed but concentrated at the big toe (T1), metatarsal heads (especially, M2 and M3), and heel (MH and LH); these areas showed a significantly ($p < 0.001$, $d > 1.3$) higher difference than the others. Toes 2 to 5 (T2,3,4,5), fifth metatarsal head (M5), and the midfoot (MF) showed the smallest difference between gait and stance of all areas ($p < 0.001$, $d > 0.98$ for all comparisons).

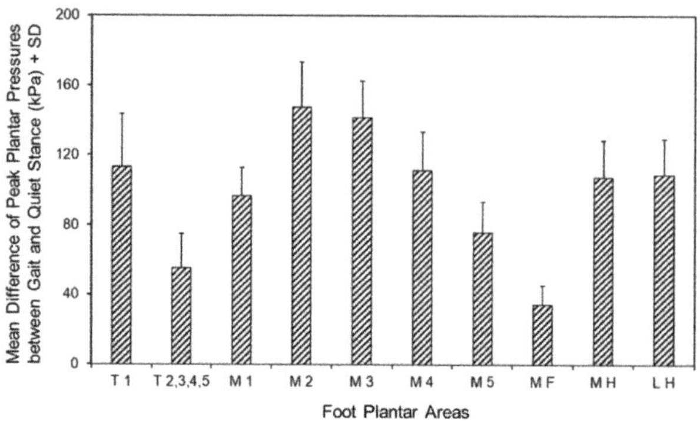

Figure 4. Mean + SD of the difference in peak plantar pressure distribution between quiet stance and gait in the ten anatomical areas of the foot sole, averaged from both feet. T1, big toe; T2,3,4,5, toes 2 to 5; M1, metatarsal 1; M2, metatarsal 2; M3, metatarsal 3; M4, metatarsal 4; M5, metatarsal 5; MF, midfoot; MH, medial half of the heel; LH, lateral half of the heel.

3.6. Relationships Between Quiet Stance, Gait, and BMI

When the average peak pressures of the ten areas of the foot sole during gait were correlated with the corresponding pressures during quiet stance, a significant positive relationship ($y = 2.1x + 64.7$, $p < 0.01$, $R^2 = 0.64$) (Figure 5) was found. On the contrary, no relationship was found between the average peak pressure during gait or stance and the following variables: BMI, gait speed, time of single and double contact, and surface of the 95% confidence ellipse of the CoP and its path (see Table S1).

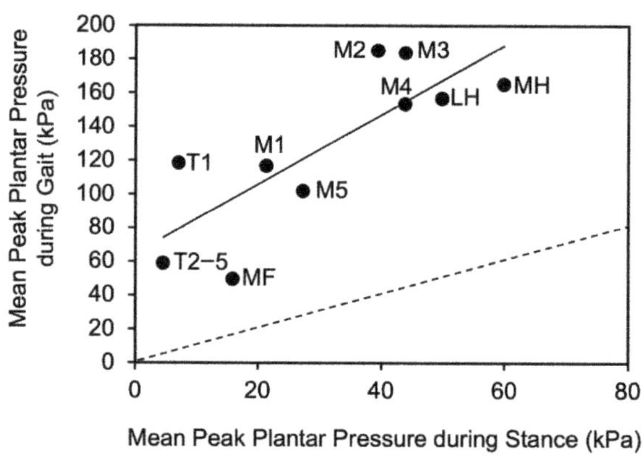

Figure 5. Relationship between the peak plantar pressure of the ten anatomical areas of the foot sole averaged from both feet during gait and quiet stance. T1, big toe; T2,3,4,5, toes 2 to 5; M1, metatarsal 1; M2, metatarsal 2; M3, metatarsal 3; M4, metatarsal 4; M5, metatarsal 5; MF, midfoot; MH, medial half of the heel; LH, lateral half of the heel. The dashed line indicates the identity line.

4. Discussion

In this study, we found that, despite the expected quantitative differences in mean plantar pressures between foot areas and between quiet stance and gait, the distribution of plantar pressures during gait is only slightly qualitatively different compared to quiet stance. During the latter condition, the regions of greatest pressure correspond to the heel and the metatarsals, from the second to the fourth. Conversely, during gait, the areas of greatest pressure correspond to the big toe and, in a similar way to quiet stance, to the heel and the metatarsals. Interestingly, a strong relationship was observed between the peak pressures at corresponding areas of the foot during stance and gait.

4.1. Plantar Pressures During Quiet Stance

In static conditions, such as quiet standing, the distribution of pressure across the foot is relatively uniform and stable. Static standing involves minimal movement and predominantly vertical forces acting on the foot. Under this condition, the body weight is distributed across both feet, primarily through the heels and the balls of the feet, but more on the heels. This phenomenon could be related to the known projection of the center of pressure (CoP) just in front of the ankle [30]. In fact, during quiet stance, the distance between the internal malleolus and the anterior–posterior position of the CoP is on average less than 6 cm, corresponding to about 24% of foot length. As suggested by Hennig and Sterzing [31] and Machado et al. [32], the midfoot may play a key role in balance control since it seems to be the most sensitive region to somatosensory stimuli. In this context, Fernández-Seguín et al. [14] have shown that during quiet stance, the areas where the greatest pressure is exerted are precisely at the level of the forefoot, second, and third metatarsal heads, as in our case. This distribution could be explained by the conformation of the foot, with the bones of the second and third metatarsal heads getting stuck between the wedge-shaped joints and therefore having less freedom of movement. As a result, they are less able to distribute the load they receive [33].

4.2. Plantar Pressures During Gait

As shown by Merry et al. [23], in comparing static and dynamic foot support, the overall pressure distribution appears similar in both conditions, with higher pressures at the heel and forefoot regions. During gait, the dynamic nature of the task leads to constantly changing pressure distribution across the foot [2]. Indeed, smooth progression of the body over the supporting foot during the stance phase is achieved by the actions of three functional rockers: the heel, the ankle, and the forefoot [17,18]. During foot transitions through the rocker phases, pressure shifts and concentrates in specific areas. In the heel strike phase (MH, LH), initial contact generates high pressure. During the ankle rocker phase, pressure moves toward the midfoot (MF), facilitating dorsiflexion and propulsion. In the forefoot rocker phase (M2, M3, M4), pressure concentrates under the metatarsal heads, enabling push-off (T1) [17]. Consequently, the temporal characteristics of pressure change significantly, and these differences in pressure distribution between static and dynamic conditions can be attributed to the functional demands of gait [34]. In fact, during walking, the foot must act as a flexible structure that absorbs shock, adapts to uneven terrain, and generates propulsive forces. The three rocker phases represent a coordinated sequence of movements that optimize these functions. This dynamic loading pattern helps distribute the forces evenly across the foot, reducing the risk of localized pressure-related injuries [35].

4.3. Relationship Between Quiet Stance and Gait

The above considerations explain why the regression between the corresponding areas of foot pressure during gait and quiet stance in healthy subjects accounts for 64% of the variance of plantar pressures during gait that can be predicted by quiet stance. Therefore, it is possible to obtain a rather good estimate of foot pressure distribution during gait from its distribution during quiet stance. Overall, our results make plantar pressure collection more accessible to clinical practice, also in terms of the cost and time of evaluations and analyses. In fact, many studies have only analyzed plantar pressures under static conditions, as the dynamic analysis requires the availability of a sensorized walkway [14,36,37]. The relationship between mean plantar pressure in corresponding foot sole areas during gait and quiet stance is stronger when data points are closer to the regression line. A close alignment with the regression line suggests a well-defined, predictable relationship between pressure points, allowing for an accurate assessment of pressure distribution across the foot, enabling healthcare professionals to identify high-risk areas with greater confidence. Understanding these foot support areas is crucial for identifying patients prone to ulcers or other complications. It also facilitates the development of personalized interventions, such as insoles or orthopedic shoes, to enhance support and reduce injury risk. Additionally, monitoring plantar pressure helps evaluate treatment effectiveness in improving foot support and preventing complications [38].

4.4. Comparison with Literature Findings

In addition to these insights, our study offers a novel and clinically meaningful advancement over the existing literature. Specifically, Merry et al. (2020) [23] investigated plantar pressure characteristics to distinguish among sitting, standing, and walking. Their aim was primarily categorical classification of postures in work environments, especially concerning plantar heel pain. In contrast, our objective was to analyze whether gait pressure profiles could be inferred from static measurements in the same individuals, providing a continuous and predictive biomechanical relationship. Furthermore, our study involved a substantially large sample size to evaluate spatial and quantitative differences. Although the overall pattern of plantar pressure distribution in our study was similar to that reported by [23], one important point of divergence between the two studies lies in the absolute pressure values reported. In our study, peak plantar pressures during gait reached values well over 180 kPa in some forefoot areas (e.g., M2 and M3), while Merry et al. (2020) [23] reported substantially lower regional peak pressures. This discrepancy can be attributed to multiple methodological factors. For example, we used a resistive sensor walkway with high resolution and analyzed a well-defined cohort of 60 healthy adults, whereas Merry et al. (2020) [23] used a different system with a smaller sample size. In addition, variations in protocol, such as walking both along linear and curvilinear trajectories, barefoot versus shod conditions, or trial repetitions, may further contribute to inconsistencies in reported pressure values. These methodological differences highlight the importance of standardization in plantar pressure studies. However, it should also be noted that, while absolute values may differ between studies, similar conclusions can still be drawn.

Although several studies suggest that the peak pressure increases linearly with an increase in walking speed [19,39,40], we did not find a correlation between walking speed and plantar pressures or between plantar pressures and the sway area or path during quiet stance. The lack of correlation between gait speed and plantar pressures may be related to the different methodologies used in our study compared to others. For example, in the study by Hughes et al. [19], subjects had to walk at three different speeds, whereas in our study, subjects walked at their preferred speed. In the latter condition, we found a very small variation coefficient (13.3%) of the walking speed, which explains the small scatter of the data and presumably prevented the finding of a significant correlation between plantar pressures and walking speed.

We did not find a relationship between BMI and peak plantar pressures, either in the quiet stance or during gait. This is not surprising, since the current literature is unclear as to whether there is a relationship between peak plantar pressure and BMI during standing. For example, Lalande et al. [41] found a relationship between peak plantar pressures and subjects' weight as well as BMI during quiet stance. On the other hand, Arnold et al. [42] found a positive relationship between increasing body mass and peak and mean plantar pressure variables for most foot areas, but the relationship was highly dependent on the area of interest of the foot. However, the correlation between body mass and plantar pressure only accounted for 16% of the variance in peak plantar pressure. In addition, the same authors deliberately increased the body mass of their subjects up to 15 kg, whereas in our study, the body mass was not varied, thus preventing a sufficient scatter of data to highlight a possible linear relationship between pressure and BMI. Finally, Phetean et al. [43] found a weak degree of association between body weight, BMI, and plantar pressures. Overall, such differences could be explained by differences in the methodology used in the different studies.

4.5. Limitations

The results of this study should be considered in light of the following limitations. Firstly, due to the lack of comparable data in the literature, it was not possible to perform an a priori sample size calculation. However, the number of subjects in our study was comparable to other studies of gait and foot pressure [44]. Secondly, the number of steps required to characterize plantar pressure during gait was small (four), but this is a matter of debate in the literature [45]. In clinical analysis of gait [46], three steps are commonly used, and three to five steps are thought to be sufficient to record plantar pressure in adults aged 20 to 35 years [47]. As Kernozek et al. [48] reported for peak pressure, a minimum of two to three footfalls was needed to reach a reliability coefficient of 0.70, indicating good reliability, regardless of the foot area considered. In addition, the plantar pressure distribution obtained in our study was similar to that found in the literature, with a larger number of footprints [49] and a smaller number of subjects [23]. For example, Putti et al. [50] found that two to three steps were sufficient to capture consistent pressure values with excellent intra-subject repeatability. These studies suggest that key pressure parameters remain stable and reproducible with as few as two steps, especially when consistent walking protocols are followed.

Finally, comparison of our data with other normative references for plantar pressures is complicated by a lack of agreement on how to divide the foot and how to examine the areas under the foot. Despite the different ways of splitting the foot areas, our findings for plantar pressures are consistent with the literature [41,51,52]. Various approaches have been used, including expressing pressure as an absolute measure, or scaled to peak plantar pressure, foot length, body mass, or body mass index for ten, nine, five, or three areas of the foot [50,53,54]. Despite this variable approach, only small associations between body weight, body mass index, and plantar pressure data have been reported in the literature, suggesting that scaling to these parameters is not advantageous [43].

5. Conclusions

In summary, the present study investigated the distribution of plantar pressures in a sample of young healthy adults in two different conditions, quiet stance and gait. The results showed that the highest peak pressure was in the heel during stance, rather than in the metatarsal region and the greater toe, as occurred during gait. However, the overall similar profile of the plantar pressure distribution under static and dynamic conditions was reflected by a significant positive correlation between the corresponding areas of foot pressure during gait and those during quiet stance. This finding allows the pressure distribution during gait to be estimated to a rather good extent from its distribution during quiet stance, but, since these results are collected from healthy subjects, they need to be confirmed in a cohort of patients to be applied in a clinical setting.

The assessment of plantar pressures in healthy individuals during both standing and walking goes beyond traditional pathological studies to explore the natural biomechanics of the foot. By directly comparing static and dynamic conditions in the same subjects, this approach reveals how the foot adapts to movement, revealing important pressure shifts that might be overlooked.

Supplementary Materials: The following supporting information can be downloaded at https://www.mdpi.com/article/10.3390/jfmk10030301/s1. Table S1: Linear relationships between the average value of the ten areas of the right and the left foot sole during gait or stance and BMI, gait speed, time of single and double contact, and surface of the 95% confidence ellipse of the CoP and its path.

Author Contributions: Conceptualization, A.N. and M.M.; methodology, M.M. and S.S.; formal analysis, M.M., S.S. and V.P.; investigation, M.M., S.S. and C.P.; data curation, M.M. and S.S.; writing—original draft preparation, M.M. and A.N.; writing—review and editing, C.P., S.S. and V.P.; supervision, C.P.; project administration, A.N.; funding acquisition, A.N. All authors have read and agreed to the published version of the manuscript.

Funding: This research was partly supported by the Italian Ministry of Universities and Research under the complementary actions of the NRRP "Fit4MedRob-Fit for Medical Robotics" (Grant #PNC0000007-B53C22006890001). It did not receive any specific grant from funding agencies in the commercial or for-profit sectors.

Institutional Review Board Statement: The study was conducted in accordance with the Declaration of Helsinki and approved by the Institutional Review Board of Istituti Clinici Scientifici Maugeri of Pavia, Italy (#2461CE, approval date: 6 October 2020).

Informed Consent Statement: Informed consent was obtained from all subjects involved in the study.

Data Availability Statement: The mean data presented in this study are available on request from the corresponding author.

Acknowledgments: This research was partly supported by the Ricerca Corrente funding scheme of the Ministry of Health, Italy.

Conflicts of Interest: The authors declare no conflicts of interest.

Abbreviations

The following abbreviations are used in this manuscript:

CoP	Center of pressure
CoM	Center of mass
EO	Eyes open
kPa	Kilopascal
T1	Big toe
T2,3,4,5	Toes 2 to 5
M1	Metatarsal 1
M2	Metatarsal 2
M3	Metatarsal 3
M4	Metatarsal 4
M5	Metatarsal 5
MF	Midfoot
MH	Medial half of the heel
LH	Lateral half of the heel
SD	Standard deviation
ANOVA	Analysis of variance
BMI	Body mass index

References

1. Zulkifli, S.S.; Loh, W.P. A state-of-the-art review of foot pressure. *Foot Ankle Surg.* **2020**, *26*, 25–32. [CrossRef]
2. Cleland, L.D.; Rowland, H.M.; Mazzà, C.; Saal, H.P. Complexity of spatio-temporal plantar pressure patterns during everyday behaviours. *J. R. Soc. Interface* **2023**, *20*, 20230052. [CrossRef] [PubMed]
3. Cornwall, M.W.; McPoil, T.G. Velocity of the center of pressure during walking. *J. Am. Podiatr. Med. Assoc.* **2000**, *90*, 334–338. [CrossRef] [PubMed]
4. Winter, D.A.; Patla, A.E.; Frank, J.S. Assessment of balance control in humans. *Med. Prog. Technol.* **1990**, *16*, 31–51.
5. Winter, D.A. Human balance and posture control during standing and walking. *Gait Posture* **1995**, *3*, 193–214. [CrossRef]
6. Orlin, M.N.; McPoil, T.G. Plantar pressure assessment. *Phys. Ther.* **2000**, *80*, 399–409. [CrossRef]
7. Morton, D.J. Structural factors in static disorders of the foot. *Am. J. Surg.* **1930**, *9*, 315–328. [CrossRef]
8. Boulton, A.J.; Hardisty, C.A.; Betts, R.P.; Franks, C.I.; Worth, R.C.; Ward, J.D.; Duckworth, T. Dynamic foot pressure and other studies as diagnostic and management aids in diabetic neuropathy. *Diabetes Care* **1983**, *6*, 26–33. [CrossRef]
9. Vossen, L.E.; Bus, S.A.; Van Netten, J.J. Unlocking the multidimensionality of plantar pressure measurements for the evaluation of footwear in people with diabetes. *J. Biomech.* **2025**, *180*, 112502. [CrossRef]
10. Jandova, S.; Pazour, J.; Janura, M. Comparison of Plantar Pressure Distribution During Walking After Two Different Surgical Treatments for Calcaneal Fracture. *J. Foot Ankle Surg.* **2019**, *58*, 260–265. [CrossRef]
11. Dürr, C.; Apinun, J.; Mittlmeier, T.; Rammelt, S. Foot Function After Surgically Treated Intraarticular Calcaneal Fractures: Correlation of Clinical and Pedobarographic Results of 65 Patients Followed for 8 Years. *J. Orthop. Trauma* **2018**, *32*, 593–600. [CrossRef] [PubMed]
12. Mirando, M.; Conti, C.; Zeni, F.; Pedicini, F.; Nardone, A.; Pavese, C. Gait Alterations in Adults after Ankle Fracture: A Systematic Review. *Diagnostics* **2022**, *12*, 199. [CrossRef] [PubMed]
13. Burns, J.; Crosbie, J.; Hunt, A.; Ouvrier, R. The effect of pes cavus on foot pain and plantar pressure. *Clin. Biomech.* **2005**, *20*, 877–882. [CrossRef] [PubMed]
14. Fernández-Seguín, L.M.; Diaz Mancha, J.A.; Sánchez Rodríguez, R.; Escamilla Martínez, E.; Gómez Martín, B.; Ramos Ortega, J. Comparison of plantar pressures and contact area between normal and cavus foot. *Gait Posture* **2014**, *39*, 789–792. [CrossRef]
15. Caselli, A.; Pham, H.; Giurini, J.M.; Armstrong, D.G.; Veves, A. The forefoot-to-rearfoot plantar pressure ratio is increased in severe diabetic neuropathy and can predict foot ulceration. *Diabetes Care* **2002**, *25*, 1066–1071. [CrossRef]
16. Periyasamy, R.; Anand, S. The effect of foot arch on plantar pressure distribution during standing. *J. Med. Eng. Technol.* **2013**, *37*, 342–347. [CrossRef]
17. Perry, J.M.; Slac Thorofare, K.; Davids, J.R. Gait Analysis: Normal and Pathological Function. *J. Pediatr. Orthop.* **1992**, *12*, 815. [CrossRef]
18. Han, T.R.; Paik, N.J.; Im, M.S. Quantification of the path of center of pressure (COP) using an F-scan in-shoe transducer. *Gait Posture* **1999**, *10*, 248–254. [CrossRef]
19. Hughes, J.; Pratt, L.; Linge, K.; Clark, P.; Klenerman, L. Reliability of pressure measurements: The EM ED F system. *Clin. Biomech.* **1991**, *6*, 14–18. [CrossRef]
20. Kelly, L.A.; Kuitunen, S.; Racinais, S.; Cresswell, A.G. Recruitment of the plantar intrinsic foot muscles with increasing postural demand. *Clin. Biomech.* **2012**, *27*, 46–51. [CrossRef]
21. Schieppati, M.; Nardone, A.; Siliotto, R.; Grasso, M. Early and late stretch responses of human foot muscles induced by perturbation of stance. *Exp. Brain Res.* **1995**, *105*, 411–422. [CrossRef]
22. Drăgulinescu, A.; Drăgulinescu, A.M.; Zincă, G.; Bucur, D.; Feieș, V.; Neagu, D.M. Smart Socks and In-Shoe Systems: State-of-the-Art for Two Popular Technologies for Foot Motion Analysis, Sports, and Medical Applications. *Sensors* **2020**, *20*, 4316. [CrossRef]
23. Merry, K.; MacPherson, M.; Macdonald, E.; Ryan, M.; Park, E.J.; Sparrey, C.J. Differentiating Sitting, Standing, and Walking Through Regional Plantar Pressure Characteristics. *J. Biomech. Eng.* **2020**, *142*. [CrossRef]
24. Penati, R.; Sozzi, S.; Mirando, M.; Nardone, A. Qualitative and quantitative differences in plantar pressure distribution during quiet stance and gait in healthy individuals. In Proceedings of the Congresso SIAMOC, online, 30 September 2021; p. 86.
25. Vasileiou, K.; Barnett, J.; Thorpe, S.; Young, T. Characterising and justifying sample size sufficiency in interview-based studies: Systematic analysis of qualitative health research over a 15-year period. *BMC Med. Res. Methodol.* **2018**, *18*, 148. [CrossRef]
26. De Blasiis, P.; Caravaggi, P.; Fullin, A.; Leardini, A.; Lucariello, A.; Perna, A.; Guerra, G.; De Luca, A. Postural stability and plantar pressure parameters in healthy subjects: Variability, correlation analysis and differences under open and closed eye conditions. *Front. Bioeng. Biotechnol.* **2023**, *11*, 1198120. [CrossRef]

27. Fullin, A.; Caravaggi, P.; Picerno, P.; Mosca, M.; Caravelli, S.; De Luca, A.; Lucariello, A.; De Blasiis, P. Variability of Postural Stability and Plantar Pressure Parameters in Healthy Subjects Evaluated by a Novel Pressure Plate. *Int. J. Environ. Res. Public Health* **2022**, *19*, 2913. [CrossRef]
28. Scoppa, F.; Gallamini, M.; Belloni, G.; Messina, G. Clinical stabilometry standardization: Feet position in the static stabilometric assessment of postural stability. *Acta Med. Mediterr.* **2017**, *33*, 707–713.
29. Kim, J.; Kim, K.; Gubler, C. Comparisons of Plantar Pressure Distributions between the Dominant and Non-dominant Sides of Older Women during Walking. *J. Phys. Ther. Sci.* **2013**, *25*, 313–315. [CrossRef]
30. Schieppati, M.; Hugon, M.; Grasso, M.; Nardone, A.; Galante, M. The limits of equilibrium in young and elderly normal subjects and in parkinsonians. *Electroencephalogr. Clin. Neurophysiol.* **1994**, *93*, 286–298. [CrossRef] [PubMed]
31. Hennig, E.M.; Sterzing, T. Sensitivity mapping of the human foot: Thresholds at 30 skin locations. *Foot Ankle Int.* **2009**, *30*, 986–991. [CrossRef] [PubMed]
32. Machado, Á.S.; Bombach, G.D.; Duysens, J.; Carpes, F.P. Differences in foot sensitivity and plantar pressure between young adults and elderly. *Arch. Gerontol. Geriatr.* **2016**, *63*, 67–71. [CrossRef] [PubMed]
33. De Doncker, E.; Kowalski, C.; Coeur, P.L. *Cinésiologie et Rééducation du Pied*; Masson: Issy-les-Moulineaux, France, 1979.
34. Ten Wolde, I.Y.; van Kouwenhove, L.; Dekker, R.; Hijmans, J.M.; Greve, C. Effects of rocker radii with two longitudinal bending stiffnesses on plantar pressure distribution in the forefoot. *Gait Posture* **2021**, *90*, 457–463. [CrossRef]
35. Reints, R.; Hijmans, J.M.; Burgerhof, J.G.M.; Postema, K.; Verkerke, G.J. Effects of flexible and rigid rocker profiles on in-shoe pressure. *Gait Posture* **2017**, *58*, 287–293. [CrossRef]
36. Pomarino, D.; Pomarino, A. Plantar Static Pressure Distribution in Healthy Individuals. *Foot Ankle Spec.* **2014**, *7*, 293–297. [CrossRef]
37. Patel, H.M.; Balaganapathy, M. Normative values of static-dynamic plantar pressure and its cutoff values. *Indian J. Med. Spec.* **2024**, *15*, 4–11. [CrossRef]
38. Tang, W.H.; Zhao, Y.N.; Cheng, Z.X.; Xu, J.X.; Zhang, Y.; Liu, X.M. Risk factors for diabetic foot ulcers: A systematic review and meta-analysis. *Vascular* **2024**, *32*, 661–669. [CrossRef] [PubMed]
39. Jonely, H.; Brismée, J.M.; Sizer, P.S.; James, C.R. Relationships between clinical measures of static foot posture and plantar pressure during static standing and walking. *Clin. Biomech.* **2011**, *26*, 873–879. [CrossRef]
40. Tse, C.T.F.; Ryan, M.B.; Dien, J.; Scott, A.; Hunt, M.A. An exploration of changes in plantar pressure distributions during walking with standalone and supported lateral wedge insole designs. *J. Foot Ankle Res.* **2021**, *14*, 55. [CrossRef]
41. Lalande, X.; Vie, B.; Weber, J.P.; Jammes, Y. Normal Values of Pressures and Foot Areas Measured in the Static Condition. *J. Am. Podiatr. Med. Assoc.* **2016**, *106*, 265–272. [CrossRef]
42. Arnold, J.B.; Causby, R.; Pod, G.D.; Jones, S. The impact of increasing body mass on peak and mean plantar pressure in asymptomatic adult subjects during walking. *Diabet Foot Ankle* **2010**, *1*, 5518. [CrossRef]
43. Phethean, J.; Nester, C. The influence of body weight, body mass index and gender on plantar pressures: Results of a cross-sectional study of healthy children's feet. *Gait Posture* **2012**, *36*, 287–290. [CrossRef]
44. Yan, Y.; Ou, J.; Shi, H.; Sun, C.; Shen, L.; Song, Z.; Shu, L.; Chen, Z. Plantar pressure and falling risk in older individuals: A cross-sectional study. *J. Foot Ankle Res.* **2023**, *16*, 14. [CrossRef]
45. Zammit, G.V.; Menz, H.B.; Munteanu, S.E. Reliability of the TekScan MatScan(R) system for the measurement of plantar forces and pressures during barefoot level walking in healthy adults. *J. Foot Ankle Res.* **2010**, *3*, 11. [CrossRef]
46. Bus, S.A.; de Lange, A. A comparison of the 1-step, 2-step, and 3-step protocols for obtaining barefoot plantar pressure data in the diabetic neuropathic foot. *Clin. Biomech.* **2005**, *20*, 892–899. [CrossRef]
47. McPoil, T.G.; Cornwall, M.W.; Dupuis, L.; Cornwell, M. Variability of plantar pressure data. A comparison of the two-step and midgait methods. *J. Am. Podiatr. Med. Assoc.* **1999**, *89*, 495–501. [CrossRef] [PubMed]
48. Kernozek, T.W.; LaMott, E.E.; Dancisak, M.J. Reliability of an in-shoe pressure measurement system during treadmill walking. *Foot Ankle Int.* **1996**, *17*, 204–209. [CrossRef]
49. Turcato, A.M.; Godi, M.; Giordano, A.; Schieppati, M.; Nardone, A. The generation of centripetal force when walking in a circle: Insight from the distribution of ground reaction forces recorded by plantar insoles. *J. Neuroeng. Rehabil.* **2015**, *12*, 4. [CrossRef]
50. Putti, A.B.; Arnold, G.P.; Cochrane, L.A.; Abboud, R.J. Normal pressure values and repeatability of the Emed ST4 system. *Gait Posture* **2008**, *27*, 501–505. [CrossRef] [PubMed]
51. Yuan, X.N.; Liang, W.D.; Zhou, F.H.; Li, H.T.; Zhang, L.X.; Zhang, Z.Q.; Li, J.J. Comparison of walking quality variables between incomplete spinal cord injury patients and healthy subjects by using a footscan plantar pressure system. *Neural. Regen. Res.* **2019**, *14*, 354–360. [CrossRef]
52. McKay, M.J.; Baldwin, J.N.; Ferreira, P.; Simic, M.; Vanicek, N.; Wojciechowski, E.; Mudge, A.; Burns, J. Spatiotemporal and plantar pressure patterns of 1000 healthy individuals aged 3–101 years. *Gait Posture* **2017**, *58*, 78–87. [CrossRef] [PubMed]

53. Liu, X.C.; Thometz, J.G.; Tassone, C.; Barker, B.; Lyon, R. Dynamic plantar pressure measurement for the normal subject: Free-mapping model for the analysis of pediatric foot deformities. *J. Pediatr. Orthop.* **2005**, *25*, 103–106. [CrossRef] [PubMed]
54. Bosch, K.; Gerss, J.; Rosenbaum, D. Preliminary normative values for foot loading parameters of the developing child. *Gait Posture* **2007**, *26*, 238–247. [CrossRef] [PubMed]

Journal of
Functional Morphology and Kinesiology

MDPI

Article

The Predictive Capacity of the 3-Meter Backward Walk Test for Falls in Older Adults: A Case–Control Analysis

Luis Polo-Ferrero [1,2,*], Javier Torres-Alonso [1], María Carmen Sánchez-Sánchez [1,2], Ana Silvia Puente-González [1,2], Fausto J. Barbero-Iglesias [1,2] and Roberto Méndez-Sánchez [1,2]

1 Department of Nursing and Physiotherapy, University of Salamanca, 37007 Salamanca, Spain; javiertorres@usal.es (J.T.-A.); csanchez@usal.es (M.C.S.-S.); silviapugo@usal.es (A.S.P.-G.); fausbar@usal.es (F.J.B.-I.); ro_mendez@usal.es (R.M.-S.)

2 Institute of Biomedical Research of Salamanca (IBSAL), 37007 Salamanca, Spain

* Correspondence: pfluis@usal.es

Abstract: Background: The early detection of fall risk in older adults is crucial for prevention. This study assessed the 3-Meter Backward Walk Test (3m-BWT) as a predictor of falls. **Methods**: A retrospective observational case–control study was conducted with 483 community-dwelling participants (mean age 76.3 ± 6.5 years), including 101 individuals with a history of falls in the previous 12 months. A standardized battery of functional assessments was applied. **Results**: Significant differences were observed between fallers and non-fallers across all functional variables ($p < 0.001$), with fallers demonstrating slower performance on the 3m-BWT (6.8 ± 3.4 s vs. 5.1 ± 1.3 s). The 3m-BWT showed moderate correlations with Short Physical Performance Battery, 5-repetition Sit-to-Stand, gait speed, and 4-Square Step Test, and a moderate-to-strong correlation with Timed Up-and-Go (r = 0.632), even after adjusting for age, sex, and BMI. Although the 3m-BWT exhibited superior discriminative ability compared to other tests (AUC = 0.655), its predictive power in isolation remains limited. The optimal cut-off point was identified at 5.5 s (sensitivity: 59.5%; specificity: 68.6%), while a threshold of <3.5 s yielded high sensitivity (98%) but low specificity, supporting its use in fall risk screening. **Conclusions**: These findings support the integration of the 3m-BWT as a complementary tool within comprehensive geriatric assessments, particularly in contexts requiring high sensitivity. Given the multifactorial nature of falls, combining the 3m-BWT with other clinical evaluations and fall history is recommended to enhance risk stratification and inform preventive strategies.

Keywords: older adults; aging; frailty; falls; fall risk; backward walking; 3 m backward walk; functional assessment; geriatric evaluation; physical performance

1. Introduction

Aging is a complex process involving structural, functional, and psychological changes, leading to cellular and organ deterioration, reduced responsiveness, and increased disease susceptibility [1,2]. This process contributes to geriatric syndromes, particularly frailty, which is prevalent among older adults and heightens the demand for social and healthcare services [3,4]. Frailty results from declines in physiological reserve, increasing vulnerability to stressors, and is characterized by symptoms such as exhaustion, low physical activity, unintentional weight loss, weakness, and slow gait [5,6]. It is a precursor to disability and a significant risk factor for falls in older adults [7,8].

Falls are common among older adults, with about 30% of those over 65 experiencing a fall each year, and the rate increases after age 75 [9,10]. The risk of recurrence within a year is approximately 66% [11]. Falls in older adults are caused by a combination of intrinsic and extrinsic factors, including underlying diseases, medications, psychological factors, and environmental conditions [12]. Between 10% and 25% of falls result in serious injury, making them the leading cause of fatal injury and trauma-related hospital admissions in this population [9,13]. In the United States, the average cost of hospital treatment for a fall injury exceeds USD 30,000 [14], underscoring the importance of fall prevention and early risk detection in older adults.

Fall prevention efforts have utilized medical records, questionnaires, and functional tests to assess patient risk, with such tests being essential in comprehensive geriatric evaluations. The Timed Up and Go Test (TUG) and 5 Times Sit-to-Stand Test (5STS) are two of the most widely used functional tests predictive of falls and are widely supported in the literature. However, none have demonstrated high discriminative accuracy in isolation [15]. Specifically, a TUG time greater than 12 s and a 5STS time greater than 15 s are commonly used cut-off points to indicate increased fall risk, while gait speed (GS) values below 0.7 to 1.0 m/s, depending on the source, and Short Physical Performance Battery (SPPB) scores below 8 have also been associated with a higher likelihood of falling in older adults [16–21]. Other tests, such as Hand Grip Strength (HG) and the 4-Square Step Test (4SST), have also been linked to frailty and fall risk, though without widely accepted cut-off thresholds for predicting falls [22,23]. These tests primarily assess forward motion or turning, whereas walking backward, which demands greater neuromuscular and proprioceptive control [24], is less studied [25]. Thus, exploring functional tests that assess backward walking and their predictive power for falls in older adults is necessary.

The 3-Meter Backward Walk Test (3m-BWT) is a clinical assessment that measures the ability to walk backward. It is an innovative functional measure that has been the subject of studies since 2019 [26]. A recent systematic review, which covered studies published between 2019 and 2023, evaluated the measurement properties of the test. The results confirmed its validity and reliability in patients with various clinical conditions, including community-dwelling older adults, and demonstrated its sensitivity to change, providing normative data for these populations. However, the authors noted that many of the included studies had limited sample sizes (less than 100 participants), which restricts the generalizability of the findings. Therefore, they recommended further research involving larger samples to obtain more robust evidence regarding the predictive validity of the 3m-BWT in the assessment of fall risk [27]. This study aims to address that gap by evaluating the discriminative capacity of the 3m-BWT and establishing optimal cut-off points with adequate sensitivity and specificity. A 3.5 s threshold has been proposed in older adults, which may enhance its clinical applicability in fall risk screening [26].

By comparing fallers and non-fallers, this study aims to identify the functional characteristics that most clearly differentiate these groups, thereby enhancing the clinical utility of the 3m-BWT in fall risk assessment. It also seeks to provide more robust and accurate information on the predictive ability of the 3m-BWT in older adults, using a larger sample than previous studies. By strengthening the evidence on its predictive validity, we seek to support the integration of this test as a potential tool for identifying fall risk within comprehensive geriatric assessments and to contribute to the development of effective fall prevention strategies.

2. Materials and Methods

2.1. Study Design

A retrospective observational case–control study was conducted among older adults to establish reference values for the 3m-BWT in predicting falls. This study is part of a research project approved by the Ethics Committee for Drug Research of the Salamanca

Health Area (Protocol Code: PI 2024061702), conducted in accordance with the Declaration of Helsinki [28], and registered on ClinicalTrials.gov on 23 May 2024 (Registration No.: NCT06434857). This study also adheres to the CONSORT 2010 guidelines [29].

2.2. Study Population

Participants were recruited annually through the Geriatric Revitalization Program (GRP) coordinated by the University of Salamanca, a community-based initiative aimed at promoting healthy aging. Recruitment was conducted through open calls in local media and community centers, and all participants enrolled voluntarily. Inclusion criteria comprised community-dwelling adults aged 60 years and older who were able to provide informed consent, complete functional and physical assessments, and follow verbal instructions adequately. Cognitive status was screened through a brief clinical interview conducted by trained personnel; individuals with suspected cognitive impairment or a prior diagnosis of dementia were excluded. Additional exclusion criteria included the presence of central nervous system disorders associated with neurological deficits (e.g., Parkinson's disease, stroke), a history of major surgery or traumatic injury in the previous six months, and any musculoskeletal or cardiorespiratory condition contraindicating exercise. Individuals with visual, auditory, or sensory impairments that could compromise test performance and those with clinically diagnosed orthostatic hypotension were not included. The use of medication was not a criterion for exclusion, and pharmacological profiles were not analyzed in the present study. Participants were classified as cases or controls based on self-reported history of one or more falls within the 12 months prior to assessment.

2.3. Assessment and Outcomes

The evaluation was conducted under standardized and controlled conditions at the Research Unit of the Faculty of Nursing and Physiotherapy, University of Salamanca. For this study, the recruitment period took place between May and August 2024, and all testing sessions were conducted during the second half of September 2024. A pre-trained research team with over three years of experience in geriatrics was responsible for data collection. Each test was consistently administered by the same researcher throughout the study to ensure procedural uniformity and minimize inter-rater variability. Although multiple researchers participated in the evaluation process, each was assigned a specific test and conducted only that test across all participants. All assessments followed a standardized internal protocol (Table S1). To minimize bias, participants were anonymized using coded identifiers, and group allocation (fallers vs. non-fallers) was determined based on self-reported falls within the previous 12 months. Prior to participation, all individuals received detailed verbal and written information and provided written informed consent.

During the structured personal interview, sociodemographic variables (e.g., age and sex), relevant medical history, and selection criteria were collected. Body composition was assessed using bioelectrical impedance analysis (TANITA BC-418), recording weight, height, body mass index (BMI; weight/height^2), appendicular skeletal muscle mass (ASM), and skeletal muscle mass index (SMI; ASM/height^2).

Functional performance was assessed using the 3m-BWT as the main test, alongside other established functional tests commonly used to predict falls, and evaluated in this study based on their respective cut-off points. For the 3m-BWT, participants stood with their backs to a marked line and were instructed to walk backward until both feet had crossed a second marked line. They were allowed to look back but not to run [26]. The test was performed three times, and the best time was recorded using a smartphone stopwatch.

In addition to the 3m-BWT, this study included the TUG, which measures the time needed to rise from a chair, walk 3 m, turn around, return, and sit down; the 5STS, which assesses lower limb strength through five consecutive sit-to-stand repetitions; the GS, calculated from a 4 m walk at usual pace; and the SPPB, a composite score based on balance, gait speed, and chair rise performance. The HG test evaluates upper limb strength using a dynamometer, and the 4SST assesses dynamic balance through timed multidirectional stepping. Full protocols for all tests are available in Supplementary Table S1.

2.4. Sample Size

The sample size was determined using the GRANMO tool version 8, tailored for case–control studies. Given that the prevalence of falls among older adults is approximately 30%, a 3:1 ratio between controls and cases was anticipated [9]. To achieve an alpha risk of 0.05 and a statistical power greater than 0.8 in a bilateral contrast, 101 cases (fallers) and 353 controls (non-fallers) were needed to detect a minimum Odds Ratio of 2, accounting for an estimated 5% loss to follow-up.

2.5. Statistical Analysis

The data were analyzed using IBM SPSS Statistics 28.0, employing descriptive measures and frequencies with a significance level of 0.05. The normality of the data was verified using box plots and the Kolmogorov–Smirnov test. A descriptive analysis of the baseline characteristics was conducted for the faller and non-faller groups. The Chi-square test was employed for categorical variables with a normal distribution, while the McNemar test was used for those with a non-normal distribution. Quantitative variables were analyzed with the *t*-test for independent samples when they were normally distributed; otherwise, the Mann–Whitney U-test was used.

The correlation analysis examined the relationship between the 3m-BWT, other functional variables that predict falls (TUG, 5STS, GS, SPPB), and others related to frailty status (HG and 4SST) using the Pearson correlation coefficient when the data were normally distributed and the Spearman coefficient when they were not. In addition, a partial correlation analysis (r_p) was performed, controlling for the possible effect of age, sex, and BMI. Correlations were classified as weak (0.1–0.3), moderate (0.4–0.6), and strong (0.7–1.0), following Cohen's classification [30].

The area under the curve (AUC) of the receiver operating characteristic (ROC) curve was calculated to assess the discriminative ability of the functional tests in identifying falls. AUC values were interpreted according to established criteria: 0.5–0.6 (fail), 0.6–0.7 (poor), 0.7–0.8 (acceptable), 0.8–0.9 (excellent), and >0.9 (outstanding) [31]. Sensitivity and specificity were determined at different cut-off points on the ROC curve, as described in the scientific literature. A detailed analysis of the 3m-BWT test at various cut-off points was performed to identify the optimal value for detecting falls in older adults, evaluating its sensitivity and specificity. For each cut-off point, sensitivity, which reflects the model's ability to correctly identify positive cases, and specificity, which assesses its ability to identify negative cases, were calculated. In addition, discriminative capacity was quantified using the Youden Index (J), providing a comprehensive measure of test accuracy at each threshold.

3. Results

3.1. Participant Characteristics

In this study, 483 older adults were included with no participant loss, achieving the expected case–control proportions. Table 1 presents demographic and anthropometric data for fallers (n = 101) and non-fallers (n = 382). Non-parametric tests were used due to the non-normal distribution of variables.

Table 1. Comparison of characteristics between non-fallers and fallers.

Variable	Non-Fallers (n = 382)	Fallers (n = 101)	p-Value
Female, (n, %)	328 (85.9%)	92 (91.1%)	<0.001
Age (years)	75.9 ± 6.4	77.6 ± 6.8	0.150
Height (m)	1.54 ± 0.08	1.54 ± 0.06	0.610
Weight (kg)	64.7 ± 11.6	66.9 ± 11.6	0.151
BMI (kg/m^2)	27.2 ± 4.3	28.3 ± 4.6	0.038
SMI (kg/m^2)	7.5 ± 0.9	6.2 ± 0.9	<0.001
3m-BWT (s)	5.1 ± 1.3	6.8 ± 3.4	<0.001
TUG (s)	8.6 ± 1.8	10.1 ± 3.3	<0.001
5STS (s)	9.5 ± 2.2	11.4 ± 4.6	<0.001
GS (m/s)	1.20 ± 0.3	1.07 ± 0.26	<0.001
SPPB	11.6 ± 0.9	10.9 ± 1.8	<0.001
HG (Kg)	22.6 ± 6.2	21 ± 5.4	0.018
4SST (s)	6.4 ± 1.5	7.4 ± 2.4	<0.001

Values expressed as means ± standard deviation (SD) and frequencies (n, %).

No statistically significant differences were observed in age between fallers (77.6 ± 6.8 years) and non-fallers (75.9 ± 6.4 years; $p = 0.150$). Although a significant difference in sex distribution was identified ($p < 0.001$), the absolute difference was minimal (5.2%) and likely of limited clinical relevance. Similarly, no significant differences were found in body weight ($p = 0.151$) or height ($p = 0.610$). However, when analyzing body composition variables, a statistically significant difference was observed in the body mass index (BMI; $p = 0.038$) and skeletal muscle mass index (SMI; $p < 0.001$), with fallers showing higher BMI and lower SMI values, indicating a potential imbalance between fat and lean mass components.

Functional tests showed significant differences between fallers and non-fallers. Fallers took longer in the 3m-BWT (6.8 ± 3.4 s vs. 5.1 ± 1.3 s; $p < 0.001$), 5STS (11.4 ± 4.6 s vs. 9.5 ± 2.2 s; $p < 0.001$), and especially in TUG (10.1 ± 3.3 s vs. 8.6 ± 1.8 s; $p < 0.001$) tests, demonstrating the effectiveness of these tests in identifying fall risk. Additional significant differences were also observed in GS (1.07 ± 0.26 m/s vs. 1.20 ± 0.3 m/s; $p < 0.001$), SPPB (10.9 ± 1.8 vs. 11.6 ± 0.9; $p < 0.001$), HG (21 ± 5.4 kg vs. 22.6 ± 6.2 kg; $p = 0.018$), and 4SST (7.4 ± 2.4 s vs. 6.4 ± 1.5 s; $p < 0.001$).

3.2. Correlation of 3m-BWT with Functional Variables

A simple correlation analysis (r) and a partial correlation analysis (r_p) adjusted for age, sex, and BMI were performed. The 3m-BWT showed a weak correlation with HG (r = −0.199; 95% CI: −0.283, −0.112; r_p = −0.168), suggesting only a slight inverse association between faster 3m-BWT and higher HG, even when adjusted for age, sex, and BMI. Moderate correlations were identified with the SPPB (r = −0.511, 95% CI: −0.574, −0.442; r_p = −0.477), 5STS (r = 0.528, 95% CI: 0.460, 0.589; r_p = 0.505), GS (r = −0.517, 95% CI: −0.579, −0.448; r_p = −0.469), and 4SST (r = 0.596, 95% CI: 0.547, 0.644; r_p = 0.571), indicating that better functional performance on these measures is associated with faster 3m-BWT times, even after adjustment for sex, age, and BMI. A correlation between moderate and strong was observed with the TUG (r = 0.632, 95% CI: 0.575, 0.682; r_p = 0.581). All of these correlations were statistically significant ($p < 0.001$), highlighting the significant association of the 3m-BWT with several functional tests and emphasizing its value in assessing fall risk in older adults, even when controlling for the effect of age, sex, and BMI (Table 2).

Table 2. Correlation of 3m-BWT with functional variables predictors of falls.

Functional Variables	r (CI 95%)	r_p	p-Value
TUG [a]	0.632 (0.575, 0.682)	0.581	<0.001
5STS [a]	0.528 (0.460, 0.589)	0.505	<0.001
GS [a]	−0.517 (−0.579, −0.448)	−0.469	<0.001
SPPB [a]	−0.511 (−0.574, −0.442)	−0.477	<0.001
HG [a]	−0.199 (−0.283, −0.112)	−0.168	<0.001
4SST [a]	0.596 (0.547, 0.644)	0.571	<0.001

Values expressed as correlation coefficients and the confidence interval (r CI 95%), partial correlation (age, sex, and BMI), and p-value (p). [a]: Spearman correlation coefficient. p-value of r.

3.3. Discriminative Capacity of Functional Tests

Regarding the discriminative capacity of functional tests in older adults who experience falls compared to those who do not, significant results were observed in all variables ($p = 0.001$), except for HG ($p = 0.18$; AUC = 0.424; 95% CI 0.363–0.484) (Table 3). The findings indicate that the 3m-BWT is the most effective test for identifying falls, with an AUC of 0.655 (95% CI: 0.592–0.719) and a p-value of 0.001 (Figure 1). However, this AUC still reflects limited discriminative ability, and its clinical use as a standalone predictor should be considered with caution.

Table 3. Global discriminative capacity of functional tests to identify falls in older adults.

Functional Variable	AUC	95% CI for AUC	p-Value
3m-BWT	0.655	0.592–0.719	<0.001
TUG	0.637	0.573–0.702	0.011
5STS	0.636	0.573–0.699	<0.001
GS	0.362	0.303–0.422	<0.001
SPPB	0.415	0.349–0.482	0.013
4SST	0.630	0.566–0.694	<0.001
HG	0.424	0.363–0.484	0.180

The values express the discriminatory capacity of the model according to the AUC, its confidence interval (95% CI), standard error, and p-value.

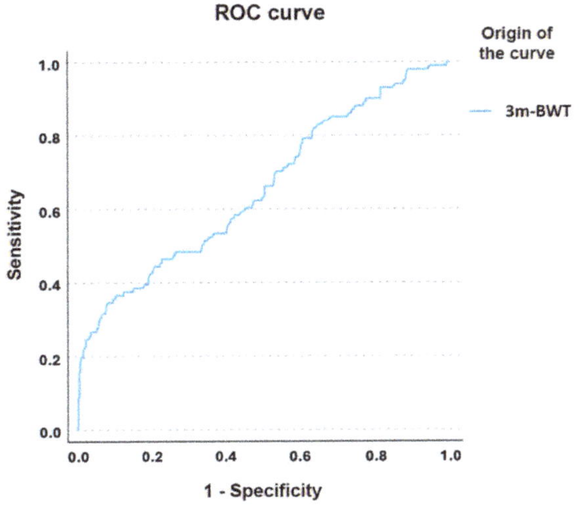

Figure 1. ROC curve of the 3m-BWT for identifying falls in older adults.

The TUG demonstrated the second highest discriminative ability, with an AUC of 0.637 (95% CI: 0.573–0.699). The 5STS had an AUC of 0.636 (95% CI: 0.573–0.699), and the 4SST showed an AUC of 0.630 (95% CI: 0.566–0.694). The SPPB, a composite measure of physical performance, exhibited an AUC of 0.415 (95% CI: 0.349–0.482), indicating a moderate capacity to discriminate fallers, with a p-value of 0.013. In contrast, the HG test demonstrated limited discriminatory power, with an AUC of 0.424 (95% CI: 0.363–0.484) and a non-significant p-value of 0.18. The GS had the lowest discriminative capacity among the significant tests, with an AUC of 0.362 (95% CI: 0.303–0.422) and a p-value of 0.001.

3.4. Sensitivity and Specificity of Various Cut-Off Points

Various cut-off points of the 3m-BWT were analyzed to detect fall risk in older adults. The lowest cut-off points (3.0–4.5 s) showed high sensitivity (99.0% to 79.2%) but low specificity (2.1% to 37.7%), reflecting high fall detection but with numerous false positives and limited discriminative ability (J = 0.011 to 0.169). As the cut-off time increased, sensitivity decreased (46.5% at 6.0 s to 26.7% at 7.5 s), while specificity improved significantly (50.0% to 95.5%). The optimal cut-off point, with a low discriminative ability, was observed at 5.5 s (J = 0.280), balancing sensitivity (59.5%) and specificity (68.6%). Thus, in order to consider the predictive value, it is more optimal to consider the cut-off point with the highest sensitivity (3.5 s) and thus be able to identify people who may be at higher risk of falling. However, these results highlight the possibility of adjusting the cut-off point depending on the clinical context and objective. The full data are presented in Table 4.

Table 4. Discriminative capacity of falls at different cut-off points of the 3m-BWT.

Cut-Off Points	Sensitivity (%)	Specificity (%)	Youden's Index (J)
3.0 s	99.0	2.1	0.011
3.5 s	98.0	9.8	0.079
4.0 s	89.1	22.8	0.119
4.5 s	79.2	37.7	0.169
5.0 s	63.4	50.0	0.134
5.5 s	59.5	68.6	0.280
6.0 s	46.5	76.4	0.230
6.5 s	37.6	86.1	0.237
7.0 s	34.7	92.1	0.268
7.5 s	26.7	95.5	0.222

The values in real numbers represent the sensitivity, specificity, and discriminatory capacity (J) of different cut-off points.

4. Discussion

4.1. Main Findings

In this study, we evaluated the 3m-BWT as a practical and alternative functional assessment tool to predict fall risk in older adults. By analyzing data from 483 participants, we demonstrated its potential for identifying individuals at a high risk of falls, offering a simple yet effective option for clinical and community settings. The proportion of fallers in our sample (18.95%; n = 101) was slightly lower than previously reported (30%) [9]. Our results do not align with previous studies reporting an increased incidence of falls with advancing age [32,33], as no statistically significant age differences were found between fallers and non-fallers in our sample. However, we did confirm the association between a lower SMI and higher fall risk, consistent with previous research [34,35]. Significant differences in functional variables such as the TUG, 5STS, GS, SPPB, HG, and 4SST indicate that poorer performance in these components—reflected by slower times, lower strength, or reduced scores—is associated with increased fall risk. Among these, the 3m-BWT showed the largest difference between fallers and non-fallers, suggesting it may offer superior discriminative ability. However, despite being the best-performing test in our study, its overall discriminative capacity remains modest, and it should not be used as a standalone tool for fall prediction. These findings underscore the need for interventions focused on maintaining muscle mass and functionality to prevent falls in older adults, consistent with prior research [36].

The 3m-BWT reveals a significant difference of 1.71 s between fallers and non-fallers, which is statistically notable since the minimum detectable change in this population is 1.52 s [37]. This suggests that the 3m-BWT could be a valid tool for identifying and predicting fall risk, as it detects greater time differences in those who fall compared to those who do not. The 3m-BWT shows moderate correlations with other functional tests used for fall detection, such as the 5STS, SPPB, GS, and 4SST. It has a particularly strong relationship with the TUG, the most commonly used fall predictor [38]. Despite the different movements emphasized by the TUG and 3m-BWT, studies report similar correlations between them [27]. These findings support the potential use of the 3m-BWT as an additional fall prediction tool, as walking backward challenges postural control systems [24].

4.2. Clinical Implications

Backward walking with assistance from a parallel has been shown to be an important functional predictor of falls, surpassing even forward walking speed or the TUG in independent community-dwelling older adults [39,40]. These findings have been supported by performing the same movement unassisted by the 3m-BWT in our study. Although the 3m-BWT demonstrated the highest discriminative capacity among the tests evaluated in this study, its AUC of 0.655 still reflects poor overall discriminative ability. Therefore, it should not be used as a standalone tool to predict fall risk in older adults. Instead, its value lies in its potential as a complementary screening measure, especially in settings where high sensitivity is prioritized. For example, a cut-off point below 3.5 s shows high sensitivity but low specificity, making it useful to identify individuals at higher risk of falling, despite the risk of false positives. Conversely, specific populations such as those with Parkinson's disease or multiple sclerosis may require adjusted thresholds, as indicated in previous research [41–43]. However, it is important to note that the different cut-off values explored in this study (e.g., 3.5 s and 5.5 s) have not yet been validated across specific clinical subgroups or in prospective designs. Future research should aim to confirm the predictive validity of these thresholds in relation to incident falls in diverse populations. Our findings support the integration of the 3m-BWT within a broader battery of functional assessments to help detect mobility limitations, rather than relying on it in isolation. These results are not surprising, as other commonly used tests, such as the TUG, SPPB, GS, HG, or 4SST, also do not show adequate discriminative ability to predict falls in older adults when used in isolation [44–47]. Further research is needed to develop a comprehensive fall risk assessment tool that can accurately identify common and individual risk factors. Falls are multifactorial, suggesting the need to explore other associated factors that may not influence performance on a balance test [44].

In settings where it is crucial to detect the highest number of individuals at risk, a cut-off point of 3.5 s identifies 98% of positive cases, albeit with a high false positive rate. This result reinforces previous findings, where the same cut-off point was reported but with a lower sensitivity (74%) than in our study [26]. If the aim is to find a more balanced cut-off point, we propose adjusting it to 5.5 s (0.72 m/s), taking advantage of the larger sample size. This threshold has sufficient sensitivity (59.5%) and specificity (68.6%), achieving balanced values comparable to previous studies, reducing false positives, and improving accuracy [25,26].

When interpreting the results, it is important to acknowledge this study's limitations and consider recommendations for future research. The sample may not be fully representative of the general population, as it excludes institutionalized or hospitalized individuals, potentially affecting the generalizability of the findings. Additionally, this study did not account for all factors influencing falls, such as environmental, physiological, and psychological factors. Key aspects of physical performance, including stride length, proprioception, and attention, which might impact test results, were also not assessed. Falls were identified based on participants' self-reports over the past year, which could be affected by memory issues or biases, and whether the individual had fallen one or more times was not recorded.

4.3. Limitations, Recommendations, and Future Perspectives

To address these limitations, future research should include more representative samples across various ages, genders, and health statuses, including institutionalized and hospitalized individuals. It should also be noted that participants in this study were recruited from a voluntary healthy aging program, which may have introduced a selection bias toward a more functional and motivated population. This may limit the generalizability of the findings to more frail, institutionalized, or hospitalized populations. Longitudinal studies are needed to evaluate the test's effectiveness over time, track predictive changes in risk variables, and measure the impact of preventive interventions. Moreover, future studies should distinguish between single and recurrent falls, as this may improve the clinical relevance of the 3m-BWT and allow for more detailed analyses. Although partial correlations were adjusted for age, sex, and BMI, other potential confounders—such as comorbidities, medication use, cognitive status, and physical activity levels—were not controlled for. This represents an important limitation, and future studies should consider multivariate analyses that account for these variables to strengthen the validity of the findings. Additionally, relevant functional domains such as proprioception, cognitive function, dual-task gait performance, and reaction time—which are known to influence fall risk—were not evaluated in this study. It should also be acknowledged that the sample included a higher proportion of non-fallers than fallers, which could affect the generalizability of the group comparisons; however, this distribution is expected in community-dwelling older adult populations, where the prevalence of falls typically ranges from 20% to 30%. These omissions should be acknowledged as limitations, and future research is encouraged to incorporate these measures to enhance the comprehensiveness of fall risk assessments.

The results suggest that older adults who complete the 3m-BWT in less than 3.5 s are less likely to have a history of falls, while the risk appears to increase significantly above this time. However, as this is a cross-sectional study, these results should not be interpreted as predictive of future fall risk. Although the 5.5 s point offers a reasonable balance, its limitations highlight the need for further research in diverse populations to optimize predictive accuracy. Furthermore, the 3m-BWT should not be considered as a sole diagnostic tool but as part of a comprehensive geriatric assessment, combining it with other instruments and considering factors such as history of falls, individual characteristics, and other functional tests [44–47]. This will allow for a more accurate and personalized assessment of fall risk. Developing personalized fall risk protocols with specific interventions and ongoing follow-up could further enhance fall prevention efforts.

5. Conclusions

The findings of this study support the potential of the 3m-BWT as a complementary functional tool in the assessment of fall risk in older adults, highlighting its superior discriminatory ability compared to widely used tests such as the TUG, GS, and SPPB. However, its limited sensitivity and specificity underscore that it should not be used as a sole method, given the multifactorial nature of falls.

Test execution time emerges as a relevant indicator: Values below 3.5 s suggest minimal risk, while exceeding 5.5 s could signal greater vulnerability, albeit with predictive limitations. These results reinforce the need to integrate the 3m-BWT within a multidimensional approach, combining it with clinical assessments, falls history, and other functional tests to improve risk stratification.

Future research should explore the optimization of cut-off points, their validity in heterogeneous populations, and their interaction with other risk factors. In the meantime, the application of personalized protocols, accompanied by targeted interventions and continuous monitoring, could enhance more effective preventive strategies in the geriatric population. The 3m-BWT thus represents a promising advance, but its clinical utility will depend on a contextualized and holistic implementation.

Supplementary Materials: The following supporting information can be downloaded at https://www.mdpi.com/article/10.3390/jfmk10020154/s1, Table S1: Standardized measurement of the result variables.

Author Contributions: L.P.-F., R.M.-S. and F.J.B.-I. conceived the study; L.P.-F. and J.T.-A. wrote the original draft; A.S.P.-G. and M.C.S.-S. critically reviewed the manuscript for relevant intellectual content. L.P.-F. and R.M.-S. analyzed the data. All authors participated in the methodology and assessments. All authors have read and agreed to the published version of the manuscript.

Funding: The participants' assessments were funded by the Salamanca City Council through an agreement with the University of Salamanca (Project code: L9AB). The funder had no influence on the analysis of the results or the decision to publish them. No funding was received by any of the authors for the conduct of this study.

Institutional Review Board Statement: This study was approved on 22 July 2024 by the Ethics Committee for Drug Research of the Salamanca Health Area (Protocol Code: PI 2024061702), conducted in accordance with the Declaration of Helsinki, and registered on ClinicalTrials.gov on 23 May 2024 (Registration No: NCT06434857). Before participating in the study, participants were informed about the research procedure, and informed consent was obtained from all participants involved.

Informed Consent Statement: Informed consent was obtained from all subjects involved in this study.

Data Availability Statement: The data sets used and/or analyzed during the present study are available from the corresponding author upon request.

Acknowledgments: The research team extends its gratitude to all the patients who participated in this study and to the Salamanca City Council for funding the assessment.

Conflicts of Interest: The authors declare no competing interests.

Abbreviations

The following abbreviations are used in this manuscript:

3m-BWT	3-Meter Backward Walk Test
4SST	4-Square Step Test
5STS	5 Times Sit-to-Stand Test
ASM	Appendicular Skeletal Muscle Mass
AUC	Area Under the Curve
BMI	Body Mass Index
GRP	Geriatric Revitalization Program
GS	Gait Speed
HG	Hand Grip Strength

ROC	Receiver Operating Characteristic
SMI	Skeletal Muscle Mass Index
SPPB	Short Physical Performance Battery
TUG	Timed Up and Go Test

References

1. da Costa, J.P.; Vitorino, R.; Silva, G.M.; Vogel, C.; Duarte, A.C.; Rocha-Santos, T. A synopsis on aging—Theories, mechanisms and future prospects. *Ageing Res. Rev.* **2016**, *29*, 90–112. [PubMed]
2. Kennedy, B.K.; Berger, S.L.; Brunet, A.; Campisi, J.; Cuervo, A.M.; Epel, E.S.; Franceschi, C.; Lithgow, G.J.; Morimoto, R.I.; Pessin, J.E.; et al. Geroscience: Linking aging to chronic disease. *Cell* **2014**, *159*, 709–713. [PubMed]
3. Fong, B.Y.F. Ageing and frailty. *Hong Kong Med. J.* **2022**, *28*, 344–346. [PubMed]
4. Brivio, P.; Paladini, M.S.; Racagni, G.; Riva, M.A.; Calabrese, F.; Molteni, R. From healthy aging to frailty: In search of the underlying mechanisms. *Curr. Med. Chem.* **2019**, *26*, 3685–3701.
5. Nascimento, C.M.; Ingles, M.; Salvador-Pascual, A.; Cominetti, M.R.; Gomez-Cabrera, M.C.; Viña, J. Sarcopenia, frailty and their prevention by exercise. *Free Radic. Biol. Med.* **2019**, *132*, 42–49.
6. Fried, L.P.; Tangen, C.M.; Walston, J.; Newman, A.B.; Hirsch, C.; Gottdiener, J.; Seeman, T.; Tracy, R.; Kop, W.J.; Burke, G.; et al. Frailty in older adults: Evidence for a phenotype. *J. Gerontol. A Biol. Sci. Med. Sci.* **2001**, *56*, M146–M156.
7. Taguchi, C.K.; Menezes, P.d.L.; Melo, A.C.S.; de Santana, L.S.; Conceição, W.R.S.; de Souza, G.F.; Araújo, B.C.L.; da Silva, A.R. Frailty syndrome and risks for falling in the elderly community. *CoDAS* **2022**, *34*, e20210025.
8. Yang, Z.-C.; Lin, H.; Jiang, G.-H.; Chu, Y.-H.; Gao, J.-H.; Tong, Z.-J.; Wang, Z.-H. Frailty is a risk factor for falls in the older adults: A systematic review and meta-analysis. *J. Nutr. Health Aging* **2023**, *27*, 487–495.
9. Bergen, G.; Stevens, M.R.; Burns, E.R. Falls and fall injuries among adults aged ≥65 years—United States, 2014. *MMWR Morb. Mortal. Wkly. Rep.* **2016**, *65*, 993–998.
10. Morrison, A.; Fan, T.; Sen, S.S.; Weisenfluh, L. Epidemiology of falls and osteoporotic fractures: A systematic review. *Clinicoecon. Outcomes Res.* **2013**, *5*, 9–18.
11. Vieira, E.R.; Palmer, R.C.; Chaves, P.H.M. Prevention of falls in older people living in the community. *BMJ* **2016**, *353*, i1419. [PubMed]
12. Callis, N. Falls prevention: Identification of predictive fall risk factors. *Appl. Nurs. Res.* **2016**, *29*, 53–58. [PubMed]
13. Rubenstein, L.Z. Falls in older people: Epidemiology, risk factors and strategies for prevention. *Age Ageing* **2006**, *35* (Suppl. S2), ii37–ii41. [PubMed]
14. Burns, E.R.; Stevens, J.A.; Lee, R. The direct costs of fatal and non-fatal falls among older adults—United States. *J. Saf. Res.* **2016**, *58*, 99–103.
15. Lusardi, M.M.; Fritz, S.; Middleton, A.; Allison, L.; Wingood, M.; Phillips, E.; Criss, M.; Verma, S.; Osborne, J.; Chui, K.K. Determining risk of falls in community dwelling older adults: A systematic review and meta-analysis using posttest probability. *J. Geriatr. Phys. Ther.* **2017**, *40*, 1–36.
16. Mishra, A.K.; Skubic, M.; Despins, L.A.; Popescu, M.; Keller, J.; Rantz, M.; Abbott, C.; Enayati, M.; Shalini, S.; Miller, S. Explainable fall risk prediction in older adults using gait and geriatric assessments. *Front. Digit. Health* **2022**, *4*, 869812.
17. Cruz-Jentoft, A.J.; Bahat, G.; Bauer, J.; Boirie, Y.; Bruyère, O.; Cederholm, T.; Cooper, C.; Landi, F.; Rolland, Y.; Sayer, A.A.; et al. Sarcopenia: Revised European consensus on definition and diagnosis. *Age Ageing* **2019**, *48*, 16–31.
18. Gould, H.; Brennan, S.L.; Kotowicz, M.A.; Nicholson, G.C.; Pasco, J.A. Total and appendicular lean mass reference ranges for Australian men and women: The Geelong osteoporosis study. *Calcif. Tissue Int.* **2014**, *94*, 363–372.
19. Álvarez, M.N.; Rodríguez-Sánchez, C.; Huertas-Hoyas, E.; García-Villamil-Neira, G.; Espinoza-Cerda, M.T.; Pérez-Delgado, L.; Reina-Robles, E.; Martin, I.B.; Del-Ama, A.J.; Ruiz-Ruiz, L.; et al. Predictors of fall risk in older adults using the G-STRIDE inertial sensor: An observational multicenter case–control study. *BMC Geriatr.* **2023**, *23*, 379.
20. Buatois, S.; Perret-Guillaume, C.; Gueguen, R.; Miget, P.; Vançon, G.; Perrin, P.; Benetos, A. A simple clinical scale to stratify risk of recurrent falls in community-dwelling adults aged 65 years and older. *Phys. Ther.* **2010**, *90*, 550–560.
21. Beaudart, C.; McCloskey, E.; Bruyère, O.; Cesari, M.; Rolland, Y.; Rizzoli, R.; Araujo De Carvalho, I.; Amuthavalli Thiyagarajan, J.; Bautmans, I.; Bertière, M.-C.; et al. Sarcopenia in daily practice: Assessment and management. *BMC Geriatr.* **2016**, *16*, 10.
22. Neri, S.G.R.; Lima, R.M.; Ribeiro, H.S.; Vainshelboim, B. Poor handgrip strength determined clinically is associated with falls in older women. *J. Frailty Sarcopenia Falls* **2021**, *6*, 43. [PubMed]
23. de Aquino, M.P.M.; de Oliveira Cirino, N.T.; Lima, C.A.; de Miranda Ventura, M.; Hill, K.; Perracini, M.R. The Four Square Step Test is a useful mobility tool for discriminating older persons with frailty syndrome. *Exp. Gerontol.* **2022**, *161*, 111699. [PubMed]
24. Laufer, Y. Age- and gender-related changes in the temporal-spatial characteristics of forwards and backwards gaits. *Physiother. Res. Int.* **2003**, *8*, 131–142.

25. Fritz, N.E.; Worstell, A.M.; Kloos, A.D.; Siles, A.B.; White, S.E.; Kegelmeyer, D.A. Backward walking measures are sensitive to age-related changes in mobility and balance. *Gait Posture* **2013**, *37*, 593–597.
26. Carter, V.; Jain, T.; James, J.; Cornwall, M.; Aldrich, A.; De Heer, H.D. The 3-m backwards walk and retrospective falls: Diagnostic accuracy of a novel clinical measure. *J. Geriatr. Phys. Ther.* **2019**, *42*, 249–255.
27. Hao, J.; Pu, Y.; He, Z.; Remis, A.; Yao, Z.; Li, Y. Measurement properties of the backward walk test in people with balance and mobility deficits: A systematic review. *Gait Posture* **2024**, *110*, 1–9.
28. Association, W.M. World Medical Association Declaration of Helsinki: Ethical principles for medical research involving human subjects. *JAMA* **2013**, *310*, 2191–2194.
29. Moher, D.; Hopewell, S.; Schulz, K.F.; Montori, V.; Gøtzsche, P.C.; Devereaux, P.; Elbourne, D.; Egger, M.; Altman, D.G. CONSORT 2010 explanation and elaboration: Updated guidelines for reporting parallel group randomised trials. *Int. J. Surg.* **2012**, *10*, 28–55.
30. Cohen, J. *Statistical Power Analysis for the Behavioral Sciences*; Routledge: London, UK, 2013.
31. Swets, J.A. Measuring the accuracy of diagnostic systems. *Science* **1988**, *240*, 1285–1293.
32. Gale, C.R.; Westbury, L.D.; Cooper, C.; Dennison, E.M. Risk factors for incident falls in older men and women: The English longitudinal study of ageing. *BMC Geriatr.* **2018**, *18*, 141.
33. Talbot, L.A.; Musiol, R.J.; Witham, E.K.; Metter, E.J. Falls in young, middle-aged and older community dwelling adults: Perceived cause, environmental factors and injury. *BMC Public Health* **2005**, *5*, 86.
34. Sinaki, M.; Brey, R.H.; Hughes, C.A.; Larson, D.R.; Kaufman, K.R. Balance disorder and increased risk of falls in osteoporosis and kyphosis: Significance of kyphotic posture and muscle strength. *Osteoporos. Int.* **2005**, *16*, 1004–1010. [PubMed]
35. Kaufman-Cohen, Y.; Ratzon, N.Z. Correlation between risk factors and musculoskeletal disorders among classical musicians. *Occup. Med.* **2011**, *61*, 90–95.
36. Sherrington, C.; Michaleff, Z.A.; Fairhall, N.; Paul, S.S.; Tiedemann, A.; Whitney, J.; Cumming, R.G.; Herbert, R.D.; Close, J.C.T.; Lord, S.R. Exercise to prevent falls in older adults: An updated systematic review and meta-analysis. *Br. J. Sports Med.* **2017**, *51*, 1749–1757.
37. Özden, F.; Özkeskin, M.; Bakırhan, S.; Şahin, S. The test–retest reliability and concurrent validity of the 3-m backward walk test and 50-ft walk test in community-dwelling older adults. *Ir. J. Med. Sci.* **2022**, *191*, 921–928.
38. Barry, E.; Galvin, R.; Keogh, C.; Horgan, F.; Fahey, T. Is the Timed Up and Go test a useful predictor of risk of falls in community dwelling older adults: A systematic review and meta-analysis. *BMC Geriatr.* **2014**, *14*, 14.
39. Taulbee, L.; Yada, T.; Graham, L.; O'Halloran, A.; Saracino, D.; Freund, J.; Vallabhajosula, S.; Balasubramanian, C.K. Use of backward walking speed to screen dynamic balance and mobility deficits in older adults living independently in the community. *J. Geriatr. Phys. Ther.* **2021**, *44*, 189–197.
40. Edwards, E.M.; Daugherty, A.M.; Nitta, M.; Atalla, M.; Fritz, N.E. Backward walking sensitively detects fallers in persons with multiple sclerosis. *Mult. Scler. Relat. Disord.* **2020**, *45*, 102390.
41. Söke, F.; Demirkaya, Ş.; Yavuz, N.; Gülşen, E.Ö.; Tunca, Ö.; Gülşen, Ç.; Karakoç, S.; Koçer, B.; Aydin, F.; Yücesan, C. The 3-m backward walk test: Reliability and validity in ambulant people with multiple sclerosis. *Int. J. Rehabil. Res.* **2022**, *45*, 209–214.
42. Kocer, B.; Soke, F.; Ataoglu, N.E.E.; Ersoy, N.; Gulsen, C.; Gulsen, E.O.; Yasa, M.E.; Uysal, I.; Comoglu, S.S.; Bora, H.A.T. The reliability and validity of the 3-m backward walk test in people with Parkinson's disease. *Ir. J. Med. Sci.* **2023**, *192*, 3063–3071. [PubMed]
43. Carter, V.A.; Farley, B.G.; Wing, K.; De Heer, H.D.; Jain, T.K. Precisión diagnóstica de la prueba de marcha atrás de 3 metros en personas con enfermedad de Parkinson. *Temas Rehabil. Geriátrica* **2020**, *36*, 140–145.
44. Moreland, B.; Kakara, R.; Henry, A. Trends in nonfatal falls and fall-related injuries among adults aged ≥65 years—United States, 2012–2018. *MMWR Morb. Mortal. Wkly. Rep.* **2023**, *69*, 875–881.
45. Lee, Y.C.; Chang, S.F.; Kao, C.Y.; Tsai, H.C. Muscle strength, physical fitness, balance, and walking ability at risk of fall for prefrail older people. *BioMed Res. Int.* **2022**, *2022*, 4581126.
46. Li, W.; Rao, Z.; Fu, Y.; Schwebel, D.C.; Li, L.; Ning, P.; Huang, J.; Hu, G. Value of the short physical performance battery (SPPB) in predicting fall and fall-induced injury among old Chinese adults. *BMC Geriatr.* **2023**, *23*, 290.
47. Adam, C.E.; Fitzpatrick, A.L.; Leary, C.S.; Hajat, A.; Ilango, S.D.; Park, C.; Phelan, E.A.; Semmens, E.O. Change in gait speed and fall risk among community-dwelling older adults with and without mild cognitive impairment: A retrospective cohort analysis. *BMC Geriatr.* **2023**, *23*, 890.

Journal of
Functional Morphology and Kinesiology

MDPI

Article

Wearable Sensor Assessment of Gait Characteristics in Individuals Awaiting Total Knee Arthroplasty: A Cross-Sectional, Observational Study

Elina Gianzina [1], Christos K. Yiannakopoulos [1,*], Elias Armenis [1] and Efstathios Chronopoulos [2]

[1] School of Physical Education and Sport Science, National and Kapodistrian University of Athens, 17232 Athens, Greece

[2] Laboratory for Research of the Musculoskeletal System, "Th. Garofalidis", KAT General Hospital, Medical School, National and Kapodistrian University of Athens, 14561 Athens, Greece

* Correspondence: c.yiannakopoulos@phed.uoa.gr

Abstract

Background: Gait impairments are common in individuals with knee osteoarthritis awaiting total knee arthroplasty, affecting their mobility and quality of life. This study aimed to assess and compare biomechanical gait features between individuals awaiting total knee arthroplasty and healthy, non-arthritic controls, focusing on less-explored variables using sensor-based measurements. **Methods:** A cross-sectional observational study was conducted with 60 participants: 21 individuals awaiting total knee arthroplasty and 39 nonarthritic controls aged 64–85 years. Participants completed a standardized 14 m walk, and 17 biomechanical gait parameters were measured using the BTS G-Walk inertial sensor. Key variables, such as stride duration, cadence, symmetry indices, and pelvic angles, were analyzed for group differences. **Results:** The pre-total knee arthroplasty group exhibited significantly longer gait cycles and stride durations ($p < 0.001$), reduced cadence ($p < 0.001$), and lower gait cycle symmetry index ($p < 0.001$) than the control group. The pelvic angle symmetry indices for tilt ($p = 0.014$), rotation ($p = 0.002$), and obliquity ($p < 0.001$) were also lower. Additionally, the pre-total knee arthroplasty group had lower propulsion indices for both legs ($p < 0.001$) and a lower walking quality index on the right leg ($p = 0.005$). The number of elaborated steps was significantly greater in the pre-total knee arthroplasty group (left, $p < 0.001$, right: $p < 0.001$). No significant differences were observed in any other gait parameters. **Conclusions:** This study revealed significant gait impairment in individuals awaiting total knee arthroplasty. Although direct evidence for prehabilitation is lacking, future research should explore whether targeted approaches, such as strengthening exercises or gait retraining, can improve gait and functional outcomes before surgery.

Keywords: gait impairments; knee osteoarthritis; total knee arthroplasty; wearable sensors; gait biomechanics

1. Introduction

Knee osteoarthritis is a common chronic degenerative joint disease characterized by stiffness, discomfort, and reduced joint function. In its advanced stages, knee osteoarthritis leads to significant physical impairment, pain, and disability, severely restricting daily activities such as walking, standing, and climbing stairs [1–3]. Consequently, the burden of knee osteoarthritis is not only felt physically but also socially and psychologically, affecting overall well-being and productivity [4]

Total knee arthroplasty (TKA) is regarded as the most effective treatment for individuals with advanced knee osteoarthritis, as it alleviates symptoms and improves mobility [5–7]. However, patients awaiting TKA often experience substantial gait impairment, which compromises their mobility, balance, and stability [8,9]. These gait disturbances include reduced walking speed, prolonged gait cycle duration, and increased asymmetry, all of which contribute to an elevated risk of falls and decreased independence in performing activities of daily living [10–12].

Recent systematic reviews have emphasized the critical role of gait impairment as an indicator of functional decline in patients with knee osteoarthritis. For example, Favre and Jolles [13] provided a reference dataset on lower limb biomechanics in knee osteoarthritis, underscoring the importance of gait analysis in understanding the disease progression. Meta-analyses have also shown that reduced walking speed and asymmetry correlate with knee osteoarthritis severity and can predict outcomes after TKA [14].

Wearable sensor technology has emerged as a valuable tool for assessing and quantifying gait biomechanics in clinical and research settings. Devices such as the BTS G-Walk inertial sensor provide noninvasive, real-time evaluations of gait parameters, including cadence, gait cycle duration, stride length, and symmetry [15–19]. These sensors allow for detailed gait analysis, enabling clinicians to track gait abnormalities over time and develop targeted prehabilitation and rehabilitation strategies to improve functional outcomes before surgery [20,21].

The primary aim of this study was to evaluate the biomechanical gait features of pre-TKA individuals and compare them with those of healthy, nonarthritic controls using inertial sensor-based measurements. While previous studies have explored general gait impairments in patients with knee osteoarthritis, they have primarily concentrated on basic parameters such as gait speed and cadence [10,11,14,21,22]. This study further investigated less-studied parameters, particularly pelvic motion asymmetries (e.g., pelvic tilt, rotation, and obliquity) and the propulsion index, which provide new insights into the compensatory strategies employed by individuals before TKA. By using advanced wearable technology to track these parameters, we aimed to uncover compensatory movement patterns and biomechanical dysfunctions in the pre-TKA group before surgery. These findings may inform the development of targeted presurgical interventions to optimize postoperative recovery.

2. Materials and Methods

2.1. Participants

The study included 21 patients with primary knee osteoarthritis (3 males and 18 females) with a mean age of 73.57 $\pm$ 6.44 years and 39 volunteers without arthritis (10 males and 29 females) with a mean age of 71.59 $\pm$ 4.81 years. Cases and controls were matched individually based on age, sex, and body mass index (BMI), with each knee osteoarthritis patient paired with approximately 1.9 non-arthritic controls. Matching criteria were selected to control for potential confounding factors, such as age, sex, and BMI, which are known to affect gait performance and may influence study outcomes. Patients with end-stage unilateral primary knee osteoarthritis scheduled for TKA were recruited. The inclusion criteria required participants to walk independently without the use of ambulatory aids. Individuals with neurological, cardiorespiratory, or severe orthopedic conditions that impaired mobility were excluded. The normal non-arthritic group comprised healthy individuals with no history of orthopedic or neurological disorders, recent injuries, surgeries, or medications that could affect their gait or balance.

Before participation, all participants provided written informed consent after receiving a detailed explanation of the study objectives. This study adhered to the principles of the Declaration of Helsinki and was approved by the Institutional Review Board (IRB) of the School of Physical Education and Sport Science at the National and Kapodistrian University of Athens, Greece (Approval Number: 1306/22-09-2021).

2.2. Instrumentations

Gait analysis was conducted using the G-Walk wireless inertial sensor (BTS Bioengineering S.p.A., Milan, Italy), which integrates a triaxial accelerometer, gyroscope, and magnetometer. The G-Walk system has demonstrated high test–retest reliability (ICCs > 0.90) and strong agreement with motion capture systems for parameters such as gait cycle duration, cadence, and step length [15–19]. The algorithms used primarily rely on accelerometer and gyroscope data, with the magnetometer contributing to orientation tracking, particularly for pelvic rotation. All trials were performed on flat, nonmetallic indoor surfaces to minimize magnetic interference.

The triaxial accelerometer offers multiple sensitivity settings with dynamic ranges of ±2, ±4, ±8, and ±16 g, operating within a bandwidth of 4–1000 Hz and providing 16-bit precision per axis. The magnetometer features a 13-bit resolution, dynamic range of ±1200 μT, and bandwidth of up to 100 Hz. The gyroscope also provides 16-bit precision per axis, with sensitivity options of ±250, ±500, ±1000, and ±2000°/s and a bandwidth range of 4–8000 Hz.

Additionally, the module is equipped with a GPS receiver that ensures high positional accuracy, offering 2.5 m accuracy at up to 5 Hz or 3 m accuracy at up to 10 Hz with a bandwidth of up to 10 Hz.

In terms of dimensions, the device measures 70 mm × 40 mm × 18 mm (2.75 × 1.57 × 0.7 in) and supports acquisition frequencies of up to 1000 Hz. For data collection, it was connected to a laptop via Bluetooth 3.0, with a transmission range of up to 60 m in a direct line of sight.

2.3. Data Collection Protocol

During testing, the sensor was secured inside a semi-elastic black belt positioned over the participants' S1–S2 vertebrae. This study was conducted in three sequential phases: (1) data collection, (2) analysis, and (3) interpretation of the results. These steps were completed without strict time tracking.

During the data collection phase, the participants followed a 14 m walking protocol. Prior to the test, they received clear instructions to ensure the consistency and reliability of the results. The test began with the participants standing still for a moment to allow for stabilization. Upon receiving a signal, the participants walked along a straight path at a steady and moderate pace. The objective was to complete at least five full gait cycles over a 14 m distance before turning around.

Before each turn, the participants paused for at least one second to regain stability and then turned and paused again for another second before proceeding in the opposite direction. This approach helps minimize variability while preserving natural walking patterns.

Each participant completed at least two trials of the 14 m walk, with additional trials permitted to ensure reliable data and confirm gait pattern consistency. As this was a cross-sectional study, no follow-up was required, and all data were collected at a single time point.

2.4. Data Analysis

Gait data were collected using Bluetooth 3.0 and transmitted in real time to a computer for further processing. G-Studio software (version 1.3.0) was used to analyze the data, applying automated filters to eliminate noise and correct inconsistencies in the walking patterns. The software then uses built-in algorithms to calculate the various spatiotemporal gait parameters. These algorithms transform raw motion sensor signals into clinically relevant gait metrics. Their accuracy was confirmed through internal calibration procedures and validation studies against gold-standard motion capture systems. Previous studies have also shown strong correlations between parameters calculated from wearable sensors and directly measured joint kinematics, supporting the reliability of this approach [15–19].

The extracted gait parameters were categorized into three main groups:

1. Global analysis parameters

These parameters provide an overview of the walking pattern and include the following:

- Cadence (steps/min): number of steps taken per minute.
- Speed (m/s): average walking velocity.
- Symmetry index of the gait cycle: this index measures the percentage of symmetry between the anterior and posterior acceleration curves during the right and left gait cycles.
- Symmetry index of pelvic angles (tilt, obliquity, rotation): This index assesses the percentage similarity or difference in pelvic movements recorded during the right and left gait cycles. These angles were measured in three anatomical planes—sagittal (tilt), frontal (obliquity), and transverse (rotation) planes.

2. Side-specific parameters (Left and Right)

These parameters focus on the individual foot movements and gait cycle dynamics for each leg:

- Stride length (m): the average distance covered between consecutive initial contacts of the same foot.
- Stride length as a percentage of height (% height): normalized stride length relative to the participant's height.
- Gait cycle duration (s): time interval between two consecutive heel strikes of the same foot.
- Step length (% stride length): the average distance between the initial foot contact and the next contact made by the opposite foot.
- Stance phase (% cycle): percentage of the gait cycle during which the foot remains in contact with the ground.
- Swing phase (% cycle): the percentage of the gait cycle during which the foot is in motion and not in contact with the ground.
- Double support phase (% cycle): percentage of the gait cycle in which both feet are simultaneously in contact with the ground.
- Single support phase (% cycle): percentage of the gait cycle in which only one foot is in contact with the ground.
- Elaborated steps: total number of strides considered in the analysis.
- Propulsion index: represents the inclination of the line following the rising edge of the acceleration pattern.

3. Walk quality index

The walk quality index is a composite measure that evaluates gait efficiency, stability, and symmetry by integrating key gait parameters such as step length, cadence, symmetry, and variability. A higher score indicates a more efficient, stable, and symmetrical walking pattern, whereas a lower score indicates a less efficient, unstable, or more variable gait.

2.5. Statistical Analysis

All statistical analyses were performed using IBM SPSS Statistics version 29.0 (IBM Corporation, Somers, NY, USA). Data are presented as mean $\pm$ standard deviation (SD) or, for non-normally distributed variables, as the median with interquartile range (IQR).

The Kolmogorov–Smirnov and Shapiro–Wilk tests were used to assess the normality of the data.

To compare the groups, an independent samples *t*-test and Fisher's exact test were used to evaluate homogeneity between the groups. If the normality assumptions were violated, the Mann–Whitney U test was used to analyze the differences between the groups. Effect sizes were reported alongside *p*-values: Cohen's d for *t*-tests and rank-biserial correlation (r) for Mann–Whitney U tests, providing a more comprehensive understanding of the practical significance of the observed differences.

A priori power analysis was conducted using GPower (version 3.1) to determine the required sample size for detecting large effect sizes (Cohen's d $\approx$ 0.8) at a significance level of $p < 0.05$, with a target power of 80%. All statistical tests were two-tailed, with significance set at $p < 0.05$.

3. Results

The demographic characteristics of the participants are presented in Table 1. The pre-TKA group had a mean age of 73.57 ± 6.44 years, whereas the normal non-arthritic group had a mean age of 71.59 ± 4.81 years, with no significant difference between the groups ($p = 0.229$). Similarly, no significant differences were observed in weight (pre-TKA: 82.29 ± 16.92 kg, normal: 77.96 ± 9.66 kg; $p = 0.270$), height (pre-TKA: 165.52 ± 7.23 cm, normal: 163.81 ± 7.45 cm; $p = 0.429$), BMI (pre-TKA: 30.01 ± 5.75, normal: 29.15 ± 3.97; $p = 0.541$), or shoe size (pre-TKA: 39.76 ± 2.26, normal: 39.81 ± 3.98; $p = 0.332$). Sex distribution was comparable among the groups ($p = 0.704$).

Table 1. The demographic characteristics of the participants included in this study are presented as means and standard deviations for normally distributed variables and medians with interquartile ranges for non-normally distributed variables.

	Knee Osteoarthritis (n = 21)	Controls (n = 39)	p Value
Age (years)	73.57 ± 6.44	71.59 ± 4.81	0.229
Weight (kg)	82.29 ± 16.92	77.96 ± 9.66	0.270
Height (cm)	165.52 ± 7.23	163.81 ± 7.45	0.429
BMI	30.01 ± 5.75	29.15 ± 3.97	0.541
Shoe size (EU)	39.76 ± 2.26	39.81 ± 3.98	0.332 [a]
Gender, Male/Female, N (%)	3 (14.3)/18 (85.7)	10 (25.6)/29 (74.4)	0.704

[a] *p*-value based on Mann–Whitney U test; shoe size reported as median (IQR) due to non-normal distribution.

Table 2 summarizes the gait parameters of the two groups. Significant differences were observed in several gait parameters. First, the gait cycle duration was significantly longer in the pre-TKA group than in the normal group for both the left (1.36 ± 0.14 vs. 1.11 ± 0.06 s, $p < 0.001$, Cohen's d = 2.17) and right (1.35 ± 0.14 vs. 1.11 ± 0.07 s, $p < 0.001$, Cohen's d = 2.17) sides, with large effect sizes, indicating substantial differences. Similarly, stride duration was significantly longer in the pre-TKA group for both the left (1.37 ± 0.16 vs. 1.11 ± 0.06 s, $p < 0.001$, Cohen's d = 2.15) and right (1.36 ± 0.16 vs. 1.11 ± 0.07 s, $p < 0.001$, Cohen's d = 2.02) legs.

In addition, cadence was significantly lower in the pre-TKA group (91.12 ± 9.02 vs. 108.78 ± 6.64 steps/min, $p < 0.001$, Cohen's d = −2.23) with a large effect size. Similarly, walking speed was significantly slower in the pre-TKA group (0.87 ± 0.16 vs. 1.11 ± 0.14 m/s, $p < 0.001$, Cohen's d = −1.60).

Table 2. Gait parameters in patients with severe knee osteoarthritis prior to total knee arthroplasty and in the non-arthritic control group are presented as means and standard deviations (SDs) for normally distributed variables and as medians with interquartile ranges (IQRs) for non-normally distributed variables.

Parameter	Knee Osteoarthritis	Controls		
	Mean ± SD	**Mean ± SD**	***p* Value**	**Effect Size (Cohen's d)**
Left gait cycle duration (s)	1.36 ± 0.14	1.11 ± 0.06	0.000	2.17
Right gait cycle duration (s)	1.35 ± 0.14	1.11 ± 0.07	0.000	2.17
Cadence (steps/min)	91.12 ± 9.02	108.78 ± 6.64	0.000	−2.23
Speed (m/s)	0.87 ± 0.16	1.11 ± 0.14	0.000	−1.60
Left stride duration (s)	1.37 ± 0.16	1.11 ± 0.06	0.000	2.15
Right stride duration (s)	1.36 ± 0.16	1.11 ± 0.07	0.000	2.02
Left stance duration (%)	60.95 ± 5.16	60.80 ± 2.34	0.892	0.04
Right stance duration (%)	60.66 ± 5.07	60.15 ± 2.90	0.663	0.12
Left stride length (m)	1.18 ± 0.20	1.23 ± 0.15	0.274	−0.28
Right stride length (m)	1.18 ± 0.19	1.23 ± 0.15	0.277	−0.29
First left double support (%)	11.18 ± 2.02	10.26 ± 2.38	0.163	0.42
Left single support (%)	39.14 ± 4.88	39.65 ± 2.67	0.646	−0.13
Right single support (%)	38.79 ± 5.22	39.10 ± 1.91	0.773	−0.08
Right swing duration (%)	39.34 ± 5.07	39.85 ± 2.90	0.663	−0.12
Left propulsion index	3.78 ± 1.47	6.45 ± 1.30	0.000	−1.92
Right propulsion index	4.01 ± 1.58	6.45 ± 1.42	0.000	−1.62
Right walk quality index	91.47 ± 5.30	94.91 ± 2.65	0.005	−0.82
	Median ± IQR	**Median ± IQR**	***p* value**	**Effect Size (r)**
Left elaborated steps (s)	11.0 ± 6.0	8.0 ± 2.0	0.000	0.66
Right elaborated steps (s)	11.0 ± 5.0	8.0 ± 2.0	0.000	0.69
Symmetry index of gait cycle	92.7 ± 14.85	97.0 ± 2.4	0.000	0.71
% Left stride length (% height)	69.1 ± 18.25	75.9 ± 11.7	0.143	0.17
% Right stride length (% height)	69.5 ± 17.65	75.4 ± 10.9	0.132	0.18
Left swing duration (%)	39.3 ± 6.6	38.5 ± 3.2	0.893	0.01
First right double support (%)	10.2 ± 3.1	11.8 ± 4.3	0.417	0.08
Left walk quality index	93.5 ± 6.8	95.9 ± 4.3	0.036	0.21
Tilt—symmetry index of pelvic angles	50.5 ± 49.1	74.2 ± 27.4	0.014	0.28
Obliquity—symmetry index of pelvic angles	90.3 ± 9.8	98.7 ± 0.8	0.000	0.52
Rotation—symmetry index of pelvic angles	94.8 ± 4.1	98.1 ± 2.4	0.002	0.40

However, no significant differences were observed in stance duration for the left (60.95 ± 5.16 vs. 60.80 ± 2.34%, $p = 0.892$, Cohen's d = 0.04) or right (60.66 ± 5.07 vs. 60.15 ± 2.90%, $p = 0.663$, Cohen's d = 0.12) side, with very small effect sizes. Likewise, no significant differences were found in stride length for the left (1.18 ± 0.20 vs. 1.23 ± 0.15 m, $p = 0.274$, Cohen's d = −0.28) or right (1.18 ± 0.19 vs. 1.23 ± 0.15 m, $p = 0.277$, Cohen's d = −0.29) sides.

Moreover, the first left double support was not significantly different between the groups (11.18 ± 2.02 vs. 10.26 ± 2.38%, $p = 0.163$, Cohen's d = 0.42). Similarly, no significant differences were found in the left single support (39.14 ± 4.88 vs. 39.65 ± 2.67%, $p = 0.646$, Cohen's d = −0.13) or right single support (38.79 ± 5.22 vs. 39.10 ± 0.91%, $p = 0.773$, Cohen's d = −0.08) times. The right swing duration was not significantly different between the groups (39.34± 5.07 vs. 39.85 ± 2.90%, $p = 0.663$, Cohen's d = −0.12).

In contrast, the left (3.78 ± 1.47 vs. 6.45 ± 1.30, $p < 0.001$, Cohen's d = −1.92) and right (4.01 ± 1.58 vs. 6.45 ± 1.42, $p < 0.001$, Cohen's d = −1.62) propulsion indices were significantly lower in the pre-TKA group, with large effect sizes. Furthermore, the right walk quality index was significantly lower in the pre-TKA group (91.47 ± 5.30 vs. 94.91 ± 2.65, $p = 0.005$, Cohen's d = −0.82).

The elaborated steps were significantly longer in the pre-TKA group for both the left (11.00 ± 6.00 vs. 8.00 ± 2.00 s, $p < 0.001$, r = 0.66) and right (11.00 ± 5.00 vs. 8.00 ± 2.00 s, $p < 0.001$, r = 0.69) sides, with moderate effect sizes. However, the symmetry index of the gait cycle was significantly lower in the pre-TKA group (92.7 ± 14.85 vs. 97.0 ± 2.4, $p < 0.001$, r = 0.71), indicating more asymmetrical gait patterns in the pre-TKA group.

Regarding stride length as a percentage of height, there were no significant differences between the left (69.1 ± 18.25 vs. 75.9 ± 11.7%, $p = 0.143$, r = 0.17) and right (69.5 ± 17.65 vs. 75.4 ± 10.9%, $p = 0.132$, r = 0.18). Similarly, the left swing duration showed no significant difference (39.3 ± 6.6 vs. 38.5 ± 3.2%, $p = 0.893$, r = 0.01). The first right double support was not significantly different (10.2 ± 3.1 vs. 11.8 ± 4.3%, $p = 0.417$, r = 0.08).

Finally, the left walk quality index was significantly lower in the pre-TKA group (93.5 ± 6.8 vs. 95.9 ± 4.3, $p = 0.036$, r = 0.21). In addition, significant differences were observed in the symmetry indices of pelvic angles for tilt (50.5 ± 49.1 vs. 74.2 ± 27.4, $p = 0.014$, r = 0.28), obliquity (90.3 ± 9.8 vs. 98.7 ± 0.8, $p < 0.001$, r = 0.52), and rotation (94.8 ± 4.1 vs. 98.1 ± 2.4, $p = 0.002$, r = 0.40), with moderate-to-large effect sizes, indicating more asymmetrical gait patterns in the pre-TKA group.

4. Discussion

This study compared the gait characteristics between individuals pre-TKA and those in a normal non-arthritic group, providing valuable baseline data for future research. The findings revealed significant differences in gait cycle duration, cadence, stride duration, propulsion indices, symmetry, and other gait phase alterations, with large effect sizes for many variables, indicating substantial gait impairment in the pre-TKA group. These results underscore the significant gait impairments in pre-TKA individuals, which could affect their mobility and functional performance [23].

In particular, the pre-TKA group exhibited significantly longer gait cycle and stride durations ($p < 0.001$), indicating a slower walking pattern, which is consistent with previous findings in patients with knee osteoarthritis [24,25]. These results support the view that individuals with knee osteoarthritis often adopt cautious and pain-avoiding gait strategies. However, stride length did not differ significantly between the groups (left, $p = 0.274$; right, $p = 0.277$), implying that the slower pace is primarily driven by reduced cadence rather than altered step length [26,27].

Indeed, cadence was significantly lower in the pre-TKA group (91.12 ± 9.02 vs. 108.78 ± 6.64 steps/min, $p < 0.001$, Cohen's d = −2.23), reinforcing the trend toward a more cautious walking pattern to minimize joint strain [28,29]. Gait speed was also significantly lower (0.87 ± 0.16 m/s vs. 1.11 ± 0.14 m/s, Cohen's d = −1.60), reflecting further functional decline before surgery. These observations point to meaningful mobility limitations in this population, although the causal benefits of prehabilitation remain to be established.

Pelvic angle symmetry was significantly reduced in the pre-TKA group, with lower symmetry indices for tilt ($p = 0.014$, d = −0.28), obliquity ($p < 0.001$, d = −0.52), and rotation ($p = 0.002$, d = −0.40). These asymmetries likely reflect compensatory adaptations to offloading the affected limbs. Such strategies may lead to muscular imbalance and joint overloading, contributing to postoperative dysfunction [30,31]. Gait cycle symmetry was also significantly compromised (92.7 ± 14.85 vs. 97.0 ± 2.4, $p = 0.000$, r = 0.71), indicating widespread gait irregularities that could predispose patients to further musculoskeletal problems.

Additionally, the significantly lower propulsion index in the pre-TKA group for both the left (Cohen's d = −1.92) and right (Cohen's d = −1.62) limbs further support the idea that individuals with knee osteoarthritis have compromised gait mechanics. Reduced propulsion reflects diminished force generation during the push-off phase, indicating impaired walking dynamics [32,33]. The walk quality index also showed significant reductions on the right side (p = 0.005, Cohen's d = −0.82) and a marginal reduction on the left side (p = 0.036, Cohen's d = −0.21), further emphasizing the impaired overall gait quality in the pre-TKA group.

Notably, the elaborated steps (left, p = 0.000, Cohen's r = 0.66; right, p = 0.000, Cohen's r = 0.69) were significantly longer in the pre-TKA group, suggesting altered stepping strategies possibly linked to pain or compensation for mobility impairment.

No significant differences were observed in stance duration, single support phase, or stride length between the pre-TKA and control groups. These nonsignificant findings suggest that gait impairments in the pre-TKA group may be primarily due to reduced cadence rather than changes in step length or gait phase duration.

The findings of reduced cadence, propulsion, and pelvic symmetry in this study are consistent with previous evidence that individuals with knee osteoarthritis adopt compensatory gait patterns to mitigate pain and maintain stability [22,26]. These maladaptive patterns can lead to muscle imbalances, reduced mobility, and elevated fall risk, underscoring the importance of early targeted intervention. Evidence supports the effectiveness of strengthening exercises, particularly of the quadriceps and hip abductors, in improving gait biomechanics in this population [34]. In addition, wearable sensor-based biofeedback, such as real-time gait monitoring using inertial measurement units, may help to personalize rehabilitation and improve motor learning [20,21].

Although the current study did not assess the impact of prehabilitation, the observed biomechanical deficits provide a strong rationale for future studies. Recommended strategies include pelvic stabilization and trunk control exercises to address asymmetries in tilt, obliquity, and rotation; strengthening of the hip musculature to enhance stance phase stability; and eccentric quadriceps training to support deceleration and propulsion during gait transitions [35]. Real-time biofeedback can further enhance outcomes by providing visual or auditory cues to correct asymmetry and improve temporal parameters. Collectively, these findings support the prioritization of individualized prehabilitation programs to optimize mobility in patients awaiting TKA.

5. Limitations

Although the findings of this study provide valuable insights into gait mechanics in individuals with severe knee osteoarthritis awaiting TKA, several limitations should be acknowledged.

The pre-TKA and non-arthritic control groups comprised 21 and 39 participants, respectively. Although the sample sizes were adequate for detecting large effect sizes (Cohen's d $\approx$ 0.8) with 80% power, the unequal sample sizes between the groups may limit the statistical robustness of certain comparisons, especially for subgroup analyses (e.g., those based on sex). Future research should aim for larger and more balanced sample sizes to enhance statistical power, improve generalizability, and reduce potential bias.

The cross-sectional design of this study restricts the ability to infer causal relationships and observe longitudinal changes over time. Although this study provides a snapshot of gait characteristics in a specific population, it does not allow us to assess how gait patterns evolve with the progression of knee osteoarthritis, after surgery, or in response to rehabilitation intervention. Longitudinal studies are needed to understand how gait mechanics change over time and in response to clinical treatments.

The study sample consisted of patients with knee osteoarthritis awaiting total knee arthroplasty and a nonarthritic control group, which may not fully represent the general population. The findings may be specific to individuals with knee osteoarthritis awaiting surgery and may not apply to other populations with different health conditions, ethnic backgrounds, or lifestyle factors. Future studies should consider diverse groups to increase the generalizability of their findings.

Although the BTS G-Walk sensor system is a reliable tool for gait analysis, its placement on the lower back may not fully capture lower limb kinematics, particularly joint-specific data. This limitation affects the comprehensiveness of the gait analysis. Future studies using multisensor systems, including sensors on the foot or knee, could provide a more detailed and accurate understanding of gait mechanics and asymmetries.

Additionally, despite the BTS G-Walk sensor system offering a convenient and reliable method for assessing gait, pelvic rotation measurements may be influenced by magnetic disturbances in indoor environments, especially when metallic objects are present. Although data were collected on a clear, non-metallic indoor surface to minimize this risk, some variability in the rotation symmetry measures may persist. Future studies should consider applying magnetometer calibration procedures or comparing alternative sensor placements to enhance accuracy.

While the use of Welch's *t*-test helped correct for violations of the assumption of equal variances, some assumptions of the *t*-tests (such as normality) may still have influenced the effect size estimates and statistical conclusions. Although the Kolmogorov–Smirnov and Shapiro–Wilk tests were used to assess the normality of the data, some deviations from normality could have remained, which may affect the reliability of the results. Future studies should consider employing more advanced statistical methods, such as mixed-model analyses, which can better account for variations and improve the robustness of the findings, particularly in cases where violations of the assumptions persist.

Addressing these limitations in future studies will improve the understanding of gait mechanics in individuals with knee OA and help refine clinical applications for rehabilitation, performance optimization, and postsurgical recovery.

6. Conclusions

This study highlighted significant gait impairments in individuals with knee osteoarthritis awaiting TKA, including slower walking speed, reduced cadence, and altered symmetry, compared with those in healthy controls. These findings suggest that individuals in the pre-TKA group adopt compensatory gait strategies that potentially affect their mobility and functional performance negatively. Although this study emphasizes the need to address these impairments, it remains unclear whether prehabilitation effectively improves gait. Future research should explore the potential of interventions such as strengthening exercises, gait retraining, and wearable sensor feedback to enhance gait mechanics and improve mobility in this population before surgery.

Author Contributions: Conceptualization, E.G. and C.K.Y.; methodology, E.G.; software, E.G.; validation, E.G. and C.K.Y.; formal analysis, E.G.; investigation, E.G.; resources, C.K.Y.; data curation, E.G.; writing—original draft preparation, E.G.; writing—review and editing, C.K.Y.; visualization, E.G. and C.K.Y.; supervision, C.K.Y., E.A., and E.C. All authors have read and agreed to the published version of the manuscript.

Funding: This study did not receive any external funding.

Institutional Review Board Statement: This study was conducted in accordance with the principles of the Declaration of Helsinki. The study protocol was reviewed and approved by the Research Ethics Biology Committee of the School of Physical Education and Sport Science of the National and Kapodistrian University of Athens (approval number: 1306/22 September 2021).

Informed Consent Statement: Informed consent was obtained from all the participants involved in this study.

Data Availability Statement: The original contributions presented in this study are included in this article. Further inquiries should be directed to the corresponding author.

Conflicts of Interest: The authors declare no conflicts of interest.

References

1. Gianzina, E.; Kalinterakis, G.; Delis, S.; Vlastos, I.; Platon Sachinis, N.; Yiannakopoulos, C.K. Evaluation of gait recovery after total knee arthroplasty using wearable inertial sensors: A systematic review. *Knee* **2023**, *41*, 190–203. [CrossRef]
2. Liao, T.C.; Samaan, M.A.; Popovic, T.; Neumann, J.; Zhang, A.L.; Link, T.M.; Majumdar, S.; Souza, R.B. Abnormal joint loading during gait in persons with hip osteoarthritis is associated with symptoms and cartilage lesions. *J. Orthop. Sports Phys. Ther.* **2019**, *49*, 917–924. [CrossRef]
3. Wada, S.; Murakami, H.; Tajima, G.; Maruyama, M.; Sugawara, A.; Oikawa, S.; Chida, Y.; Doita, M. Analysis of characteristics required for gait evaluation of patients with knee osteoarthritis using a wireless accelerometer. *Knee* **2021**, *32*, 37–45. [CrossRef] [PubMed]
4. Atukorala, I.; Hunter, D.J. A review of quality-of-life in elderly osteoarthritis. *Expert Rev. Pharmacoecon Outcomes Res.* **2023**, *23*, 365–381. [CrossRef] [PubMed]
5. Naili, J.E.; Iversen, M.D.; Esbjörnsson, A.C.; Hedström, M.; Schwartz, M.H.; Häger, C.K.; Broström, E.W. Deficits in functional performance and gait one year after total knee arthroplasty despite improved self-reported function. *Knee Surg. Sports Traumatol. Arthrosc.* **2016**, *25*, 3378. [CrossRef] [PubMed] [PubMed Central]
6. Rönn, K.; Reischl, N.; Gautier, E.; Jacobi, M. Current Surgical Treatment of Knee Osteoarthritis. *Arthritis* **2011**, *2011*, 454873. [CrossRef]
7. Skou, S.T.; Roos, E.M.; Laursen, M.B.; Rathleff, M.; Arendt-Nielsen, L.; Rasmussen, S.; Simonsen, O. Total knee replacement and nonsurgical treatment of knee osteoarthritis: 2-year outcome from two parallel randomized controlled trials. *Osteoarthr. Cartil.* **2018**, *26*, 1170–1180. [CrossRef]
8. Peat, G.; Thomas, M.J. Osteoarthritis year in review 2020: Epidemiology & therapy. *Osteoarthr. Cartil.* **2021**, *29*, 180–189. [CrossRef]
9. Scheuing, W.J.; Reginato, A.M.; Deeb, M.; Acer Kasman, S. The burden of osteoarthritis: Is it a rising problem? *Best Pract. Res. Clin. Rheumatol.* **2023**, *37*, 101836. [CrossRef]
10. Boekesteijn, R.J.; van Gerven, J.; Geurts, A.C.H.; Smulders, K. Objective gait assessment in individuals with knee osteoarthritis using inertial sensors: A systematic review and meta-analysis. *Gait Posture* **2022**, *98*, 109–120. [CrossRef]
11. Pollet, J.; Buraschi, R. Gait Alterations in Knee Osteoarthritis A Narrative Review on Gait Analysis Studies. *Top. Geriatr. Rehabil.* **2021**, *37*, 239–243. [CrossRef]
12. Zeng, Z.; Shan, J.; Zhang, Y.; Wang, Y.; Li, C.; Li, J.; Chen, W.; Ye, Z.; Ye, X.; Chen, Z.; et al. Asymmetries and relationships between muscle strength, proprioception, biomechanics, and postural stability in patients with unilateral knee osteoarthritis. *Front. Bioeng. Biotechnol.* **2022**, *10*, 922832. [CrossRef]
13. Favre, J.; Jolles, B.M. Gait analysis of patients with knee osteoarthritis highlights a pathological mechanical pathway and provides a basis for therapeutic interventions. *EFORT Open Rev.* **2016**, *1*, 368–374. Available online: https://eor.bioscientifica.com/view/journals/eor/1/10/2058-5241.1.000051.xml (accessed on 20 February 2025). [CrossRef] [PubMed]
14. Abbasi-Bafghi, H.; Fallah-Yakhdani, H.R.; Meijer, O.G.; de Vet, H.C.; Bruijn, S.M.; Yang, L.-Y.; Knol, D.L.; Van Royen, B.J.; van Dieën, J.H. The effects of knee arthroplasty on walking speed: A meta-analysis. *BMC Musculoskelet. Disord.* **2012**, *13*, 66. [CrossRef] [PubMed] [PubMed Central]
15. Kleiner, A.F.R.; Pacifici, I.; Vagnini, A.; Camerota, F.; Celletti, C.; Stocchi, F.; De Pandis, M.F.; Galli, M. Timed Up and Go evaluation with wearable devices: Validation in Parkinson's disease. *J. Bodyw. Mov. Ther.* **2018**, *22*, 390–395. [CrossRef] [PubMed]
16. De Ridder, R.; Lebleu, J.; Willems, T.; De Blaiser, C.; Detrembleur, C.; Roosen, P. Concurrent validity of a commercial wireless trunk triaxial accelerometer system for gait analysis. *J. Sport. Rehabil.* **2019**, *28*. [CrossRef]
17. Spina, S.; Facciorusso, S.; D'ascanio, M.C.; Morone, G.; Baricich, A.; Fiore, P.; Santamato, A. Sensor based assessment of turning during instrumented Timed Up and Go Test for quantifying mobility in chronic stroke patients. *Eur. J. Phys. Rehabil. Med.* **2023**, *59*, 6–13. [CrossRef]

18. Viteckova, S.; Horakova, H.; Polakova, K.; Krupicka, R.; Ruzicka, E.; Brozova, H. Agreement between the GAITRite R System and the Wearable Sensor BTS G-Walk R for measurement of gait parameters in healthy adults and Parkinson's disease patients. *PeerJ.* **2020**, *8*, e8835. [CrossRef]
19. Volkan-Yazici, M.; Çobanoğlu, G.; Yazici, G. Test-retest reliability and minimal detectable change for measures of wearable gait analysis system (G-Walk) in children with cerebral palsy. *Turk. J. Med. Sci.* **2022**, *52*, 658–666. [CrossRef]
20. Porciuncula, F.; Roto, A.V.; Kumar, D.; Davis, I.; Roy, S.; Walsh, C.J.; Awad, L.N. Wearable Movement Sensors for Rehabilitation: A Focused Review of Technological and Clinical Advances. *PMR* **2018**, *10*, S220–S232. [CrossRef]
21. Prasanth, H.; Caban, M.; Keller, U.; Courtine, G.; Ijspeert, A.; Vallery, H.; von Zitzewitz, J. Wearable sensor-based real-time gait detection: A systematic review. *Sensors* **2021**, *21*, 2727. [CrossRef]
22. Burnett, D.R.; Campbell-Kyureghyan, N.H.; Topp, R.V.; Quesada, P.M. Biomechanics of Lower Limbs during Walking among Candidates for Total Knee Arthroplasty with and without Low Back Pain. *Biomed. Res. Int.* **2015**, *2015*, 142562. [CrossRef] [PubMed]
23. Chughtai, M.; Shah, N.V.; Sultan, A.A.; Solow, M.; Tiberi, J.V.; Mehran, N.; North, T.; Moskal, J.T.; Newman, J.M.; Samuel, L.T.; et al. The role of prehabilitation with a telerehabilitation system prior to total knee arthroplasty. *Ann. Transl. Med.* **2019**, *7*, 68. [CrossRef] [PubMed]
24. Azaman, A.; Qahtani, I.A.M.; Puspanathan, J.; Zulkapri, I.; Soeed, K. Simulation of Lower Limb Muscle Moment and Total Muscle Fiber Force Using OpenSim for Knee Osteoarthritis. *J. Med. Device Technol.* **2023**, *2*, 38–42. [CrossRef]
25. Rana, P.; Joshi, S.; Bodwal, M. Quantitative Gait Analysis in Patients With Knee Osteoarthritis. *Int. J. Physiother. Res.* **2016**, *4*, 1684–1688. [CrossRef]
26. Akimoto, T.; Kawamura, K.; Wada, T.; Ishihara, N.; Yokota, A.; Suginoshita, T.; Yokoyama, S. Gait cycle time variability in patients with knee osteoarthritis and its possible associated factors. *J. Phys. Ther. Sci.* **2022**, *34*, 140–145. [CrossRef]
27. Franz, A.; Ji, S.; Bittersohl, B.; Zilkens, C.; Behringer, M. Impact of a six-week prehabilitation with blood-flow restriction training on pre- and postoperative skeletal muscle mass and strength in patients receiving primary Total Knee Arthroplasty. *Front. Physiol.* **2022**, *13*, 881484. [CrossRef]
28. McCarthy, I.; Hodgins, D.; Mor, A.; Elbaz, A.; Segal, G. Analysis of knee flexion characteristics and how they alter with the onset of knee osteoarthritis: A case control study. *BMC Musculoskelet. Disord.* **2013**, *14*, 169. [CrossRef]
29. Simic, M.; Hinman, R.S.; Wrigley, T.V.; Bennell, K.L.; Hunt, M.A. Gait modification strategies for altering medial knee joint load: A systematic review. *Arthritis Care Res.* **2011**, *63*, 405–426. [CrossRef]
30. Kline, P.W.; Jacobs, C.A.; Duncan, S.T.; Noehren, B. Rate of torque development is the primary contributor to quadriceps avoidance gait following total knee arthroplasty. *Gait Posture* **2019**, *68*, 397–402. [CrossRef]
31. Rahman, J.; Tang, Q.; Monda, M.; Miles, J.; McCarthy, I. Gait assessment as a functional outcome measure in total knee arthroplasty: A cross-sectional study. *BMC Musculoskelet. Disord.* **2015**, *16*, 66. [CrossRef]
32. Koseki, K.; Mutsuzaki, H.; Yoshikawa, K.; Endo, Y.; Kanazawa, A.; Nakazawa, R.; Fukaya, T.; Aoyama, T.; Kohno, Y. Gait Training Using a Hip-Wearable Robotic Exoskeleton After Total Knee Arthroplasty: A Case Report. *Geriatr. Orthop. Surg. Rehabil.* **2020**, *11*, 2151459320966483. [CrossRef]
33. Su, W.; Zhou, Y.; Qiu, H.; Wu, H. The effects of preoperative rehabilitation on pain and functional outcome after total knee arthroplasty: A meta-analysis of randomized controlled trials. *J. Orthop. Surg. Res.* **2022**, *17*, 175. [CrossRef]
34. Christiansen, C.L.; Bade, M.J.; Weitzenkamp, D.A.; Stevens-Lapsley, J.E. Factors predicting weight-bearing asymmetry 1 month after unilateral total knee arthroplasty: A cross-sectional study. *Gait Posture* **2013**, *37*, 363–367. [CrossRef]
35. Baker, C.S.; McKeon, J.M. Does preoperative rehabilitation improve patient-based outcomes in persons who have undergone total knee arthroplasty? A systematic review. *PMR* **2012**, *4*, 756–767. [CrossRef]

Journal of
Functional Morphology and Kinesiology

MDPI

Brief Report

Estimation of the External Knee Adduction Moment Using Inertial Measurement Unit Sensors on the Shank and Lower Back: A Pilot Study

Tomoaki Matsuda [1,2], Junichi Watanabe [2], Tasuku Sotokawa [2], Toru Shishime [3] and Hiroshi Katoh [2,*]

1 Department of Rehabilitation, Shishime Orthopedic Hospital, Miyazaki 880-0121, Japan; hqmcb719@gmail.com
2 Graduate School of Health Sciences, Yamagata Prefectural University of Health Sciences, Yamagata 990-2212, Japan
3 Department of Orthopedic Surgery, Shishime Orthopedic Hospital, Miyazaki 880-0121, Japan
* Correspondence: hikato@yachts.ac.jp

Abstract

Background: The external knee adduction moment (KAM) is an important biomechanical parameter that reflects the load on the medial tibiofemoral compartment during gait. The KAM is typically evaluated using three-dimensional motion analysis (3DMA) systems. The present study aimed to evaluate and validate the waveform similarity between the KAM estimated using only two inertial measurement units (IMUs) sensors, attached to the shank and lower back (IMU-KAM), as a simpler method and that obtained from a 3DMA system (3DMA-KAM) under different step rate conditions. **Methods:** Three healthy adult men were included. The gait task involved walking in a straight line over a distance of approximately 10 m at three step rate conditions: 115, 100, and 85 steps/min. Data were collected using a 3DMA system, force plates, and IMUs. The primary outcome measures included the KAM waveforms for 3DMA-KAM and IMU-KAM during the early and late phases of the single-limb support (Early-SLS phase and Late-SLS phase, respectively). The coefficient of multiple correlation (CMC) was used to evaluate the waveform pattern similarity. **Results:** IMU-KAM demonstrated high similarity to 3DMA-KAM waveforms in the Early-SLS phase under 115 and 100 steps/min, with CMC values ranging from 0.66 to 0.99. However, no clear similarity was observed in the Late-SLS phase. **Conclusions:** In the Preferred and Reduced conditions, wherein the walking rate exceeded 100 steps/min, the KAM waveform pattern during the Early-SLS phase was accurately estimated using IMU sensors attached to the shank and lower back. The findings of this study suggest the potential of simplified gait analysis using IMUs for evaluating knee joint biomechanics and provide foundational data for future clinical applications.

Keywords: external knee adduction moment; IMU sensor; waveform pattern; gait; early phase of single-limb support

1. Introduction

Gait analysis is a widely used and effective method for evaluating motor function and the effects of interventions in the field of rehabilitation [1–4]. Hulleck et al. [1] reviewed various gait analysis methods and their clinical applications, including the identification and quantification of disease-specific gait impairments and the prediction of prognosis. Wren et al. [2] performed a systematic review on the clinical utility of gait analysis using measurement devices and reported that it can inform treatment decision-making and determine therapeutic effects. Furthermore, Miyashita et al. [3] suggested the potential of detecting gait impairments using a single inertial measurement unit (IMU) sensor in older adults at an early stage. Boyer et al. [4] also conducted a systematic review and meta-analysis involving both young and older adults and clarified age-related biomechanical changes during gait. In gait biomechanics studies, the estimation of joint loading is a key research topic, and its significance is particularly emphasized in the gait analysis of patients with knee osteoarthritis (OA). Among those changes, the external knee adduction moment (KAM) has attracted attention as an indicator of the load on the medial tibiofemoral compartment and has been reported as a vital biomechanical parameter [5–9]. During gait, the KAM waveform generally exhibits a bimodal pattern, with the first peak occurring in the early phase of single-limb support (SLS) after the initial contact and the subsequent reduction during midstance [10–13]. Previous studies considered both features clinically important indicators due to their association with the onset, progression, and severity of knee OA [10–13]. Three-dimensional motion analysis (3DMA) based on optical motion capture systems combined with force plates is the gold standard for gait analysis using KAM [1,8,14–16]. 3DMA enables high-precision calculation of KAM by combining joint center positions and joint angles derived from three-dimensional coordinate data obtained via optical motion capture with three-dimensional ground reaction forces directly measured using a force plate. However, these systems are expensive and require a dedicated laboratory environment, limiting their clinical application [15–17]. To address these limitations, recent studies estimated the KAM using inertial measurement units (IMUs) [16,18–20]. Iwama et al. [16] demonstrated the potential for simplified KAM estimation by showing a correlation between acceleration-based indices from a single IMU sensor and the first peak of KAM measured using 3DMA. Stetter et al. [18] reported estimation methods applicable to various locomotor tasks by combining IMU sensors on the thigh and shank with machine learning. Moreover, Akiba et al. [19] applied machine learning and a proprietary algorithm to a single IMU sensor and reported that KAM during gait can be estimated with clinically practical accuracy. Kobsar et al. [20] also reviewed multiple approaches, including the use of multiple IMU sensors combined with instrumented force shoes and methods using IMU sensors attached to the foot for estimating KAM. Nevertheless, most of these methods involve constructing full-body skeletal models with multiple IMUs or require machine learning algorithms.

By contrast, Baniasad et al. [21] investigated the relationship between the KAM and four important gait elements (i.e., ground reaction force [GRF], shank tilt angle [STA], foot progression angle [FPA], and center of pressure [COP]). The results showed that the vertical component of the GRF (GRF-VT) and frontal plane STA (FP-STA) were the most influential factors contributing to increased KAM in individuals with knee OA. Importantly, these two parameters can be estimated using IMUs, suggesting that IMU-derived data can be used to estimate the KAM [22–28].

Moreover, previous studies have shown that the peak value and waveform pattern of KAM are influenced by spatiotemporal gait parameters, including walking speed and step rate [29–31]. In particular, the step rate has been reported to exert a remarkable effect on the KAM [29–31], indicating that step rate variations need to be considered when estimating the KAM.

Therefore, the present study was conducted to investigate and validate the waveform similarity between KAM estimated using only two IMU sensors, attached to the shank and lower back (IMU-KAM), as a simpler method and KAM obtained from a 3DMA system (3DMA-KAM) under different step rate conditions. Based on previous findings indicating that the first KAM peak is primarily influenced by the GRF-VT and knee adduction angle [32], we hypothesized that the KAM waveform during the early phase of SLS could be estimated with clinically acceptable accuracy.

2. Methods

2.1. Participants

This study included three healthy adult men: participant 1 (age, 21 years; body height, 172.0 cm; body weight, 64.0 kg), participant 2 (age, 24 years; body height, 170.5 cm; body weight, 67.3 kg), and participant 3 (age, 46 years; body height, 171.0 cm; body weight, 63.0 kg). The inclusion criterion was as follows: absence of any neurological, psychiatric, or orthopedic disorders. Meanwhile, the exclusion criterion was as follows: presence of any pain during walking.

Before the study, approval was obtained from the ethics committee of our institution (Approval No. 2409-01). All participants were provided with a detailed explanation of the study's purpose and significance, and written informed consent was obtained.

2.2. Gait Task

The participants walked in a straight line over a distance of approximately 10 m under three step rate conditions. The step rate was controlled using a metronome and set at 115 steps/min (preferred step rate: Preferred), 100 steps/min (reduced step rate: Reduced), and 85 steps/min (lowest step rate: Lowest). No restrictions were imposed on the step length. The step rate conditions were based on previous studies [33–37]. The gait task was performed in the following fixed order: Preferred, Reduced, and Lowest. Two trials were performed for each condition, yielding a total of six trials per participant. The changes in step rate were manually implemented for each condition.

2.3. Data Collection

An optical motion capture system (optical system) was used for the measurements. This system comprised a 3DMA device (VICON MX-T, VICON Motion Systems Ltd., Oxford, UK) with 16 cameras and six force plates (OR6-7-2000, Advanced Mechanical Technology Inc., Watertown, MA, USA), as shown in Figure 1.

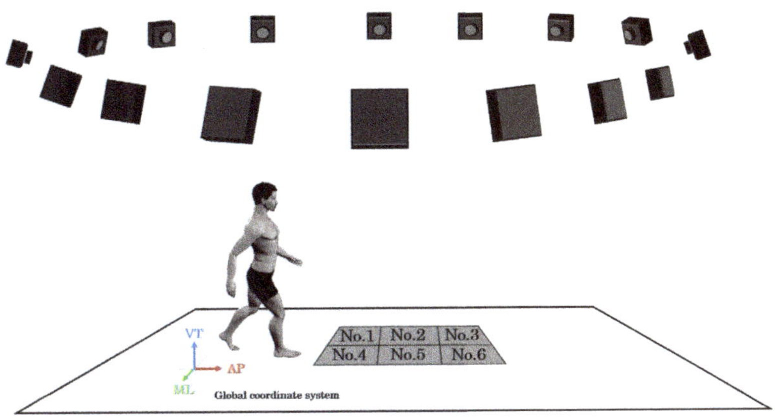

Figure 1. Measurement environment.

In addition, an inertial motion capture system (inertial system) comprising two IMU sensors (SS-MS-HMA5G3A2YZ, Sports Sensing Inc., Fukuoka, Japan) and one wireless synchronization unit (Sports Sensing Inc., Fukuoka, Japan), which was synchronized with the optical system, was used.

During the measurements using the optical system, a seven-segment rigid body model, which comprised the foot, shank, thigh, and pelvis segments, was constructed by attaching 33 infrared reflective markers (14 mm in diameter) to the participant's body, in accordance with the method of Kito et al. [38]. For the inertial system, two sensors were attached: one to the spinous process of the third lumbar vertebra (L3) and the other to the lower lateral shank (LLS) of the right leg [39]. The axes of both IMU sensors were aligned as closely as possible with the global coordinate system. The L3 IMU sensor was oriented with the X-, Y-, and Z-axes in the mediolateral, vertical, and anteroposterior direction, respectively. Conversely, the LLS IMU sensor was oriented with the X-, Y-, and Z-axes in the anteroposterior, vertical, and mediolateral direction, respectively (Figure 2). The sampling frequency of the 3DMA device and force plates was set to 100 Hz, whereas that of the IMU sensors was set to 200 Hz.

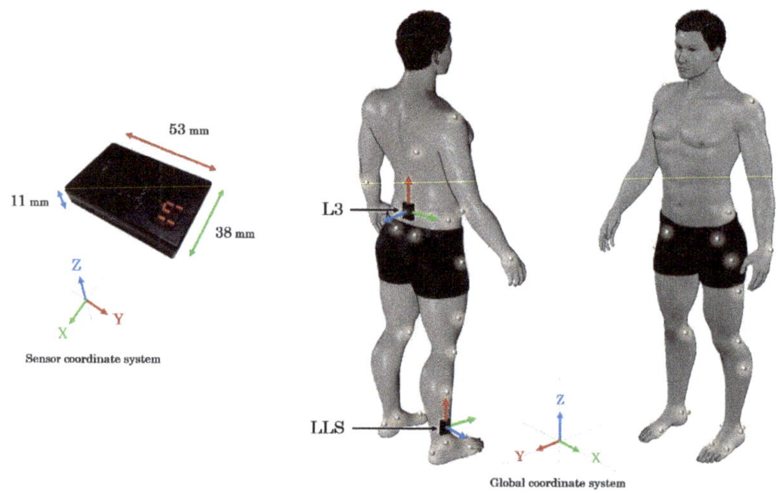

Figure 2. Placement of the infrared reflective markers and IMU sensors. The IMU sensor, which measured 53 mm in length, 38 mm in width, and 11 mm in thickness, equipped with an eight-axis sensor system comprising a three-axis accelerometer (±16 G), a two-axis accelerometer (±200 G), and a three-axis gyroscope (±1500 deg/s). The global coordinate system was defined as follows: X-axis in the mediolateral direction; Y-axis in the anteroposterior direction; and Z-axis in the vertical direction. L3: spinous process of the third lumbar vertebra; LLS: lower lateral shank (7 cm proximal to the lateral malleolus).

2.4. Data Analysis

The primary outcome measures included the 3DMA-KAM and the IMU-KAM of the right lower limb. Meanwhile, the secondary outcome measures included the GRF-VT and the FP-STA of the right lower limb, which were calculated using the optical and inertial systems, respectively. Before data processing, a low-pass Butterworth filter was used to reduce noise. For 3DMA data, the cutoff frequencies were set at 6 and 10 Hz for the marker coordinate data and GRF data, respectively. Meanwhile, for the IMU data, a cutoff frequency of 10 Hz was applied to the vertical component of the acceleration data. This value was based on the report by Jiang et al., which indicated that most of the GRF signal lies below 10 Hz [40]. A cutoff frequency of 12 Hz was applied to the angular velocity data. This value was based on the report by Tadano et al., which provided preliminary validation using quaternions to reduce integration errors in angle estimation [41].

2.4.1. Optical System

The 3DMA-KAM and center of mass were calculated using Vicon Nexus 2.12 (Vicon Motion Systems Ltd., Oxford, UK). Next, the walking speed, step length, and step rate were calculated from the center of mass, right heel marker, and GRF-VT.

2.4.2. Inertial System

The calculation of IMU-KAM was conducted in accordance with the method of Bani-asad et al. [21] (Figure 3). In this approach, the GRF-VT was estimated from the L3 IMU sensor, whereas the FP-STA was derived from the LLS IMU sensor. First, the inclination angles of both IMU sensors relative to the global coordinate system were calculated using data collected during quiet standing on the basis of a previous study [41]. Then, the GRF-VT was obtained by converting the vertical axis component from the inclination angles using trigonometric functions and multiplying it by body weight (N). Meanwhile, the FP-STA was defined as the frontal plane tilt angle of the LLS IMU sensor, which was adjusted at the initial value to match the STA calculated from the 3DMA system. Finally, IMU-KAM was estimated as the product of the GRF-VT and the lever arm derived from FP-STA (labeled as "Lever Arm" in Figure 3). The lever arm was calculated using trigonometric functions (sine) based on FP-STA and the shank length obtained from 3DMA [21].

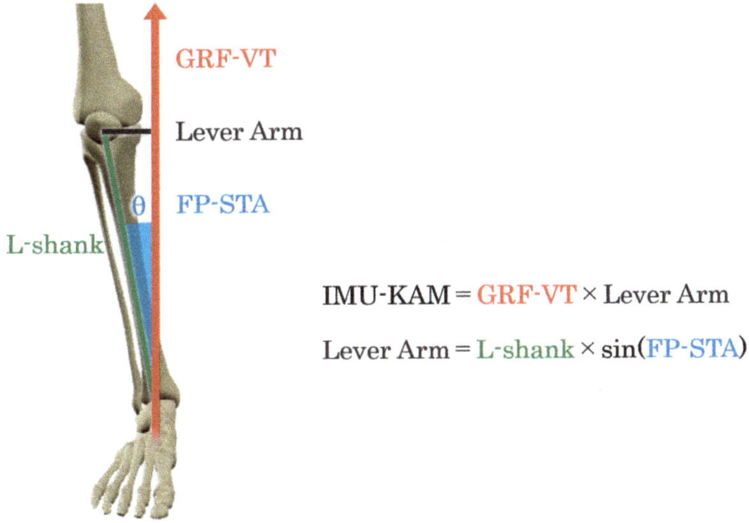

Figure 3. Method for estimating IMU-KAM based on the GRF-VT and FP-STA. IMU-KAM: knee adduction moment estimated using inertial measurement units (IMUs); GRF-VT: vertical component of the ground reaction force (GRF); FP-SPA: frontal plane (FP) shank tilt angle (STA); L-shank: shank length.

2.4.3. Analysis Interval

The analysis interval was defined as the SLS phase of the right lower limb. In this study, a single SLS phase was analyzed per trial. Specifically, the left lower limb toe-off, right lower limb stance phase, and left lower limb initial contact were identified using force plate Nos. 1, 5, and 3, respectively (Figure 1). The SLS phase was identified as the period from the point at which the GRF-VT on the left leg dropped below 10 N to just before it rose above 10 N again. This interval was time-normalized to 100%. Moreover, the SLS phase was further divided into two segments (i.e., early phase of SLS [Early-SLS phase] and late phase of SLS [Late-SLS phase]) in accordance with the method of Thorp et al. [42].

2.5. Statistical Analysis

The similarity of the waveform patterns between IMU-KAM and 3DMA-KAM was assessed using the coefficient of multiple correlation (CMC) [43–45]. Meanwhile, the similarity of the waveform patterns between GRF-VT and FP-STA estimated using IMU sensors and those measured by 3DMA was examined using CMC. The similarity was categorized into four levels based on the CMC values: moderate (0.65–0.75), good (0.75–0.85), very good (0.85–0.95), and excellent (0.95–1.00) [45].

3. Results

3.1. Walking Speed, Step Length, and Step Rate Under Different Gait Conditions

The walking speed ranged from 1.02 m/s to 1.30 m/s, 0.88 m/s to 1.08 m/s, and 0.77 m/s to 0.85 m/s under the Preferred, Reduced, and Lowest conditions, respectively. The step length ranged from 0.56 m to 0.69 m, 0.56 m to 0.65 m, and 0.56 m to 0.62 m, respectively. The step rate ranged from 111.11 steps/min to 120.00 steps/min, 100.00 steps/min to 107.14 steps/min, and 83.33 steps/min to 90.91 steps/min, respectively.

3.2. IMU-KAM and 3DMA-KAM

The mean and standard deviation of the IMU-KAM and 3DMA-KAM waveform patterns under each condition are shown in Figure 4, and the CMC values between the IMU-KAM and 3DMA-KAM during Early-SLS phase and Late-SLS phase is shown in Table 1.

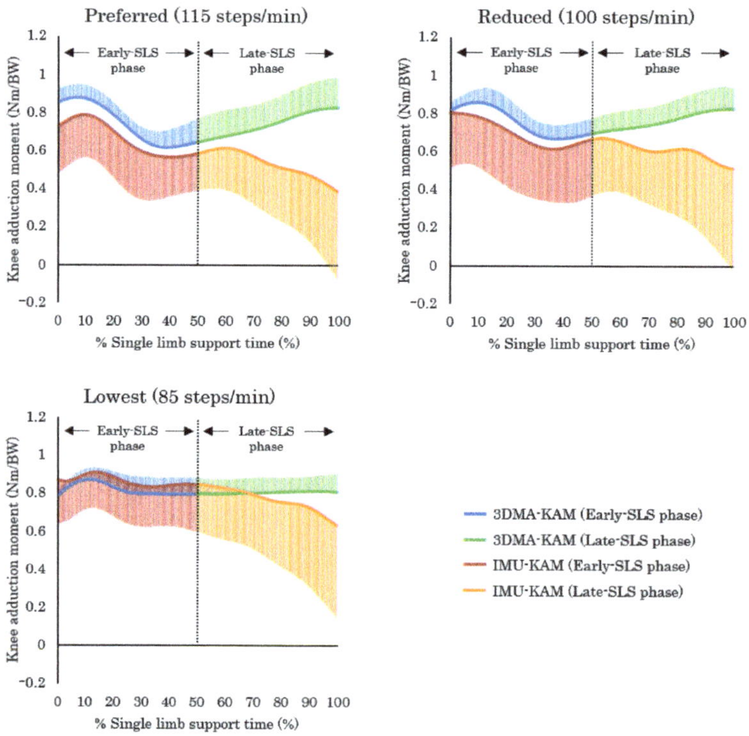

Figure 4. Mean and standard deviation of waveform patterns under each condition. Preferred: preferred step rate (115 steps/min); Reduced: reduced step rate (100 steps/min); Lowest: lowest step rate (85 steps/min); Early-SLS phase: early phase of single-limb support; Late-SLS phase: late phase of single-limb support; 3DMA-KAM: knee adduction moment calculated from three-dimensional motion analysis; IMU-KAM: knee adduction moment estimated using inertial measurement units (IMUs).

Table 1. CMC values between IMU-KAM and 3DMA-KAM waveform patterns.

		CMC					
		Preferred		Reduced		Lowest	
		Early-SLS Phase	Late-SLS Phase	Early-SLS Phase	Late-SLS Phase	Early-SLS Phase	Late-SLS Phase
Participant 1	Trial 1	0.98	NaN	0.74	NaN	0.62	0.77
	Trial 2	0.99	0.29	0.86	NaN	0.80	NaN
Participant 2	Trial 1	0.97	0.55	0.83	NaN	0.82	NaN
	Trial 2	0.67	NaN	0.89	NaN	0.43	0.23
Participant 3	Trial 1	0.83	NaN	0.66	NaN	0.52	NaN
	Trial 2	0.93	NaN	0.75	NaN	0.48	NaN

IMU-KAM: knee adduction moment estimated using inertial measurement units (IMUs); 3DMA-KAM: knee adduction moment calculated from three-dimensional motion analysis; CMC: coefficient of multiple correlation; Preferred: preferred step rate (115 steps/min); Reduced: reduced step rate (100 steps/min); Lowest: lowest step rate (85 steps/min); Early-SLS phase: early phase of single-limb support; Late-SLS phase: late phase of single-limb support; NaN: not a number (indicates that the CMC is a complex number).

3.2.1. Early-SLS Phase

Under the Preferred condition, the CMC values between the IMU-KAM and 3DMA-KAM ranged from 0.67 to 0.99, indicating moderate to excellent similarity. In the Reduced condition, the CMC values ranged from 0.66 to 0.89, indicating moderate to very good similarity. Meanwhile, under the Lowest condition, two trials showed CMC values of 0.80 and 0.82, indicating good similarity. However, the values were below 0.65 in the remaining four trials, indicating no clear similarity in waveform patterns.

3.2.2. Late-SLS Phase

Under the Preferred condition, four trials resulted in complex numbers, represented as not a number (NaN), and the remaining two trials yielded CMC values below 0.65, indicating no clear waveform similarity. In the Reduced condition, all trials produced NaN values. Meanwhile, under the Lowest condition, only one trial yielded a CMC value of 0.77, indicating good similarity, whereas the remaining five trials showed no evident waveform similarity.

3.3. GRF-VT and FP-STA

For GRF-VT, the CMC during the Early-SLS phase under the Preferred and Reduced conditions ranged from 0.67 to 0.99, with most trials rated as excellent (Table 2). Meanwhile, for the Early-SLS phase under the Lowest condition and Late-SLS phase across all conditions, some trials showed CMC values below 0.65. Moreover, no clear waveform similarity was observed. For FP-STA, the CMC values were below 0.65 in most trials across all conditions, indicating no clear waveform similarity (Table 3).

Table 2. CMC values between GRF-VT estimated using IMU and GRF-VT measured using 3DMA.

		CMC					
		Preferred		Reduced		Lowest	
		Early-SLS Phase	Late-SLS Phase	Early-SLS Phase	Late-SLS Phase	Early-SLS Phase	Late-SLS Phase
Participant 1	Trial 1	0.85	0.74	0.91	0.89	0.68	0.97
	Trial 2	0.99	0.94	0.93	0.92	0.46	0.69

Table 2. *Cont.*

		CMC					
		Preferred		Reduced		Lowest	
		Early-SLS Phase	Late-SLS Phase	Early-SLS Phase	Late-SLS Phase	Early-SLS Phase	Late-SLS Phase
Participant 2	Trial 1	0.97	0.89	0.91	0.57	NaN	NaN
	Trial 2	0.99	0.82	0.85	NaN	0.54	NaN
Participant 3	Trial 1	0.77	NaN	0.86	0.77	0.04	0.71
	Trial 2	0.67	0.13	0.84	0.44	0.84	0.81

GRF-VT: vertical component of the ground reaction force; CMC: coefficient of multiple correlation; Preferred: preferred step rate (115 steps/min); Reduced: reduced step rate (100 steps/min); Lowest: lowest step rate (85 steps/min); Early-SLS phase: early phase of single-limb support; Late-SLS phase: late phase of single-limb support; NaN: not a number (indicates that the CMC is a complex number).

Table 3. CMC values between FP-STA estimated using IMU and FP-STA measured using 3DMA.

		CMC					
		Preferred		Reduced		Lowest	
		Early-SLS Phase	Late-SLS Phase	Early-SLS Phase	Late-SLS Phase	Early-SLS Phase	Late-SLS Phase
Participant 1	Trial 1	0.70	0.96	0.30	0.59	NaN	NaN
	Trial 2	0.56	0.90	NaN	0.89	NaN	0.69
Participant 2	Trial 1	NaN	0.35	NaN	NaN	0.89	NaN
	Trial 2	NaN	0.56	NaN	0.72	NaN	NaN
Participant 3	Trial 1	NaN	NaN	NaN	NaN	NaN	NaN
	Trial 2	NaN	NaN	NaN	NaN	NaN	NaN

FP-SPA: frontal plane shank tilt angle; CMC: coefficient of multiple correlation; Preferred: preferred step rate (115 steps/min); Reduced: reduced step rate (100 steps/min); Lowest: lowest step rate (85 steps/min); Early-SLS phase: early phase of single-limb support; Late-SLS phase: late phase of single-limb support; NaN: not a number (indicates that the CMC is a complex number).

4. Discussion

4.1. Changes in Spatiotemporal Parameters Under Different Gait Conditions

Walking speed tended to vary according to the step rate conditions. Although step length varied slightly among participants, it exhibited little change across conditions. Step rate was generally similar to the values set for each condition. In this context, Sekiya et al. [46] examined how changing walking speed, step length, or step rate individually affects the other two parameters. They reported that when only step rate was altered, walking speed changed accordingly, whereas step length remained largely unchanged. These findings support the validity of the spatiotemporal changes observed under the conditions set in the present study.

4.2. Characteristics of IMU-KAM and 3DMA-KAM

This study examined the similarity between the KAM waveform patterns estimated from IMU sensors attached to the shank and lower back and those obtained from 3DMA measurements, with the SLS phase divided into the Early-SLS phase and Late-SLS phase. The hypothesis was that KAM estimation using IMU sensors could be achieved with clinically applicable accuracy during the Early-SLS phase. Our results supported the hypothesis under the condition of ≥100 steps/min but not under the condition of a low step rate, such as 85 steps/min.

4.2.1. Characteristics of the Early-SLS Phase

This study considered the influence of the step rate on the KAM waveform patterns by analyzing three walking conditions. No clear similarity in the KAM waveform patterns was observed under the Lowest condition. KAM typically exhibits a bimodal waveform pattern; however, studies have reported that reducing the step rate or walking speed alters KAM to a unimodal pattern [31,47]. In our study, it cannot be ruled out that such changes in the waveform pattern may have affected the accuracy of KAM estimation. In patients with knee OA, lower step rates are reportedly associated with greater radiographic severity [48–50]. Consistent with this finding, a recent large-scale cohort study of 1600 participants grouped by step rate found that approximately 25% of individuals, classified in the lowest group, had a mean step rate of 97.6 ± 4.6 steps/min [51]. On the basis of the findings of the present study, the proposed method may be applicable for estimating the KAM waveform patterns when the step rate is 100 steps/min or higher. Therefore, this method may be applicable to the majority of patients with knee OA, except for cases with extremely reduced step rates.

With regard to the estimation accuracy of the KAM during gait, previous studies have reported Pearson's correlation coefficients of 0.71 for waveform patterns during the stance phase, 0.58 for peak values, and 0.69 for impulse [18,19]. Existing guidelines for interpreting correlation coefficients categorize the correlation as weak ($r \leq 0.35$), moderate ($0.35 < r \leq 0.67$), strong ($0.67 < r \leq 0.90$), and excellent ($r > 0.90$) [18]. On the basis of this classification, the strength of the correlations determined in our study can be interpreted as ranging from moderate to strong. Although the proposed method estimated the KAM only in the limited interval of the Early-SLS phase, its estimation accuracy was better compared with those of previous reports.

4.2.2. Characteristics of the Late-SLS Phase

In the Late-SLS phase, little to no similarity in the KAM waveform patterns was observed across nearly all trials under all conditions. One possible reason is that factors that were not considered in the present method (e.g., COP and FPA) may influence the second peak of the KAM, which generally occurs during this phase [21,47,52]. Baniasad et al. [21] reported that the anterior–posterior position of COP and FPA particularly affects the second peak of KAM in patients with knee OA. Furthermore, Kim et al. [52] demonstrated that experimentally altering FPA in patients with knee OA modifies the second peak of KAM. Moreover, Rutherford et al. [47] conducted a cross-sectional study and reported that FPA was associated with the second peak of KAM, whereas its effect on the first peak was minimal. Moreover, previous studies on the KAM estimation accuracy have reported reduced accuracy during the late stance phase, corresponding to the Late-SLS phase, compared with the early and mid-stance phases. This reduction may result from the increased difficulty in estimating the ankle joint position and orientation during this period [53,54]. During the terminal stance phase, the COP shifts toward the forefoot as the ankle transitions from dorsiflexion to plantarflexion, accompanied by subtle inversion and eversion of the foot [55,56]. This complex three-dimensional motion likely contributes to decreased accuracy in estimating KAM during the terminal stance, although other factors cannot be ruled out.

4.3. Characteristics of GRF-VT and FP-STA

In the present study, the waveform similarity of GRF-VT and FP-STA was examined using CMC to identify the factors that contribute to the estimation accuracy of IMU-KAM. High CMC values were obtained for GRF-VT during the Early-SLS phase under both the Preferred and Reduced conditions. However, in the Early-SLS phase under the Lowest condition, CMC tended to be lower than that under the other two conditions. We consider that this tendency is consistent with the degree of waveform similarity observed in KAM. Although studies have reported that GRF-VT can be estimated with high accuracy using IMUs [25–28], considering that a similar trend in estimation accuracy was observed for both KAM and GRF-VT under the Lowest condition, it can be inferred that GRF-VT may contribute more substantially to the estimation of the KAM waveform pattern in the Early-SLS phase. In contrast, for FP-STA, many of the CMC values resulted in NaN, and no reliable consistency could be obtained. Regarding the estimation of joint angle waveform patterns, it has been reported that accuracy is high in the sagittal plane but lower in the frontal plane [57,58]. We also consider that this tendency was more pronounced in our study. Regarding the Late-SLS phase, our results suggest the difficulty of estimating accurate KAM waveforms using only GRF-VT and FP-STA information, as used in our study, indicating a potential limitation. Therefore, future studies must incorporate other related factors, such as COP and FPA, to enable a more comprehensive and multifactorial approach.

4.4. Strengths, Limitations, Future Directions, and Practical Applications

The strength of this study lies in the ability to accurately estimate the waveform pattern of KAM during the Early-SLS phase using only two IMU sensors, without the need for machine learning. A limitation of this study is the small sample size, due to which statistical validation was difficult. In particular, the KAM waveform pattern during the Late-SLS phase could not be clarified in detail, possibly due to the limited number of participants. Moreover, the ages of three participants were variable, resulting in an insufficient evaluation of age-related effects. Future studies should ensure an adequate sample size for each age group to allow systematic evaluation.

Regarding future directions, although this study estimated KAM using two parameters, GRF-VT and FP-STA, the agreement of the FP-STA waveform pattern was insufficient. Therefore, other relevant gait parameters should be incorporated in the analysis to improve the accuracy of estimation. Furthermore, because the present study manipulated only the step rate, considering additional factors such as step length and walking speed may further improve the accuracy and applicability of the estimation. It is also necessary to investigate other mechanical parameters, such as the external knee flexion moment.

Overall, the method described in our study can estimate KAM waveform patterns with clinically acceptable accuracy using a minimal number of IMU sensors, provided that the analysis is limited to the Early-SLS phase, thereby suggesting potential applications in clinical gait analysis and the evaluation of treatment effects.

5. Conclusions

This study examined whether IMU-KAM estimated using IMU sensors on the shank and lower back exhibits similar waveform patterns to those of 3DMA-KAM. The results showed that the waveform similarity was high during the Early-SLS phase under conditions with a step rate of 100 steps/min or higher, suggesting the utility of simple IMU-based estimation. By contrast, the waveform agreement decreased during the Late-SLS phase or when the step rate decreased, indicating limitations in estimation accuracy.

Author Contributions: T.M., J.W., T.S. (Tasuku Sotokawa), T.S. (Toru Shishime) and H.K. contributed to the conception and design of this study; T.M. wrote the manuscript; H.K. supervised the data analysis, advised on the data analysis and contributed to the interpretation of the results. All authors have read and agreed to the published version of the manuscript.

Funding: This research received no external funding.

Institutional Review Board Statement: This study was approved by the Ethics Committee of Shishime Orthopedic Hospital (Approval No. 2409-01). Approval date 26 September 2024. The participants received a detailed description of the study, including a brief description of the protocol. Before participation, the participants provided written informed consent. The participants confirmed that participation was voluntary and understood that they could withdraw from the study at any time without penalty. They also understood that the study adhered to the ethical principles outlined in the Declaration of Helsinki.

Informed Consent Statement: Informed consent was obtained from all study participants. After the initial screening, consent was provided by the participants to participate in this study.

Data Availability Statement: The original data presented in this study are openly available at the institutional repository of Yamagata Prefectural University of Health Sciences: https://yachts.repo.nii.ac.jp/records/2000074, accessed on 13 September 2025.

Acknowledgments: We sincerely thank Hiroshi Katoh for his invaluable guidance throughout this study. We also sincerely appreciate all volunteers who kindly participated in this research.

Conflicts of Interest: The authors declare no conflicts of interest.

References

1. Hulleck, A.A.; Menoth Mohan, D.; Abdallah, N.; El Rich, M.; Khalaf, K. Present and Future of Gait Assessment in Clinical Practice: Towards the Application of Novel Trends and Technologies. *Front. Med. Technol.* **2022**, *4*, 901331. [CrossRef]
2. Wren, T.A.L.; Tucker, C.A.; Rethlefsen, S.A.; Gorton, G.E.; Õunpuu, S. Clinical Efficacy of Instrumented Gait Analysis: Systematic Review 2020 Update. *Gait Posture* **2020**, *80*, 274–279. [CrossRef]
3. Miyashita, T.; Kudo, S.; Maekawa, Y. Assessment of Walking Disorder in Community-Dwelling Japanese Middle-Aged and Elderly Women Using an Inertial Sensor. *PeerJ* **2021**, *9*, e11269. [CrossRef] [PubMed]
4. Boyer, K.A.; Johnson, R.T.; Banks, J.J.; Jewell, C.; Hafer, J.F. Systematic Review and Meta-Analysis of Gait Mechanics in Young and Older Adults. *Exp. Gerontol.* **2017**, *95*, 63–70. [CrossRef]
5. Kutzner, I.; Trepczynski, A.; Heller, M.O.; Bergmann, G. Knee Adduction Moment and Medial Contact Force–Facts about Their Correlation during Gait. *PLoS ONE* **2013**, *8*, e81036. [CrossRef]
6. Zhao, D.; Banks, S.A.; Mitchell, K.H.; D'Lima, D.D.; Colwell, C.W.; Fregly, B.J. Correlation between the Knee Adduction Torque and Medial Contact Force for a Variety of Gait Patterns. *J. Orthop. Res.* **2007**, *25*, 789–797. [CrossRef] [PubMed]
7. Hall, M.; Bennell, K.L.; Wrigley, T.V.; Metcalf, B.R.; Campbell, P.K.; Kasza, J.; Paterson, K.L.; Hunter, D.J.; Hinman, R.S. The Knee Adduction Moment and Knee Osteoarthritis Symptoms: Relationships According to Radiographic Disease Severity. *Osteoarthr. Cartil.* **2017**, *25*, 34–41. [CrossRef] [PubMed]
8. Favre, J.; Jolles, B.M. Gait Analysis of Patients with Knee Osteoarthritis Highlights a Pathological Mechanical Pathway and Provides a Basis for Therapeutic Interventions. *EFORT Open Rev.* **2016**, *1*, 368–374. [CrossRef]
9. Bennell, K.L.; Bowles, K.-A.; Wang, Y.; Cicuttini, F.; Davies-Tuck, M.; Hinman, R.S. Higher Dynamic Medial Knee Load Predicts Greater Cartilage Loss over 12 Months in Medial Knee Osteoarthritis. *Ann. Rheum. Dis.* **2011**, *70*, 1770–1774. [CrossRef]
10. D'Souza, N.; Charlton, J.; Grayson, J.; Kobayashi, S.; Hutchison, L.; Hunt, M.; Simic, M. Are Biomechanics during Gait Associated with the Structural Disease Onset and Progression of Lower Limb Osteoarthritis? A Systematic Review and Meta-Analysis. *Osteoarthr. Cartil.* **2022**, *30*, 381–394. [CrossRef]
11. Foroughi, N.; Smith, R.; Vanwanseele, B. The Association of External Knee Adduction Moment with Biomechanical Variables in Osteoarthritis: A Systematic Review. *Knee* **2009**, *16*, 303–309. [CrossRef]
12. Astephen, J.L.; Deluzio, K.J.; Caldwell, G.E.; Dunbar, M.J. Biomechanical Changes at the Hip, Knee, and Ankle Joints during Gait Are Associated with Knee Osteoarthritis Severity. *J. Orthop. Res.* **2008**, *26*, 332–341. [CrossRef]
13. Hatfield, G.L.; Stanish, W.D.; Hubley-Kozey, C.L. Three-Dimensional Biomechanical Gait Characteristics at Baseline Are Associated with Progression to Total Knee Arthroplasty. *Arthritis Care Res.* **2015**, *67*, 1004–1014. [CrossRef]
14. Hutabarat, Y.; Owaki, D.; Hayashibe, M. Recent Advances in Quantitative Gait Analysis Using Wearable Sensors: A Review. *IEEE Sens. J.* **2021**, *21*, 26470–26487. [CrossRef]
15. Boswell, M.A.; Uhlrich, S.D.; Kidziński, Ł.; Thomas, K.; Kolesar, J.A.; Gold, G.E.; Beaupre, G.S.; Delp, S.L. A Neural Network to Predict the Knee Adduction Moment in Patients with Osteoarthritis Using Anatomical Landmarks Obtainable from 2D Video Analysis. *Osteoarthr. Cartil.* **2021**, *29*, 346–356. [CrossRef]
16. Iwama, Y.; Harato, K.; Kobayashi, S.; Niki, Y.; Ogihara, N.; Matsumoto, M.; Nakamura, M.; Nagura, T. Estimation of the External Knee Adduction Moment during Gait Using an Inertial Measurement Unit in Patients with Knee Osteoarthritis. *Sensors* **2021**, *21*, 1418. [CrossRef]

17. Salisu, S.; Ruhaiyem, N.I.R.; Eisa, T.A.E.; Nasser, M.; Saeed, F.; Younis, H.A. Motion Capture Technologies for Ergonomics: A Systematic Literature Review. *Diagnostics* **2023**, *13*, 2593. [CrossRef]
18. Stetter, B.J.; Krafft, F.C.; Ringhof, S.; Stein, T.; Sell, S. A Machine Learning and Wearable Sensor Based Approach to Estimate External Knee Flexion and Adduction Moments During Various Locomotion Tasks. *Front. Bioeng. Biotechnol.* **2020**, *8*, 9. [CrossRef] [PubMed]
19. Akiba, A.; Harato, K.; Yoshihara, H.; Iwama, Y.; Nishizawa, K.; Nagura, T.; Nakamura, M. Development of a Wearable System to Estimate Knee Adduction Moment of Patients with Knee Osteoarthritis During Gait Using a Single Inertial Measurement Unit. *J. Jt. Surg. Res.* **2025**, *3*, 84–89. [CrossRef]
20. Kobsar, D.; Masood, Z.; Khan, H.; Khalil, N.; Kiwan, M.Y.; Ridd, S.; Tobis, M. Wearable Inertial Sensors for Gait Analysis in Adults with Osteoarthritis—A Scoping Review. *Sensors* **2020**, *20*, 7143. [CrossRef] [PubMed]
21. Baniasad, M.; Martin, R.; Crevoisier, X.; Pichonnaz, C.; Becce, F.; Aminian, K. Knee Adduction Moment Decomposition: Toward Better Clinical Decision-Making. *Front. Bioeng. Biotechnol.* **2022**, *10*, 1017711. [CrossRef]
22. Favre, J.; Jolles, B.M.; Aissaoui, R.; Aminian, K. Ambulatory Measurement of 3D Knee Joint Angle. *J. Biomech.* **2008**, *41*, 1029–1035. [CrossRef]
23. Favre, J.; Luthi, F.; Jolles, B.M.; Siegrist, O.; Najafi, B.; Aminian, K. A New Ambulatory System for Comparative Evaluation of the Three-Dimensional Knee Kinematics, Applied to Anterior Cruciate Ligament Injuries. *Knee Surg. Sports Traumatol. Arthr.* **2006**, *14*, 592–604. [CrossRef]
24. Carcreff, L.; Payen, G.; Grouvel, G.; Massé, F.; Armand, S. Three-Dimensional Lower-Limb Kinematics from Accelerometers and Gyroscopes with Simple and Minimal Functional Calibration Tasks: Validation on Asymptomatic Participants. *Sensors* **2022**, *22*, 5657. [CrossRef]
25. Ancillao, A.; Tedesco, S.; Barton, J.; O'Flynn, B. Indirect Measurement of Ground Reaction Forces and Moments by Means of Wearable Inertial Sensors: A Systematic Review. *Sensors* **2018**, *18*, 2564. [CrossRef]
26. Shahabpoor, E.; Pavic, A. Measurement of Walking Ground Reactions in Real-Life Environments: A Systematic Review of Techniques and Technologies. *Sensors* **2017**, *17*, 2085. [CrossRef]
27. Karatsidis, A.; Bellusci, G.; Schepers, H.M.; de Zee, M.; Andersen, M.S.; Veltink, P.H. Estimation of Ground Reaction Forces and Moments During Gait Using Only Inertial Motion Capture. *Sensors* **2016**, *17*, 75. [CrossRef] [PubMed]
28. Mohamed Refai, M.I.; van Beijnum, B.-J.F.; Buurke, J.H.; Veltink, P.H. Portable Gait Lab: Estimating Over-Ground 3D Ground Reaction Forces Using Only a Pelvis IMU. *Sensors* **2020**, *20*, 6363. [CrossRef] [PubMed]
29. Hart, H.F.; Birmingham, T.B.; Primeau, C.A.; Pinto, R.; Leitch, K.; Giffin, J.R. Associations Between Cadence and Knee Loading in Patients with Knee Osteoarthritis. *Arthritis Care Res.* **2021**, *73*, 1667–1671. [CrossRef] [PubMed]
30. James, K.A.; Corrigan, P.; Yen, S.-C.; Hasson, C.J.; Davis, I.S.; Stefanik, J.J. Effects of Increasing Walking Cadence on Gait Biomechanics in Adults with Knee Osteoarthritis. *J. Biomech.* **2024**, *177*, 112394. [CrossRef]
31. Robbins, S.M.K.; Maly, M.R. The Effect of Gait Speed on the Knee Adduction Moment Depends on Waveform Summary Measures. *Gait Posture* **2009**, *30*, 543–546. [CrossRef]
32. Schmitz, A.; Noehren, B. What Predicts the First Peak of the Knee Adduction Moment? *Knee* **2014**, *21*, 1077–1083. [CrossRef] [PubMed]
33. Mobbs, L.; Fernando, V.; Fonseka, R.D.; Natarajan, P.; Maharaj, M.; Mobbs, R.J. Normative Database of Spatiotemporal Gait Metrics Across Age Groups: An Observational Case–Control Study. *Sensors* **2025**, *25*, 581. [CrossRef] [PubMed]
34. Murtagh, E.M.; Mair, J.L.; Aguiar, E.; Tudor-Locke, C.; Murphy, M.H. Outdoor Walking Speeds of Apparently Healthy Adults: A Systematic Review and Meta-Analysis. *Sports Med.* **2021**, *51*, 125–141. [CrossRef] [PubMed]
35. Tudor-Locke, C.; Han, H.; Aguiar, E.J.; Barreira, T.V.; Schuna, J.M., Jr.; Kang, M.; Rowe, D.A. How Fast Is Fast Enough? Walking Cadence (Steps/Min) as a Practical Estimate of Intensity in Adults: A Narrative Review. *Br. J. Sports Med.* **2018**, *52*, 776–788. [CrossRef]
36. Urbanek, J.K.; Roth, D.L.; Karas, M.; Wanigatunga, A.A.; Mitchell, C.M.; Juraschek, S.P.; Cai, Y.; Appel, L.J.; Schrack, J.A. Free-Living Gait Cadence Measured by Wearable Accelerometer: A Promising Alternative to Traditional Measures of Mobility for Assessing Fall Risk. *J. Gerontol. A Biol. Sci. Med. Sci.* **2022**, *78*, 802–810. [CrossRef]
37. Lordall, J.; Oates, A.R.; Lanovaz, J.L. Spatiotemporal Walking Performance in Different Settings: Effects of Walking Speed and Sex. *Front. Sports Act. Living* **2024**, *6*, 1277587. [CrossRef]
38. Kito, N.; Shinkoda, K.; Yamasaki, T.; Kanemura, N.; Anan, M.; Okanishi, N.; Ozawa, J.; Moriyama, H. Contribution of Knee Adduction Moment Impulse to Pain and Disability in Japanese Women with Medial Knee Osteoarthritis. *Clin. Biomech.* **2010**, *25*, 914–919. [CrossRef]
39. Niswander, W.; Wang, W.; Kontson, K. Optimization of IMU Sensor Placement for the Measurement of Lower Limb Joint Kinematics. *Sensors* **2020**, *20*, 5993. [CrossRef]
40. Jiang, X.; Napier, C.; Hannigan, B.; Eng, J.J.; Menon, C. Estimating Vertical Ground Reaction Force during Walking Using a Single Inertial Sensor. *Sensors* **2020**, *20*, 4345. [CrossRef]
41. Tadano, S.; Takeda, R.; Miyagawa, H. Three Dimensional Gait Analysis Using Wearable Acceleration and Gyro Sensors Based on Quaternion Calculations. *Sensors* **2013**, *13*, 9321–9343. [CrossRef]

42. Thorp, L.E.; Sumner, D.R.; Block, J.A.; Moisio, K.C.; Shott, S.; Wimmer, M.A. Knee Joint Loading Differs in Individuals with Mild Compared with Moderate Medial Knee Osteoarthritis. *Arthritis Rheum* **2006**, *54*, 3842–3849. [CrossRef]
43. Ferrari, A.; Cutti, A.G.; Cappello, A. A New Formulation of the Coefficient of Multiple Correlation to Assess the Similarity of Waveforms Measured Synchronously by Different Motion Analysis Protocols. *Gait Posture* **2010**, *31*, 540–542. [CrossRef] [PubMed]
44. Kadaba, M.P.; Ramakrishnan, H.K.; Wootten, M.E.; Gainey, J.; Gorton, G.; Cochran, G.V.B. Repeatability of Kinematic, Kinetic, and Electromyographic Data in Normal Adult Gait. *J. Orthop. Res.* **1989**, *7*, 849–860. [CrossRef] [PubMed]
45. Ino, T.; Samukawa, M.; Ishida, T.; Wada, N.; Koshino, Y.; Kasahara, S.; Tohyama, H. Validity of AI-Based Gait Analysis for Simultaneous Measurement of Bilateral Lower Limb Kinematics Using a Single Video Camera. *Sensors* **2023**, *23*, 9799. [CrossRef] [PubMed]
46. Sekiya, N.; Nagasaki, H.; Ito, H.; Furuna, T. The invariant relationship between step length and step rate during free walking. *J. Hum. Mov. Stud.* **1996**, *30*, 241–257.
47. Rutherford, D.J.; Hubley-Kozey, C.L.; Deluzio, K.J.; Stanish, W.D.; Dunbar, M. Foot Progression Angle and the Knee Adduction Moment: A Cross-Sectional Investigation in Knee Osteoarthritis. *Osteoarthr. Cartil.* **2008**, *16*, 883–889. [CrossRef]
48. Tas, S. Effects of Severity of Osteoarthritis on the Temporospatial Gait Parameters in Patients with Knee Osteoarthritis. *Acta Orthop. Traumatol. Turc.* **2014**, *48*, 635–641. [CrossRef]
49. Elbaz, A.; Mor, A.; Segal, G.; Debi, R.; Shazar, N.; Herman, A. Novel Classification of Knee Osteoarthritis Severity Based on Spatiotemporal Gait Analysis. *Osteoarthr. Cartil.* **2014**, *22*, 457–463. [CrossRef]
50. Mills, K.; Hunt, M.A.; Ferber, R. Biomechanical Deviations during Level Walking Associated with Knee Osteoarthritis: A Systematic Review and Meta-Analysis. *Arthritis Care Res.* **2013**, *65*, 1643–1665. [CrossRef]
51. James, K.A.; Neogi, T.; Felson, D.T.; Corrigan, P.; Lewis, C.L.; Davis, I.S.; Bacon, K.L.; Torner, J.C.; Lewis, C.E.; Nevitt, M.C.; et al. Association of Walking Cadence to Changes in Knee Pain and Physical Function: The Multicenter Osteoarthritis Study. *Osteoarthr. Cartil. Open* **2025**, *7*, 100575. [CrossRef] [PubMed]
52. Kim, Y. Influence of Internal and External Foot Rotation on Peak Knee Adduction Moments and Ankle Moments during Gait in Individuals with Knee Osteoarthritis: A Cross-Sectional Study. *Bioengineering* **2024**, *11*, 696. [CrossRef]
53. van den Noort, J.J.C.; van der Esch, M.; Steultjens, M.P.M.; Dekker, J.; Schepers, M.H.M.; Veltink, P.H.; Harlaar, J. Ambulatory Measurement of the Knee Adduction Moment in Patients with Osteoarthritis of the Knee. *J. Biomech.* **2013**, *46*, 43–49. [CrossRef]
54. van den Noort, J.C.; van der Esch, M.; Steultjens, M.P.M.; Dekker, J.; Schepers, H.M.; Veltink, P.H.; Harlaar, J. The Knee Adduction Moment Measured with an Instrumented Force Shoe in Patients with Knee Osteoarthritis. *J. Biomech.* **2012**, *45*, 281–288. [CrossRef]
55. Brockett, C.L.; Chapman, G.J. Biomechanics of the Ankle. *Orthop. Trauma* **2016**, *30*, 232–238. [CrossRef] [PubMed]
56. Jeon, E.; Cho, H. A Novel Method for Gait Analysis on Center of Pressure Excursion Based on a Pressure-Sensitive Mat. *Int. J. Environ. Res. Public Health* **2020**, *17*, 7845. [CrossRef] [PubMed]
57. Yin, L.; Chen, P.; Xu, J.; Gong, Y.; Zhuang, Y.; Chen, Y.; Wang, L. Validity and Reliability of Inertial Measurement Units for Measuring Gait Kinematics in Older Adults across Varying Fall Risk Levels and Walking Speeds. *BMC Geriatr.* **2025**, *25*, 336. [CrossRef]
58. Zeng, Z.; Liu, Y.; Li, P.; Wang, L. Validity and Reliability of Inertial Measurement Units Measurements for Running Kinematics in Different Foot Strike Pattern Runners. *Front. Bioeng. Biotechnol.* **2022**, *10*, 1005496. [CrossRef]

Journal of
Functional Morphology and Kinesiology

MDPI

Article

Preoperative Clinical Phenotyping for Individualised Rehabilitation in End-Stage Knee Osteoarthritis

Marisa Coetzee [1,*], Amanda Marie Clifford [1,2], Diribsa Tsegaya Bedada [1,3], Oloff Bergh [4] and Quinette Abegail Louw [1]

[1] Division of Physiotherapy, Department of Health and Rehabilitation Sciences, Stellenbosch University, Cape Town 7599, South Africa
[2] School of Allied Health, Health Research Institute, Ageing Research Centre, University of Limerick, V94 T9PX Limerick, Ireland
[3] Department of Statistics and Actuarial Science, University of Waterloo, Waterloo, ON N2L 3G1, Canada
[4] Neuromechanics Unit, Central Analytical Facility, Stellenbosch University, Cape Town 7599, South Africa
* Correspondence: marcoetzee@sun.ac.za

Abstract

Background: Osteoarthritis (OA) of the knee is a highly prevalent and heterogeneous condition. Identifying distinct clinical phenotypes within end-stage knee OA populations may inform tailored preoperative management strategies for individuals awaiting total knee replacement (TKR) surgery. **Methods:** This cross-sectional study employed exploratory factor analysis to identify clinical presentation patterns among patients with knee OA awaiting TKR in South Africa, using modifiable variables including demographic data, physical examination findings, patient-reported outcomes, and functional measures. **Results:** Three distinct clinical phenotypes emerged: (1) gait and weight—characterised by poor gait mechanics, obesity, and low self-efficacy; (2) central pain—encompassing central sensitisation, depression, and reduced functional performance; and (3) functional factors—reflecting muscular weakness and functional limitations. **Conclusions:** This study highlights the heterogeneity in clinical presentations among patients with end-stage knee OA awaiting TKR in South Africa. The identified phenotypes suggest a need for tailored, multidisciplinary preoperative interventions incorporating weight management, pain management, psychological support, targeted exercise programs, and behavioural change strategies to optimise post-surgical outcomes and enhance overall care.

Keywords: clinical phenotype; factor analysis; chronic pain; total knee replacement; osteoarthritis; movement analysis

1. Introduction

Osteoarthritis (OA), particularly knee OA, is a highly prevalent global musculoskeletal condition, characterised by substantial heterogeneity in its clinical manifestations, disease trajectories, and underlying pathophysiological mechanisms [1]. Emerging evidence highlights significant inter-individual variability in symptom severity, disease progression, and treatment response among patients with knee OA [2]. This heterogeneity is influenced by factors such as age, sex, genetics, biomechanics, comorbidities, and lifestyle, which influence the individual response to medical management and reduce the efficacy of standardised therapeutic interventions [1].

In recent years, the field of phenotype research has gained prominence, aiming to explain the heterogeneity of knee OA through advanced imaging modalities, biomarker analysis, and data-driven analytics [3]. By identifying distinct subgroups or phenotypes within the broader knee OA population, characterised by unique clinical, radiographic, and molecular signatures, phenotype research holds promise in clarifying underlying pathogenic mechanisms, predicting disease progression, and tailoring interventions to specific phenotypic profiles [2,4–8]. Although phenotypic classification based on molecular characteristics may provide detailed insight into underlying biological pathways, cellular taxonomy, and biochemical markers [9], it requires laboratory analysis, which may be impractical in low-resource clinical settings. In contrast, phenotyping based on clinical characteristics may be less detailed [10], but more practical in clinical settings.

Clinical phenotyping involves grouping patients based on observable and modifiable clinical characteristics, such as posture, gait, physical activity levels, obesity, muscle strength, balance, and pain behaviour [5,11–13]. Commonly included variables span domains such as age, sex, body mass index (BMI), range of motion, muscle strength, gait analysis, pain severity, psychological factors (e.g., depression, anxiety), self-efficacy, and functional performance (e.g., sit-to-stand tests, physical activity levels) [11,12]. Although studies looking at the effects of phenotype-specific interventions are still in their infancy, promising results for pain and functional response to exercise interventions have identified baseline factors related to trajectories with different treatment responses [4,7,14]. By stratification of distinct clinical phenotypes, targeted management strategies can be developed to address the unique needs of each subgroup.

Current management strategies for OA include pharmacological (e.g., NSAIDs, corticosteroids), non-pharmacological (e.g., exercise, patient education), and end-stage surgical approaches. Disease-modifying OA drugs (DMOADs) targeting specific molecular pathways are also being explored, with the intention to eventually be able to slow down, halt joint degeneration, or even reverse the effects of OA [15]. Management is typically focused on relieving pain and improving joint function, as these are reported to be the most disabling symptoms [15]. In OA patients, pain severity does not always correlate with radiographic changes [16]. Emerging evidence suggests that neuroinflammation, central sensitisation, and maladaptive pain processing contribute to chronic pain in patients with OA. Patients with chronic pain are at risk of developing central sensitisation and nociplastic pain, which can lead to poor postoperative outcomes [15,17]. In addition, pain and reduced function can lead to physical deconditioning, obesity, and the development of cardiovascular and metabolic conditions, which can negatively affect the pain experience and increase the risk for poor postoperative outcomes [18].

In South Africa, the public healthcare sector is burdened by an increase in patients with end-stage knee OA awaiting TKR surgeries [19]. Average waiting times of 3.5 to 5 years have been reported, and a majority of patients were not referred for rehabilitation interventions during this time [20]. In other contexts, prolonged surgical waiting times have been shown to exacerbate functional decline, pain, and psychosocial distress, potentially compromising postoperative outcomes [21,22]. Identifying the modifiable clinical presentation patterns in patients with end-stage OA can facilitate targeted rehabilitation interventions to ensure that patients have better pre- and postoperative outcomes and that resources are allocated optimally, especially in low- and middle-income countries like South Africa [10]. However, few studies on patient clinical presentation profiles have been conducted in the South African context. Therefore, the aim of this study was to identify distinct clinical phenotypes in the South African population to inform tailored preoperative rehabilitation strategies.

2. Materials and Methods

2.1. Study Design

A descriptive cross-sectional study design was used. All the individuals on the waiting list at Tygerberg Hospital were invited to take part in a previous study [19] and those who gave consent to take part in further studies were included in the sample pool for this study.

2.2. Study Participants

Conducting sample size calculation for factor analysis is complex due to the lack of a priori hypothesis (not knowing if, what, or how many factors there will be) [23]. Rule-of-thumb estimates have been reported in the literature for use within factor analysis and informed the sample size estimation in this study. According to Hair [23], the minimum recommended ratio for sample size in factor analysis is 5:1 (at least 5 individuals per variable), which totalled 65 individuals for the 13 variables we planned to include. A stratified random sampling technique was used [24,25], and the inclusion criteria were being waitlisted for TKR and the knee OA being the primary site of concern (other joints having only mild to moderate OA). Individuals with all levels of mobility (including wheelchair bound patients) were included in this study, and the only exclusion criterion was the inability to give consent. A detailed methodology for this study is presented in Supplementary File S1.

2.3. Study Procedures

All attempts were made to minimise the direct financial cost to the participants with regard to time taken from work or their daily activities. Individuals were offered transportation to and from the assessment facility or reimbursed for any travelling costs. In addition, individuals received remuneration for their time, an education session, and a leaflet with information on symptom management. Participants were also offered the option to bring their carer/spouse with them for support. The primary researcher (an experienced physiotherapist and clinical educator) welcomed the participants, provided an overview of the study (including the latest results from the project), and explained the procedure of the session. Followed by a detailed explanation of the self-reported questionnaires, which were completed by the individuals at their own pace during their time at the facility. During the completion of the self-reported questionnaire, assistance was provided by the primary researcher or a research assistant and included reading the questions when the participant forgot their reading glasses, as well as explaining any concepts or scales on the questionnaire. The primary researcher conducted all the objective assessments. All efforts were made to always ensure the safety of participants with ample chairs for resting and the research assistants standing in close proximity at all times.

2.4. Outcome Measures

Clinical, functional, biomechanical, and self-reported outcome measures were chosen based on systematic reviews and feasibility studies on structural/functional disease progression and patient subgroups in OA [5,26,27]. In addition, the literature on supported self-management for OA and other chronic conditions was consulted for measures related to important components of self-management such as coping behaviour and self-efficacy [28,29]. Clinical measures included height and weight for body mass index (BMI) calculation; knee range of motion (ROM) flexion and extension, which were measured using a standard goniometer; and muscle strength of knee extensors, which was measured using a Lafayette Handheld Dynamometer following a standardised protocol (HHD). The standardised protocol included three measures of each ROM and muscle strength per measurement, and the average of the three measurements was used to ensure inter-tester reliability. Our functional measure was the 30 s chair stand test (30 s CST), and the biomechanical measure used was the gait deviation index (GDI) [30,31]. Seven self-reported outcome measures were used. They included the Central Sensitisation Inventory (CSI) [32], the 10-item Center for Epidemiologic Studies Depression Scale (Ces-D 10) [33], the patient specific functional scale (PSFS) [34], the Oxford knee score (OKS) [35], the Brief Cope questionnaire [36], the arthritis self-efficacy 8-item scale (ASES-8) [37], and the Global Physical Activity Questionnaire [38]. Details on the outcome measures are presented in Supplementary File S1.

2.5. Movement Analysis

All patient-reported outcome measures were printed on paper, and individuals were assisted by research assistants in completing these in their language of choice. A VICON Optical Motion Capture (OMC) system (version 2.11; Vicon Motion Systems Ltd., Oxford, UK), specifically the MX T-series with the Plug-in-Gait (PiG) model, was used for data collection. This advanced system utilises multiple high-resolution cameras to precisely capture and reconstruct marker trajectories, providing detailed information on body segment positions and orientations relative to a global coordinate system. Renowned for its accuracy and reliability, the VICON system, along with the Conventional Gait Model in PiG, is extensively validated and commonly used in clinical research [39]. The setup included eight VICON T-20 infrared cameras (Vicon Motion Systems Ltd., Oxford, UK) paired with VICON Nexus 2.9.2 software, capturing data at 200 Hz. We used thirty-six 14 mm diameter passive retro-reflective markers that were placed on key anatomical landmarks, with additional markers placed on the iliac crest of the pelvis to enhance tracking. All biomechanical outcomes were calculated using the modified lower body PiG model in the Nexus 2.9.2 software. Additionally, gait events were captured using three time-synchronised, floor-embedded force plates (one FP6090-15 and two FP6040-15 models from Bertec Corporation, Columbus, OH, USA).

2.6. Data Analysis

Both discrete and continuous numerical variables were collected, alongside nominal, binary, and ordinal categorical variables. Frequency distribution (percentages and counts) and contingency tables were used for reporting on the categorical variables from predetermined answer options, and central tendency was used for reporting numerical variables. Muscle strength percentages of the norm were calculated using normative data per age group. Stata software (StataCorp. 2023. Stata Statistical Software: Release 17. College Station, TX, USA: StataCorp LLC) was used for data management and analysis. Selected variables were subjected to exploratory factor analysis (EFA) for the identification and description of clinical presentation patterns in the population of individuals [23,40]. Missing data were subjected to full information maximum likelihood (only required for GDI, sit-to-stand, and BMI data where individuals were wheelchair bound).

2.7. Factor Extraction

As the first step in our EFA, principal component analysis (PCA) has been chosen for factor extraction as it is a frequently recommended method for pattern recognition amongst health-related variables, and it retains the total (both common and unique) variance between the original variables for analysis [23,40]. In addition, an orthogonal factor rotation (promax) was used to reduce ambiguity and improve the interpretation of our data [23]. Each variable had calculated weightings (factor loadings) which showed the relative contribution of each variable to the factor (clinical presentation pattern). Variables with a contribution of 0.3 or more were considered relevant to the factor and were retained [40] for descriptive purposes of the clinical presentation pattern. Variables with a weighting

4. Discussion

This study aimed to identify and describe distinct clinical presentation patterns among patients awaiting TKR in South Africa, using modifiable variables that could be targeted with specific management strategies. Our analysis revealed three distinct factors: (1) gait and weight, (2) central pain, and (3) functional. Each of these factors comprises variables that resemble clinical patterns observed in the existing literature.

The first factor, gait and weight, aligns with previously described biomechanical and metabolic phenotypes [12,41,42]. The gait variable, comprising the nine frontal and sagittal knee moments and angles that were calculated in the GDI, provides a numerical value of the amount of deviation from the norm in the gait. This is potentially due to the loss in functional joint range that was seen in this factor, along with the changes in joint structure, which causes deformity and changes the biomechanics of the knee joint as well as the joints above and below [43]. Patients experiencing the most deviation in their gait pattern were likely to be in this group and present with increased weight. Obesity, a significant challenge in South Africa, disproportionately affects vulnerable populations and contributes to altered joint mechanics, increased articular surface loading, and accelerated joint degeneration [42,44]. Addressing obesity requires a comprehensive approach, as outlined in South Africa's Strategy for the Prevention and Management of Obesity (2023–2028), including equitable access to healthy foods, physical activity opportunities, and a capacitated healthcare system [45]. Having poor self-efficacy was another variable identified in the gait and weight category, meaning patients felt they did not have enough confidence to manage their OA-related symptoms. Notably, research has linked obesity with poor self-efficacy, and enhancing self-efficacy through empowerment and education is critical to sustainable weight management [46]. Hence, comprehensive weight management programs incorporating dietary modifications, physical activity promotion, and self-efficacy enhancement strategies could be beneficial for patients who present with this clinical factor [47].

The central pain factor encompassed variables such as reduced functional performance (e.g., sit-to-stand), central sensitisation, and depression. Self-reported symptoms of central sensitisation, characterised by heightened pain sensitivity due to altered central nervous system processing, were prevalent in a significant proportion (40%) of our sample, higher than typically reported in end-stage knee OA populations (30%) [48–50]. Central sensitisation is a result of maladaptive pain processing mechanisms, which cause structural changes in the brain. Coupled with depression and sleep deprivation, it has been argued that the risk for falls increases due to psychomotor retardation, deconditioning, and cognitive impairments [51–53]. This subgroup may be more vulnerable to increasing disability and reduction in quality of life while awaiting surgery, as chronic pain and psychological distress can perpetuate a cycle of inactivity, deconditioning, and functional decline [54]. Addressing psychosocial factors and optimising physical function is crucial for successful surgical outcomes in this subgroup, necessitating a staged approach integrating exercise, education, functional activity, and psychological support. Therefore, individuals in this group may benefit from multidisciplinary interventions addressing pain management, psychological support, graded functional retraining, and strategies to break the cycle of inactivity and deconditioning [55–57].

The functional factor, characterised by functional limitations, aligns with typical phenotypes identified in previous research that are extra-articular in nature and not driven by molecular mechanisms, but rather as a result of ligament instability, sarcopenia, and non-use [2,3,58]. Joint pathology and degeneration contribute to muscular weakness, particularly in weight-bearing joints, leading to challenges in activities like stair climbing, kneeling, sit-to-stand transitions, and standing up from the floor [59]. Especially in older adults who do not have the upper limb strength to assist them, struggling with transitional functions may lead to falls. The inability to stand up from the floor when they are alone has serious consequences, such as dehydration and hypothermia. Prolonged waiting times may exacerbate muscle atrophy and functional decline due to limited physical activity [60]. For patients within this functional phenotype, preoperative strengthening exercises and behavioural strategies to optimise levels of physical activity and reduce sedentary behaviour may be relatively easy to implement, likely improving postoperative outcomes [61].

Our findings support the need for clinical phenotyping in end-stage knee OA populations, as we identified distinct patterns that may benefit from tailored rehabilitation management approaches. In the South African context, where access to primary care is limited and waiting times for TKR are long [19], identifying clinical phenotypes can inform the development of targeted preoperative interventions. By tailoring rehabilitation strategies to the specific clinical presentations identified through phenotyping, we can potentially optimise preoperative management, improve postoperative outcomes, and enhance overall care for end-stage knee OA patients awaiting TKR in South Africa. Furthermore, early identification of phenotypic profiles could guide timely interventions, potentially delaying disease progression and reducing the need for surgical intervention in some cases.

A Strengthening the Reporting of Observational Studies in Epidemiology (STROBE) statement, which provides guidelines for reporting observational studies, was completed for this study (Supplementary File S2). The limitations of our study include its sole focus on clinical, modifiable variables and excluding genetic, biomolecular, or advanced imaging data. Our study employed a cross-sectional design, capturing a snapshot of the clinical presentations at a single time point. Considering that OA is a progressive condition, longitudinal studies are warranted to evaluate the stability and transition of these phenotypic profiles over time, as well as their potential impact on long-term outcomes following TKR. The study population was limited to patients awaiting TKR in a large hospital in South Africa, potentially introducing selection bias and limiting the generalisability of our findings to broader knee OA populations or different geographic contexts. While we included a comprehensive set of clinical variables, there may be additional relevant factors that could further delineate distinct phenotypes or subgroups within our identified clusters. Future research should consider incorporating a broader range of variables, such as physical activity patterns, dietary habits, or social determinants of health, to provide a more holistic understanding of clinical heterogeneity. In addition, we used no quantitative sensory testing for central sensitisation; therefore, we can only comment on what patients have reported and cannot support the reported scores with sensory testing results. Despite these limitations, our study contributes to the growing body of evidence supporting the value of clinical phenotyping in end-stage knee OA management. In addition, there is potential for some of the results to be generalisable to other LMIC settings when interpreted alongside our previously published work (patient profile description). Future research addressing these limitations, as well as exploring the implementation and outcomes of phenotype-specific interventions, could further advance our understanding and improve the care of individuals living with this debilitating condition.

5. Conclusions

In conclusion, this study provides valuable insights into the clinical presentation patterns of patients awaiting TKR. Three distinct factors emerged: gait and weight, central pain, and functional factors, each comprising variables reflective of clinical patterns observed in the literature. Notably, a significant proportion of the population awaiting TKR presents with central sensitisation, depression, and functional impairments in knee range and strength. The gait and weight factor emerged as the strongest, highlighting the impact of obesity on TKR candidacy and outcomes. These findings suggest important considerations for clinical practice. While the data are cross-sectional and do not imply causation, they underscore the need for a multifaceted approach to management that addresses both physical and psychological aspects in this patient population.

Supplementary Materials: The following supporting information can be downloaded at: https://www.mdpi.com/article/10.3390/jfmk10030360/s1, Supplementary File S1, Supplementary File S2. References [62–99] are cited in the supplementary materials.

Author Contributions: Conceptualisation, M.C., Q.A.L. and A.M.C.; methodology, M.C., A.M.C. and Q.A.L.; software, M.C., D.T.B. and O.B.; formal analysis, D.T.B. and M.C.; writing—original draft preparation, M.C.; writing—review and editing, Q.A.L., A.M.C., D.T.B. and O.B.; visualisation, M.C.; supervision, Q.A.L. and A.M.C.; project administration, M.C.; funding acquisition, M.C. All authors have read and agreed to the published version of the manuscript.

Funding: This research was partly funded by the Harry Crossley Foundation.

Institutional Review Board Statement: The study was conducted in accordance with the Declaration of Helsinki, and ethical approval to conduct this study was obtained from the Human Research Ethics Committee from Stellenbosch University (reference number S20/11/315 (PhD), 8 March 2024) and permission to conduct this study at Tygerberg Hospital was obtained from the manager of medical services through the National Research Database of the Department of Health, South Africa.

Informed Consent Statement: Written informed consent for collecting the data and publishing the results in a peer-reviewed journal was obtained from participants in their language of choice (Afrikaans, English, or isiXhosa), and translators were available to participants for the entire duration of their assessment.

Data Availability Statement: The original contributions presented in this study are included in the article/Supplementary Material. Further inquiries can be directed to the corresponding author.

Acknowledgments: The authors would like to thank the participants who made themselves available for this research.

Conflicts of Interest: The authors declare no conflicts of interest.

Abbreviations

The following abbreviations are used in this manuscript:

OA	Osteoarthritis
DMOADs	Disease-modifying OA drugs
NSAIDs	Non-steroidal Anti-inflammatory Drugs
CSI	Central Sensitisation Inventory
ASES	Arthritis self-efficacy scale
ROM	Range of motion
BMI	Body mass index
HDD	Handheld Dynamometer
GDI	Gait deviation index
CST	Chair stand test
Ces-D	Center for Epidemiologic Studies Depression Scale
PSFS	Patient-specific functional scale
OKS	Oxford knee score
WHO	World Health Organization
PiG	Plug-in-Gait
EFA	Exploratory factor analysis
PCA	Principal component analysis

References

1. Allen, K.D.; Thoma, L.M.; Golightly, Y.M. Epidemiology of osteoarthritis. *Osteoarthr. Cartil.* **2022**, *30*, 184–195. [CrossRef]
2. Silverwood, V.; Blagojevic-Bucknall, M.; Jinks, C.; Jordan, J.L.; Protheroe, J.; Jordan, K.P. Current evidence on risk factors for knee osteoarthritis in older adults: A systematic review and meta-analysis. *Osteoarthr. Cartil.* **2015**, *23*, 507–515. [CrossRef]
3. Mobasheri, A.; Kapoor, M.; Ali, S.A.; Lang, A.; Madry, H. The future of deep phenotyping in osteoarthritis: How can high throughput omics technologies advance our understanding of the cellular and molecular taxonomy of the disease? *Osteoarthr. Cartil. Open* **2021**, *3*, 100144. [CrossRef]
4. Dorio, M.; Deveza, L.A. Phenotypes in Osteoarthritis: Why Do We Need Them and Where Are We At? *Clin. Geriatr. Med.* **2022**, *38*, 273–286. [CrossRef] [PubMed]
5. Luong, M.L.N.; Cleveland, R.J.; Nyrop, K.A.; Callahan, L.F. Social determinants and osteoarthritis outcomes. *Ageing Health* **2012**, *8*, 413–437. [CrossRef]
6. Nelson, F.R.T. The Value of Phenotypes in Knee Osteoarthritis Research. *Open Orthop. J.* **2018**, *12*, 105–114. [CrossRef]
7. Munugoda, I.P.; Pan, F.; Wills, K.; Mattap, S.M.; Cicuttini, F.; Graves, S.E.; Lorimer, M.; Jones, G.; Callisaya, M.L.; Aitken, D. Identifying subgroups of community-dwelling older adults and their prospective associations with long-term knee osteoarthritis outcomes. *Clin. Rheumatol.* **2020**, *39*, 1429–1437. [CrossRef] [PubMed]
8. Ye, J.; Xie, D.; Li, X.; Lu, N.; Zeng, C.; Lei, G.; Wei, J.; Li, J. Phenotypes of osteoarthritis-related knee pain and their transition over time: Data from the osteoarthritis initiative. *BMC Musculoskelet. Disord.* **2024**, *25*, 173. [CrossRef]
9. Gijon-Nogueron, G.; Balint, P.; Batalov, A.; Ostojic, P.; Sollmann, N.; van Middelkoop, M.; Agricola, R.; Naili, J.E.; Milovanovic, D.; Popova, S.; et al. Terminologies and definitions used to classify patients with osteoarthritis: A scoping review. *BMC Rheumatol.* **2025**, *9*, 32. [CrossRef] [PubMed]
10. Sougue, C.; Diallo, M.; Bayala, Y.L.T.; Ayouba Tinni, I.; Kabore, F.; Zabsonre Tiendrebeogo, W.J.S.; Dakoure, P.W.H.; Ouedraogo, D.D. Clinical phenotypes and associated factors in knee osteoarthritis in an African black population. *Osteoarthr. Cartil. Open* **2025**, *7*, 100570. [CrossRef]
11. Knoop, J.; van der Leeden, M.; Thorstensson, C.A.; Roorda, L.D.; Lems, W.F.; Knol, D.L.; Steultjens, M.P.M.; Dekker, J. Identification of phenotypes with different clinical outcomes in knee osteoarthritis: Data from the Osteoarthritis Initiative. *Arthritis Care Res.* **2011**, *63*, 1535–1542. [CrossRef] [PubMed]
12. van der Esch, M.; Knoop, J.; van der Leeden, M.; Roorda, L.D.; Lems, W.F.; Knol, D.L.; Dekker, J. Clinical phenotypes in patients with knee osteoarthritis: A study in the Amsterdam osteoarthritis cohort. *Osteoarthr. Cartil.* **2015**, *23*, 544–549. [CrossRef] [PubMed]
13. Ma, J.; Zhang, K.; Ma, X.; Wang, H.; Ma, C.; Zhang, Y.; Liu, R. Clinical phenotypes of comorbidities in end-stage knee osteoarthritis: A cluster analysis. *BMC Musculoskelet. Disord.* **2024**, *25*, 299. [CrossRef]
14. Lee, A.C.; Harvey, W.F.; Han, X.; Price, L.L.; Driban, J.B.; Bannuru, R.R.; Wang, C. Pain and functional trajectories in symptomatic knee osteoarthritis over up to 12 weeks of exercise exposure. *Osteoarthr. Cartil.* **2018**, *26*, 501–512. [CrossRef]
15. Saxer, F.; Hollinger, A.; Bjurstrom, M.F.; Conaghan, P.G.; Neogi, T.; Schieker, M.; Berenbaum, F. Pain-phenotyping in osteoarthritis: Current concepts, evidence, and considerations towards a comprehensive framework for assessment and treatment. *Osteoarthr. Cartil. Open* **2024**, *6*, 100433. [CrossRef] [PubMed]
16. Bedson, J.; Croft, P.R. The discordance between clinical and radiographic knee osteoarthritis: A systematic search and summary of the literature. *BMC Musculoskelet. Disord.* **2008**, *9*, 116. [CrossRef] [PubMed]
17. Nijs, J.; George, S.Z.; Clauw, D.J.; Fernández-de-las-Peñas, C.; Kosek, E.; Ickmans, K.; Fernández-Carnero, J.; Polli, A.; Kapreli, E.; Huysmans, E.; et al. Central sensitisation in chronic pain conditions: Latest discoveries and their potential for precision medicine. *Lancet Rheumatol.* **2021**, *3*, e383–e392. [CrossRef]
18. Narouze, S.; Souzdalnitski, D. Obesity and chronic pain: Systematic review of prevalence and implications for pain practice. *Reg. Anesth. Pain Med.* **2015**, *40*, 91–111. [CrossRef]
19. Coetzee, M.; Clifford, A.M.; Jordaan, J.D.; Louw, Q.A. Health equity profile of knee replacement patients in the South African public sector: A descriptive study. *S. Afr. J. Physiother.* **2024**, *80*, 2027. [CrossRef]
20. Agel, J.; Coetzee, J.C.; Sangeorzan, B.J.; Roberts, M.M.; Hansen, S.T. Functional limitations of patients with end-stage ankle arthrosis. *Foot Ankle Int.* **2005**, *26*, 537–539. [CrossRef]
21. Desmeules, F.; Dionne, C.E.; Belzile, E.; Bourbonnais, R.; FrÃ©mont, P.; Desmeules, F.o.; Dionne, C.E.; Belzile, E.; Bourbonnais, R.e.; FrÃ©mont, P. Waiting for total knee replacement surgery: Factors associated with pain, stiffness, function and quality of life. *BMC Musculoskelet. Disord.* **2009**, *10*, 52. [CrossRef]
22. Ackerman, I.; Graves, S.; Wicks, I.; Bennell, K.; Osborne, R. Severely compromised quality of life in women and those of lower socioeconomic status waiting for joint replacement surgery. *Arthritis Care Res.* **2005**, *53*, 653–658. [CrossRef] [PubMed]
23. Hair, J.F.; Black, W.C.; Babin, B.J.; Anderson, R.E. *Multivariate Data Analysis*; Pearson Education Limited: Harlow, UK, 2014; p. 734.
24. DeYoreo, M. Stratified random sampling. In *The SAGE Encyclopedia of Educational Research, Measurement, and Evaluation*; Frey, B.B., Ed.; SAGE Publications, Incorporated: Thousand Oaks, CA, USA, 2018; Volume 4, p. 1624. [CrossRef]

25. Setia, M.S. Methodology series module 5: Sampling strategies. *Indian J. Dermatol.* **2016**, *61*, 505–509. [CrossRef]
26. Dell'isola, A.; Wirth, W.; Steultjens, M.; Eckstein, F.; Culvenor, A.G. Knee extensor muscle weakness and radiographic knee osteoarthritis progression. *Acta Orthop.* **2018**, *89*, 406–411. [CrossRef]
27. Aytekin, E.; Sukur, E.; Oz, N.; Telatar, A.; Eroglu Demir, S.; Sayiner Caglar, N.; Ozturkmen, Y.; Ozgonenel, L. The effect of a 12 week prehabilitation program on pain and function for patients undergoing total knee arthroplasty: A prospective controlled study. *J. Clin. Orthop. Trauma* **2019**, *10*, 345–349. [CrossRef]
28. Dineen-Griffin, S.; Garcia-Cardenas, V.; Williams, K.; Benrimoj, S.I. Helping patients help themselves: A systematic review of self-management support strategies in primary health care practice. *PLoS ONE* **2019**, *14*, e0220116. [CrossRef]
29. Dube, L.; Rendall-Mkosi, K.; Van den Broucke, S.; Bergh, A.M.; Mafutha, N.G. Self-Management Support Needs of Patients with Chronic Diseases in a South African Township: A Qualitative Study. *J. Community Health Nurs.* **2017**, *34*, 21–31. [CrossRef] [PubMed]
30. Dobson, F.; Hinman, R.S.; Roos, E.M.; Abbott, J.H.; Stratford, P.; Davis, A.M.; Buchbinder, R.; Snyder-Mackler, L.; Henrotin, Y.; Thumboo, J.; et al. OARSI recommended performance-based tests to assess physical function in people diagnosed with hip or knee osteoarthritis. *Osteoarthr. Cartil.* **2013**, *21*, 1042–1052. [CrossRef]
31. Schwartz, M.H.; Rozumalski, A. The gait deviation index: A new comprehensive index of gait pathology. *Gait Posture* **2008**, *28*, 351–357. [CrossRef]
32. Mayer, T.G.; Fau, N.R.; Cohen, H.; Howard, K.J.; Choi, Y.H.; Williams, M.J.; Perez, Y.; Gatchel, R.J. The development and psychometric validation of the central sensitization inventory. *Pain. Pract.* **2012**, *4*, 276–285. [CrossRef] [PubMed]
33. Baron, E.C.; Davies, T.; Lund, C. Validation of the 10-item Centre for Epidemiological Studies Depression Scale (CES-D-10) in Zulu, Xhosa and Afrikaans populations in South Africa. *BMC Psychiatry* **2017**, *17*, 6. [CrossRef]
34. Stratford, P.; Gill, C.; Westaway, M.; Binkley, J. Assessing disability and change on individual patients: A report of a patient specific measure. *Physiother. Can.* **1995**, *47*, 258–263. [CrossRef]
35. Dawson, J.; Fitzpatrick, R.; Murray, D.; Carr, A. Questionnaire on the perceptions of patients about total hip replacement. *J. Bone Jt. Surg. Br. Vol.* **1996**, *80*, 63–69. [CrossRef]
36. Carver, C.S. You want to measure coping but your protocol's too long: Consider the brief COPE. *Int. J. Behav. Med.* **1997**, *4*, 92–100. [CrossRef] [PubMed]
37. Brady, T. Strategies to support self-management in osteoarthritis: Five categories of interventions, including education. *Orthop. Nurs.* **2012**, *31*, 124–130. [CrossRef]
38. Cleland, C.L.; Hunter, R.F.; Kee, F.; Cupples, M.E.; Sallis, J.F.; Tully, M.A. Validity of the Global Physical Activity Questionnaire (GPAQ) in assessing levels and change in moderate-vigorous physical activity and sedentary behaviour. *BMC Public Health* **2014**, *14*, 1255. [CrossRef]
39. Yong, A.G.; Pearce, S. A Beginner's Guide to Factor Analysis: Focusing on Exploratory Factor Analysis. *Tutor. Quant. Methods Psychol.* **2013**, *9*, 79–94. [CrossRef]
40. Panaretos, D.; George, T.; Malvina, V.; Demosthenes, P. Factor analysis as a tool for pattern recognition in biomedical research; a review with application in R software. *J. Data Sci.* **2017**, *16*, 615–630. [CrossRef]
41. Huang, Z.; Bucklin, M.A.; Guo, W.; Martin, J.T. Disease progression and clinical outcomes in latent osteoarthritis phenotypes: Data from the Osteoarthritis Initiative. *Res. Sq.* **2024**. *preprint*. [CrossRef]
42. Astephen Wilson, J.L.; Kobsar, D. Osteoarthritis year in review 2020: Mechanics. *Osteoarthr. Cartil.* **2021**, *29*, 161–169. [CrossRef] [PubMed]
43. Kushioka, J.; Sun, R.; Zhang, W.; Muaremi, A.; Leutheuser, H.; Odonkor, C.A.; Smuck, M. Gait Variability to Phenotype Common Orthopedic Gait Impairments Using Wearable Sensors. *Sensors* **2022**, *22*, 9301. [CrossRef]
44. Astephen, J.L.; Wilson, D.A.; Dunbar, M.J.; Deluzio, K.J. Preoperative gait patterns and BMI are associated with tibial component migration. *Acta Orthop.* **2010**, *81*, 478–486. [CrossRef]
45. Oikarinen, N.; Jokelainen, T.; Heikkilä, L.; Nurkkala, M.; Hukkanen, J.; Salonurmi, T.; Savolainen, M.J.; Teeriniemi, A.-M. Low eating self-efficacy is associated with unfavorable eating behavior tendencies among individuals with overweight and obesity. *Sci. Rep.* **2023**, *13*, 7730. [CrossRef]
46. Allison, K.; Jones, S.; Hinman, R.S.; Pardo, J.; Li, P.; DeSilva, A.; Quicke, J.G.; Sumithran, P.; Prendergast, J.; George, E.; et al. Alternative models to support weight loss in chronic musculoskeletal conditions: Effectiveness of a physiotherapist-delivered intensive diet programme for knee osteoarthritis, the POWER randomised controlled trial. *Br. J. Sports Med.* **2024**, *58*, 538–547. [CrossRef]
47. Cole, S.; Kolovos, S.; Soni, A.; Delmestri, A.; Sanchez-Santos, M.T.; Judge, A.; Arden, N.K.; Beswick, A.D.; Wylde, V.; Gooberman-Hill, R.; et al. Progression of chronic pain and associated health-related quality of life and healthcare resource use over 5 years after total knee replacement: Evidence from a cohort study. *BMJ Open* **2022**, *12*, e058044. [CrossRef]

48. van Spil, W.E.; Bierma-Zeinstra, S.M.A.; Deveza, L.A.; Arden, N.K.; Bay-Jensen, A.C.; Kraus, V.B.; Carlesso, L.; Christensen, R.; Van Der Esch, M.; Kent, P.; et al. A consensus-based framework for conducting and reporting osteoarthritis phenotype research. *Arthritis Res. Ther.* **2020**, *22*, 54. [CrossRef] [PubMed]
49. Şahin, F.; Beyaz, S.G.; Karakuş, N.; İnanmaz, M.E. Total Knee Arthroplasty Postsurgical Chronic Pain, Neuropathic Pain, and the Prevalence of Neuropathic Symptoms: A Prospective Observational Study in Turkey. *J. Pain Res.* **2021**, *14*, 1315–1321. [CrossRef] [PubMed]
50. Li, Y.; Liu, M.; Sun, X.; Hou, T.; Tang, S.; Szanton, S.L. Independent and synergistic effects of pain, insomnia, and depression on falls among older adults: A longitudinal study. *BMC Geriatr.* **2020**, *20*, 491. [CrossRef] [PubMed]
51. Sauder, N.; Brinkman, N.; Sayegh, G.E.; Moore, M.G.; Koenig, K.M.; Bozic, K.J.; Patel, J.J.; Jayakumar, P. Preoperative Symptoms of Depression are Associated with Worse Capability 6-weeks and 6-months After Total Hip Arthroplasty for Osteoarthritis. *J. Arthroplast.* **2024**, *39*, 1777–1782. [CrossRef]
52. Senba, E. A key to dissect the triad of insomnia, chronic pain, and depression. *Neurosci. Lett.* **2015**, *589*, 197–199. [CrossRef]
53. Saw, M.M.; Kruger-Jakins, T.; Edries, N.; Parker, R. Significant improvements in pain after a six-week physiotherapist-led exercise and education intervention, in patients with osteoarthritis awaiting arthroplasty, in South Africa: A randomised controlled trial. *BMC Musculoskelet. Disord.* **2016**, *17*, 236. [CrossRef]
54. Kruger-Jakins, T.; Saw, M.; Edries, N.; Parker, R. The development of an intervention to manage pain in people with late-stage osteoarthritis. *S. Afr. J. Physiother.* **2016**, *72*, a311. [CrossRef] [PubMed]
55. Previtali, D.; Andriolo, L.; Di Laura Frattura, G.; Boffa, A.; Candrian, C.; Zaffagnini, S.; Filardo, G. Pain Trajectories in Knee Osteoarthritis-A Systematic Review and Best Evidence Synthesis on Pain Predictors. *J. Clin. Med.* **2020**, *9*, 2828. [CrossRef]
56. Veronese, N.; Cooper, C.; Bruyere, O.; Al-Daghri, N.M.; Branco, J.; Cavalier, E.; Cheleschi, S.; da Silva Rosa, M.C.; Conaghan, P.G.; Dennison, E.M.; et al. Multimodal Multidisciplinary Management of Patients with Moderate to Severe Pain in Knee Osteoarthritis: A Need to Meet Patient Expectations. *Drugs* **2022**, *82*, 1347–1355. [CrossRef]
57. Segal, N.A.; Nilges, J.M.; Oo, W.M. Sex differences in osteoarthritis prevalence, pain perception, physical function and therapeutics. *Osteoarthr. Cartil.* **2024**, *32*, 1045–1053. [CrossRef]
58. Deveza, L.A.; Melo, L.; Yamato, T.P.; Mills, K.; Ravi, V.; Hunter, D.J. Knee osteoarthritis phenotypes and their relevance for outcomes: A systematic review. *Osteoarthr. Cartil.* **2017**, *25*, 1926–1941. [CrossRef]
59. Kubitza, J.; Haas, M.; Keppeler, L.; Reuschenbach, B. Therapy options for those affected by a long lie after a fall: A scoping review. *BMC Geriatr.* **2022**, *22*, 582. [CrossRef]
60. Rausch Osthoff, A.K.; Niedermann, K.; Braun, J.; Adams, J.; Brodin, N.; Dagfinrud, H.; Duruoz, T.; Esbensen, B.A.; Günther, K.P.; Hurkmans, E.; et al. 2018 EULAR recommendations for physical activity in people with inflammatory arthritis and osteoarthritis. *Ann. Rheum. Dis.* **2018**, *77*, 1251–1260. [CrossRef] [PubMed]
61. Zhang, Y.; Li, X.; Wang, Y.; Ge, L.; Pan, F.; Winzenberg, T.; Cai, G. Association of knee and hip osteoarthritis with the risk of falls and fractures: A systematic review and meta-analysis. *Arthritis Res. Ther.* **2023**, *25*, 184. [CrossRef] [PubMed]
62. Conaghan, P.G.; Dickson, J.; Grant, R.L. Guidelines: Care and management of osteoarthritis in adults: Summary of NICE guidance. *BMJ* **2008**, *336*, 502–503. [CrossRef] [PubMed]
63. Dell'Isola, A.; Allan, R.; Smith, S.L.; Marreiros, S.S.P.; Steultjens, M. Identification of clinical phenotypes in knee osteoarthritis: A systematic review of the literature. *BMC Musculoskelet. Disord.* **2016**, *17*, 425. [CrossRef]
64. Cois, A.; Day, C. Obesity trends and risk factors in the South African adult population. *BMC Obes.* **2015**, *2*, 42. [CrossRef]
65. Peer, N.; Steyn, K.; Levitt, N. Differential obesity indices identify the metabolic syndrome in Black men and women in Cape Town: The CRIBSA study. *J. Public Health* **2016**, *38*, 175–182. [CrossRef] [PubMed]
66. Collins, J.E.; Katz, J.N.; Dervan, E.E.; Losina, E. Trajectories and Risk Profiles of Pain in Persons with Radiographic, Symptomatic Knee Osteoarthritis: Data from the Osteoarthritis Initiative. *Osteoarthr. Cartil.* **2014**, *22*, 622–630. [CrossRef]
67. Holla, J.F.M.; Van Der Leeden, M.; Heymans, M.W.; Roorda, L.D.; Bierma-Zeinstra, S.M.A.; Boers, M.; Lems, W.F.; Steultjens, M.P.M.; Dekker, J. Three trajectories of activity limitations in early symptomatic knee osteoarthritis: A 5-year follow-up study. *Ann. Rheum. Dis.* **2014**, *73*, 1369–1375. [CrossRef] [PubMed]
68. Wesseling, J.; Bastick, A.N.; Ten Wolde, S.; Kloppenburg, M.; Lafeber, F.P.J.G.; Bierma-Zeinstra, S.M.A.; Bijlsma, J.W.J. Identifying trajectories of pain severity in early symptomatic knee osteoarthritis: A 5-year followup of the cohort hip and cohort knee (CHECK) study. *J. Rheumatol.* **2015**, *42*, 1470–1477. [CrossRef] [PubMed]
69. Kingsbury, S.R.; Corp, N.; Watt, F.E.; Felson, D.T.; O'Neill, T.W.; Holt, C.A.; Jones, R.K.; Conaghan, P.G.; Arden, N.K.; Adams, J.; et al. Harmonising data collection from osteoarthritis studies to enable stratification: Recommendations on core data collection from an Arthritis Research UK clinical studies group. *Rheumatology* **2016**, *55*, 1394–1402. [CrossRef]
70. Lowry, V.; Ouellet, P.; Vendittoli, P.A.; Carlesso, L.C.; Wideman, T.H.; Desmeules, F. Determinants of pain, disability, health-related quality of life and physical performance in patients with knee osteoarthritis awaiting total joint arthroplasty. *Disabil. Rehabilitation* **2018**, *40*, 2734–2744. [CrossRef]

71. Vitaloni, M.; Botto-van Bemden, A.; Sciortino Contreras, R.M.; Scotton, D.; Bibas, M.; Quintero, M.; Monfort, J.; Carné, X.; de Abajo, F.; Oswald, E.; et al. Global management of patients with knee osteoarthritis begins with quality of life assessment: A systematic review. *BMC Musculoskelet. Disord.* **2019**, *20*, 493. [CrossRef]
72. Dobson, F.; Hinman, R.S.; Hall, M.; Marshall, C.J.; Sayer, T.; Anderson, C.; Newcomb, N.; Stratford, P.W.; Bennell, K.L. Reliability and measurement error of the Osteoarthritis Research Society International (OARSI) recommended performance-based tests of physical function in people with hip and knee osteoarthritis. *Osteoarthr. Cartil.* **2017**, *25*, 1792–1796. [CrossRef]
73. Mehta, S.P.; Morelli, N.; Prevatte, C.; White, D.; Oliashirazi, A. Validation of Physical Performance Tests in Individuals with Advanced Knee Osteoarthritis. *HSS J.* **2019**, *15*, 261–268. [CrossRef]
74. Bennell, K.; Dobson, F.; Hinman, R. Measures of Physical Performance Assessments. *Arthritis Care Res.* **2011**, *63*, S350–S370. [CrossRef]
75. Roongbenjawan, N.; Siriphorn, A. Accuracy of modified 30-s chair-stand test for predicting falls in older adults. *Ann. Phys. Rehabil. Med.* **2020**, *63*, 309–315. [CrossRef]
76. Tsonga, T.; Michalopoulou, M.; Malliou, P.; Godolias, G.; Kapetanakis, S.; Gkasdaris, G.; Soucacos, P. Analyzing the History of Falls in Patients with Severe Knee Osteoarthritis. *Clin. Orthop. Surg.* **2015**, *7*, 449–456. [CrossRef]
77. Lin, Y.C.; Davey, R.C.; Cochrane, T. Tests for physical function of the elderly with knee and hip osteoarthritis. *Scand. J. Med. Sci. Sports* **2001**, *11*, 280–286. [CrossRef]
78. Ehara, Y.; Fujimoto, H.; Miyazaki, S.; Mochimaru, M.; Tanaka, S.; Yamamoto, S. Comparison of the performance of 3D camera systems II. *Gait Posture* **1997**, *5*, 251–255. [CrossRef]
79. Biggs, P.R.; Whatling, G.M.; Wilson, C.; Metcalfe, A.J.; Holt, C.A. Which osteoarthritic gait features recover following total knee replacement surgery? *PLoS ONE* **2019**, *14*, e0203417. [CrossRef]
80. Elbaz, A.; Mor, A.; Segal, G.; Debi, R.; Shazar, N.; Herman, A. Novel classification of knee osteoarthritis severity based on spatiotemporal gait analysis. *Osteoarthr. Cartil.* **2014**, *22*, 457–463. [CrossRef]
81. Mills, K.; Hunt, M.A.; Ferber, R. Biomechanical deviations during level walking associated with knee osteoarthritis: A systematic review and meta-analysis. *Arthritis Care Res.* **2013**, *65*, 1643–1665. [CrossRef] [PubMed]
82. Kobsar, D.; Charlton, J.M.; Hunt, M.A. Individuals with knee osteoarthritis present increased gait pattern deviations as measured by a knee-specific gait deviation index. *Gait Posture* **2019**, *72*, 82–88. [CrossRef] [PubMed]
83. Naili, J.E.; BrostrÃ¶m, E.W.; Clausen, B.; Holsgaard-Larsen, A. Measures of knee and gait function and radiographic severity of knee osteoarthritis—A cross-sectional study. *Gait Posture* **2019**, *74*, 20–26. [CrossRef]
84. Moss, P.; Benson, H.A.E.; Will, R.; Wright, A. Patients with Knee Osteoarthritis Who Score Highly on the PainDETECT Questionnaire Present with Multimodality Hyperalgesia, Increased Pain, and Impaired Physical Function. *Clin. J. Pain* **2018**, *34*, 15–21. [CrossRef]
85. Rice, D.A.; Kluger, M.T.; McNair, P.J.; Lewis, G.N.; Somogyi, A.A.; Borotkanics, R.; Barratt, D.T.; Walker, M. Persistent postoperative pain after total knee arthroplasty: A prospective cohort study of potential risk factors. *Br. J. Anaesth.* **2018**, *121*, 804–812. [CrossRef]
86. Wallis, J.A.; Taylor, N.F.; Bunzli, S.; Shields, N. Experience of living with knee osteoarthritis: A systematic review of qualitative studies. *BMJ Open* **2019**, *9*, e030060. [CrossRef]
87. Moreton, B.J.; Tew, V.; Das Nair, R.; Wheeler, M.; Walsh, D.A.; Lincoln, N.B. Pain phenotype in patients with knee osteoarthritis: Classification and measurement properties of painDETECT and self-report leeds assessment of neuropathic symptoms and signs scale in a cross-sectional study. *Arthritis Care Res.* **2015**, *67*, 519–528. [CrossRef] [PubMed]
88. Kim, S.H.; Yoon, K.B.; Yoon, D.M.; Yoo, J.H.; Ahn, K.R. Influence of Centrally Mediated Symptoms on Postoperative Pain in Osteoarthritis Patients Undergoing Total Knee Arthroplasty: A Prospective Observational Evaluation. *Pain Pract.* **2015**, *15*, E46–E53. [CrossRef]
89. Soni, A.; Wanigasekera, V.; Mezue, M.; Cooper, C.; Javaid, M.K.; Price, A.J.; Tracey, I. Central Sensitization in Knee Osteoarthritis: Relating Presurgical Brainstem Neuroimaging and PainDETECT-Based Patient Stratification to Arthroplasty Outcome. *Arthritis Rheumatol.* **2019**, *71*, 550–560. [CrossRef] [PubMed]
90. Nicholls, E.; Thomas, E.; van der Windt, D.A.; Croft, P.R.; Peat, G. Pain trajectory groups in persons with, or at high risk of, knee osteoarthritis: Findings from the Knee Clinical Assessment Study and theOsteoarthritis initiative. *Osteoarthr. Cartil.* **2014**, *22*, 2041–2050. [CrossRef] [PubMed]
91. Berghmans, D.D.; Lenssen, A.F.; van Rhijn, L.W.; de Bie, R.A. The Patient-Specific Functional Scale: Its Reliability and Responsiveness in Patients Undergoing a Total Knee Arthroplasty. *J. Orthop. Sports Phys. Ther.* **2015**, *45*, 550–556. [CrossRef] [PubMed]
92. Harris, K.; Dawson, J.; Doll, H.; Field, R.E.; Murray, D.W.; Fitzpatrick, R.; Jenkinson, C.; Price, A.J.; Beard, D.J. Can pain and function be distinguished in the Oxford Knee Score in a meaningful way? An exploratory and confirmatory factor analysis. *Qual. Life Res.* **2013**, *22*, 2561–2568. [CrossRef]
93. Brady, T.J. Measures of self-efficacy. *Arthritis Care Res.* **2011**, *63*, s473–s485. [CrossRef]

94. Eyles, J.P.; Hunter, D.J.; Meneses, S.R.F.; Collins, N.J.; Dobson, F.; Lucas, B.R.; Mills, K. Instruments assessing attitudes toward or capability regarding self-management of osteoarthritis: A systematic review of measurement properties. *Osteoarthr. Cartil.* **2017**, *25*, 1210–1222. [CrossRef]
95. Peters, M.; Potter, C.M.; Kelly, L.; Fitzpatrick, R. Self-efficacy and health-related quality of life: A cross-sectional study of primary care patients with multi-morbidity. *Health Qual. Life Outcomes* **2019**, *17*, 37. [CrossRef]
96. Lorig, K.; Chastain, R.L.; Ung, E.; Shoor, S.; Holman, H.R. Development and evaluation of a scale to measure perceived self-efficacy in people with arthritis. *Arthritis Rheum.* **1989**, *32*, 37–44. [CrossRef]
97. Gates, L.S.; Leyland, K.M.; Sheard, S.; Jackson, K.; Kelly, P.; Callahan, L.F.; Pate, R.; Roos, E.M.; Ainsworth, B.; Cooper, C.; et al. Physical activity and osteoarthritis: A consensus study to harmonise self-reporting methods of physical activity across international cohorts. *Rheumatol. Int.* **2017**, *37*, 469–478. [CrossRef]
98. Fernandez-Fernandez, R.; Rodriguez-Merchan, E.C. Better survival of total knee replacement in patients older than 70 years: A prospective study with 8 to 12 years follow-up. *Arch. Bone Jt. Surg.* **2015**, *3*, 22–28. [PubMed]
99. Wang, X.; Jin, X.; Han, W.; Cao, Y.; Halliday, A.; Blizzard, L.; Pan, F.; Antony, B.; Cicuttini, F.; Jones, G.; et al. Cross-sectional and Longitudinal Associations between Knee Joint Effusion Synovitis and Knee Pain in Older Adults. *J. Rheumatol.* **2016**, *43*, 121–130. [CrossRef] [PubMed]

Journal of
Functional Morphology and Kinesiology

MDPI

Article

Effects of Tactile Sensory Stimulation Training of the Trunk and Sole on Standing Balance Ability in Older Adults: A Randomized Controlled Trial

Toshiaki Tanaka [1,*], Yusuke Maeda [2] and Takahiro Miura [3]

1 Research Center for Advanced Science and Technology (RCAST), The University of Tokyo, Tokyo 113-8656, Japan
2 Department of Physical Therapy, School of Health Sciences at Odawara, International University of Health and Welfare, Odawara 250-8588, Japan; y.maeda@iuhw.ac.jp
3 National Institute of Advanced Industrial Science and Technology (AIST), Kashiwa 277-0882, Japan; miura-t@aist.go.jp
* Correspondence: t.tanaka@iog.u-tokyo.ac.jp or tanaka@bfp.rcast.u-tokyo.ac.jp; Tel.: +81-(3)-5452-5220

Abstract: Background: Aging is associated with a decline in both motor and sensory functions that destabilizes posture, increasing the risk of falls. Dynamic standing balance is strongly linked to fall risk in older adults. Sensory information from the soles and trunk is essential for balance control. Few studies have demonstrated the efficacy of targeted sensory training on balance improvement. **Objectives:** To assess vibratory sensation function in the trunk and sole using a vibration device and evaluate the effects of trunk and sole tactile sensation training on dynamic standing balance performance in older adults. **Methods:** In this randomized controlled trial, eighteen older adults were randomly assigned to three groups: control (n = 8, mean age 66.6 ± 3.4), trunk training (n = 5, mean age 71.0 ± 1.9), and sole training (n = 5, mean age 66.4 ± 3.6). The training lasted for 10 weeks, utilizing vibratory stimulation at 128 Hz through tuning forks for 15 min during each session, conducted three times a week. The primary outcomes were vibratory sensitivity, assessed with a belt-fitted device on the trunk and a plate equipped with vibrators on the soles, and dynamic balance, evaluated through force plate testing that measured limits of stability (LoS) in multiple directions. **Results:** Correct response rates for trunk vibratory stimulation significantly improved in the trunk training group ($p < 0.05$). The rate of two-stimuli discrimination improved in both training groups. Significant advancements in balance metrics were observed in the trunk and sole training groups when compared to the control group, especially regarding anterior–posterior tilts ($p < 0.05$). A positive correlation was identified between two-point vibratory discrimination and LoS test performance. **Conclusions:** Sensory training of the trunk and sole enhances balance performance in older adults, suggesting potential benefits for fall prevention. Future studies should assess long-term effects and explore optimal training duration with larger sample sizes.

Keywords: dynamic standing balance; sensory stimulation training; older adults

1. Introduction

Aging is associated with a decline in both motor and sensory functions which destabilize posture, resulting in increased risk of injury, hospitalization, and even mortality due to falls [1]. One study reported that one-third of all older adults in the United States suffer falls every year [2], while the rate of falls among older adults in Japan every year is reported to be over 20% [3]. Fractures due to falls are a particularly major risk factor for older individuals to need care, while the gait and balance disorders accompanying a decline in muscle strength are a risk factor for falls [1].

The most frequently used technique to evaluate the ability of static and dynamic postural stability is the measurement of the position and displacement of the center of pressure (COP) by using a force plate as a clinical assessment [4,5]. Static balance is the ability to maintain postural stability and orientation with the center of mass over the base of support and the body at rest. Dynamic balance is the ability to maintain postural stability and orientation with the center of mass over the base of support while the body parts are in motion [6]. Moreover, dynamic standing balance is deeply related to falls in older adults [7,8]. Regarding dynamic balance, the maximum ability to move forward, backward, leftward, and rightward while standing was used as an important evaluation of dynamic balance ability [9].

Obtaining accurate sensory information from the soles of the feet is essential for the control of standing balance [10]. In our prior study, we developed a device to evaluate vibratory sensation as a form of tactile sensation [11]. Using this device, we showed that sensory function in the toes and the soles is lower in older people than in young people, and that sensation in the soles of the feet affects standing balance [11,12]. Other studies have reported that this tactile sensation of the legs is related to standing balance performance [12–14]. Several other studies found that the vibrotactile feedback system could be used to improve postural sway [15,16]. However, these studies did not show the effect of sensory training on balance ability, nor did they clarify the supportive relationship between sensation and balance ability.

In addition to the soles of the feet, standing balance is also significantly affected by the movement of the center of gravity, which is present in the trunk (in the region of the pelvis) when standing [17]. For this reason, a number of studies have focused on the effects of trunk function on sitting and standing balance [18–20]. Just as foot sole sensation is an important element in standing balance, it may also be conjectured that the tactile sensation of the trunk would be important in standing balance. However, virtually no studies of the effects of tactile sensation of the trunk on standing balance have been performed.

Balance training is used as a means to prevent falls in older adults, and this is mainly an exercise intervention. A variety of intervention programs have been developed for muscle strength training, mainly focusing on the legs and the trunk, postural balance training, and gait training [21–23]. As such, the most common approach to preventing falls is to maintain or improve balance performance through motor function training. A few studies have found that multisensory (visual, vestibular, and somatosensory) exercise is effective at improving balance in individuals with balance disorders [24,25]. However, studies of methods to improve balance performance through training of the tactile sensory function aspect, an important element in maintaining standing balance performance, remain rare.

While vibrotactile stimulation has been explored in several studies, these approaches have predominantly utilized vibrotactile biofeedback systems [26,27] or whole-body vibration platforms [28], rather than targeted sensory training protocols designed to enhance proprioceptive and tactile acuity. For instance, Sienko et al. [26] employed vibrotactile feedback devices as balance aids but did not seek to improve the underlying sensory processing capabilities. Furthermore, previous sensory interventions have typically concentrated on the lower extremities alone [29], overlooking the essential role of trunk somatosensation in maintaining postural stability [30]. Although somatosensory information is important for postural control, existing interventions have largely overlooked the potential for targeted sensory training, instead favoring compensatory approaches or general exercises that do not specifically address the decline in sensory acuity among older adults [26–28].

The present study therefore aims to reveal the characteristics of vibratory sensation function in the regions of the trunk and sole in older people using a vibration device developed by our research group, and to verify the effects of trunk and sole tactile sensation training on dynamic standing balance performance in older people. Using our specialized vibration device, we implemented a targeted training protocol that provides precise vibratory stimulation to enhance sensitivity in these key sensory regions. Our protocol possesses the potential to bridge a gap in sensory training by targeting the trunk and soles—key areas for postural control that provide vital sensory input. These findings may assess whether targeted sensory training can improve acuity and balance in older adults, offering a novel fall prevention approach.

2. Materials and Methods

2.1. Participants

The participants comprised 18 right-handed/footed older adults (nine men, and nine women) divided randomly into three groups: the control group, and the sole and trunk training groups. General information, including age and history of falls, was collected for each group. The control, trunk, and sole groups comprised eight participants (three men, and five women, mean age: 66.6 ± 3.4, mean height: 158.8 ± 7.0 cm, and mean weight: 57.2 ± 12.5 kg), five participants (five men, mean age: 71.0 ± 1.9, mean height: 169.0 ± 2.8 cm, and mean weight: 59.2 ± 4.7 kg), and five participants (one man, and four women, mean age: 66.4 ± 3.6, mean height: 157.9 ± 5.5 cm, and mean weight: 54.6 ± 4.1 kg), respectively. All participants were independent in their activities of daily livings (ALDs). In addition, participants had no history of falls within the year prior to this study. Participants were randomly divided into three groups.

To evaluate the effects of vibratory sensation training in the trunk and sole regions on standing balance, a training period (10 weeks) was established for both training groups, and vibratory sensation and standing balance were evaluated in the same manner as in the initial evaluation.

All participants received verbal and written explanations of the study before providing their written informed consent, with an assurance that their participation would be strictly voluntary, that their non-participation would not result in any disadvantage, and that their personal information would be protected. This study was conducted with the approval of the institutional review board of The University of Tokyo (approval review no. 21-230, 21-231).

2.2. Details of the Trunk and Sole Training

The training period for both the trunk training group and the sole training group lasted 10 weeks. Three evaluations—initial, intermediate, and final—were conducted in the first week, in the middle of the fifth week, and finally in the tenth week. Trunk training groups were carried out by delivering vibratory stimulation to the back of the trunk to train sensation to vibratory stimulation. Training was performed using two vibratory sensation test tuning forks (128 Hz). Using these tuning forks, a researcher randomly applied vibratory stimulation to one or two of the twenty sites, each with an area of 5×5 cm^2, and arranged five horizontally by four vertically on the trunk region of the participant, and the participant responded when they felt the stimulation. According to the sole training, using two tuning forks, two sets of training were performed three times each on the five toes, the forefoot area from the first to the fifth toe, and the heel area. Using these tuning forks, a researcher randomly applied vibratory stimulation to one or two of the three areas, and the participant responded when they felt the stimulation. The trunk and sole trainings were carried out for 15 min at a time, three or more times a week.

2.3. Evaluation of Trunk and Sole Region Vibratory Sensation

Vibratory sensations in the trunk and sole regions were evaluated in the three groups using the developed vibratory stimulation device (Kyowa Electronic Instruments Co., Ltd., Tokyo, Japan). The main specifications of the vibrators (diameter 14 mm, thickness 3.7 mm, weight 1.6 g) included a frequency range of 150 Hz, a voltage of 3 V, and a duration of one simulation time of 1 s. The vibratory stimulation intensity was maintained at a constant level with no variation. The vibratory sensation in the trunk region was evaluated using a developed vibratory stimulation device. Vibratory stimulation was delivered to the trunk region via a belt worn around the participant's trunk, which was fitted with nine vibrators arranged in a pattern 15 cm vertically × 20 cm horizontally (Figures 1 and 2). Participants were instructed to respond to how many vibrators they could identify. Table 1 lists the trunk vibration stimulation patterns. For a single trial, the participants were presented with 26 vibratory stimuli, and one trial each was carried out on the left, center, and right sides of the trunk, yielding a total of 78 stimuli. Three vibration patterns were presented randomly: stimulation at zero sites, stimulation at one site, and simultaneous stimulation at two sites. Additionally, for simultaneous stimulation at the two sites, the two vibrators were placed vertically, horizontally, and diagonally (Table 1).

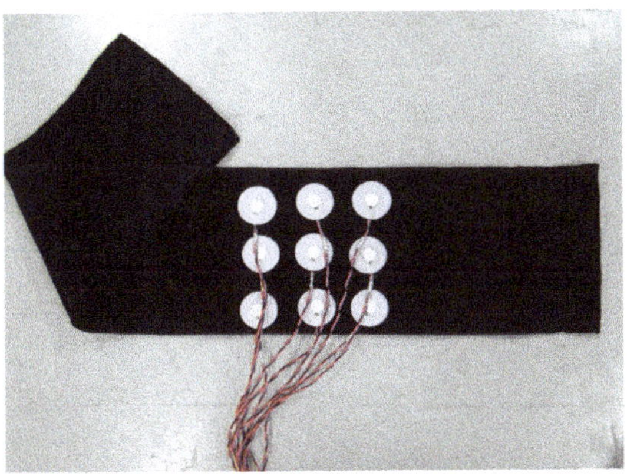

Figure 1. Image showing the placement of the trunk region vibrators in the belt.

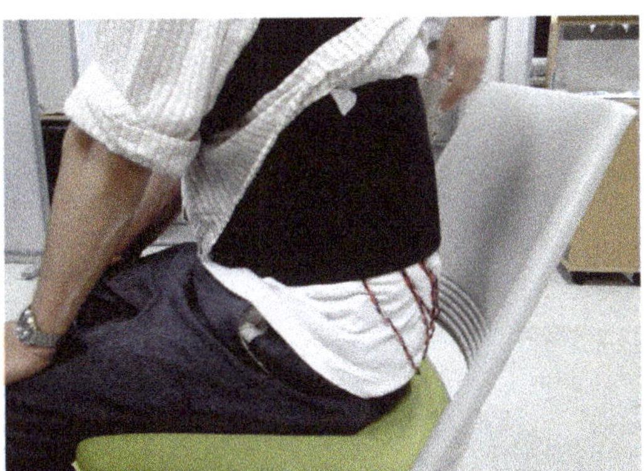

Figure 2. Image showing the experimental posture of sensory evaluation in the trunk region.

Table 1. Overview of the vibrator arrangement and vibration stimulation pattern for the trunk vibration sensation evaluation.

	Condition	Vibrators in the Trunk Position	
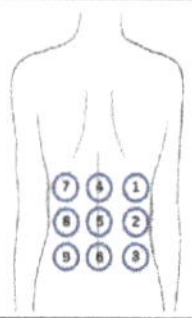	One stimulus	1, 2, 3, 4, 5, 6, 7, 8, 9	
	Two stimuli	(Vertical)	1–2, 4–5, 7–8, 2–3, 5–6, 8–9
		(Horizontal)	1–4, 4–7, 2–5, 5–8, 3–6, 6–9
		(Diagonal)	1–5, 5–9, 7–5, 5–3
	No stimulus	N/A	

The conditions for the sensory test using vibration stimulation of the sole of the foot are presented in Figures 3 and 4 and Table 2. Overall, six vibrators were placed on the sole vibration plate, with five one-point stimulations, seven two-point stimulations, and one without stimulation (Table 2). Under these conditions, vibration stimulation was randomly presented to the participants 15 times per trial. Stimulation was applied 45 times total across three trials.

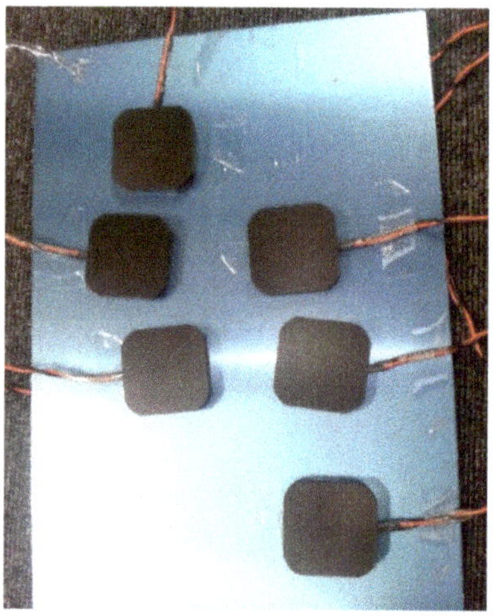

Figure 3. Image showing the placement of the sole region vibrators on a foot.

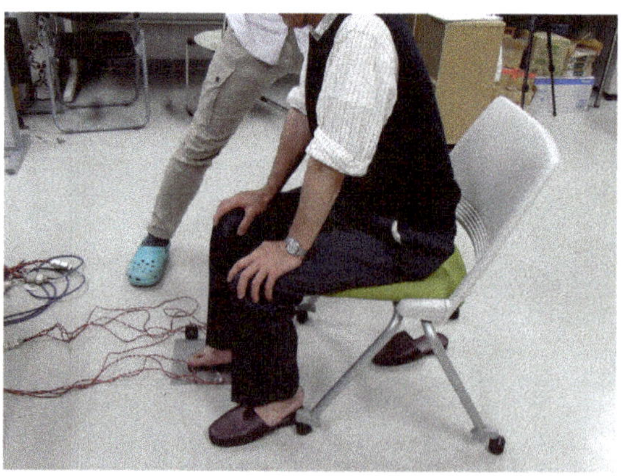

Figure 4. Image showing the experimental posture of the sensory evaluation in the sole region.

Table 2. Overview of the vibrator arrangement and vibration stimulation pattern for plantar vibration sensation evaluation. The a–f symbols in vibrators correspond to the a–f symbols on the sole shown on the left.

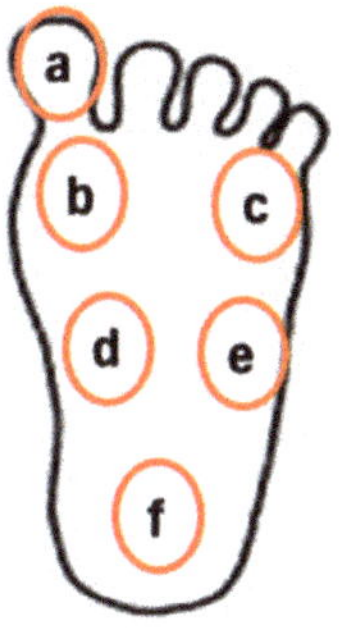

Condition	Vibrators	Plantar Position(s)	(Abbreviation)
One stimulus	a	Hallux	Hallux
	b	Thenar eminence	TE
	c	Hypothenar eminence	HE
	d	Proximal first metatarsal	P1M
	f	Heel	Heel
Two stimuli	a–b	Hallux–Thenar eminence	Hallux–TE
	a–d	Hallux–Proximal first metatarsal	Hallux–P1M
	b–d	Thenar eminence–Proximal first metatarsal	TE–P5M
	b–f	Thenar eminence–Heel	TE–Heel
	c–e	Hypothenar eminence–Proximal fifth metatarsal	HE–P5M
	c–f	Hypothenar eminence–Heel	HE–Heel
	e–f	Proximal fifth metatarsal–Heel	P5M–Heel
No stimulus	N/A	No vibration	No vibration

In both the trunk and sole sensory evaluations, participants were instructed to answer whether the stimulation was given in "zero sites", "one site", or "two sites". To avoid any visual or auditory influences, the participants were seated and wore eye masks and headphones for evaluation.

The vibrators used in the vibratory stimulation device were small vibration motors (Kyowa Electronic Instruments Co., Ltd.), commonly used in mobile telephones. The voltage of the vibrator used in this study was equal to or less than 3 V. The vibrator device did not directly touch the participants' skin. The system used a one-chip microcomputer (PIC16F84A; Microchip Technology Inc., Chandler, AZ, USA) to control all vibrators. The system could produce mechanical vibrations of up to 100 Hz. The time required for the stimulus to travel to all the points was limited to 1.0 s for all patterns.

2.4. Evaluation of Standing Balance Using a Force Plate

The measurement device for the standing balance was a force plate (Kyowa Electronic Instruments Co., Ltd.) that measured body sway parameters (Figure 5), which contained four transducers, one in each corner of the force plate, to measure the vertical forces indicating postural sway. The signals from the transducers were amplified and digitized using a computer. The computer program provided several indices of body sway calculated from the center of pressure. The accuracy and hysteresis of the force plate were ±1% and ±0.1%, respectively. The sampling rate of the force plate was 100 Hz.

To evaluate dynamic balance, the limits of stability (LoS) in the anterior, posterior, leftward, and rightward directions were measured [31]. The LoS test assessed the maximum displacement of the COP in both anteroposterior and lateral directions that participants could voluntarily maintain without altering their foot position and falling while standing upright with their knees extended. The participants performed this test standing barefoot with their arms at the sides of their bodies and eyes open, while looking at a marker placed 1.2 m in front of them. The standing position of all participants was measured barefoot under two conditions: on the force plate and on the force plate with a mattress spread over it. This method measures the sway of the body sway during standing posture where the sensation of the soles of the feet is disturbed by a mattress with maintaining the initial ankle joint position [32,33]. The study utilized a mattress (Balance pad, AIREX®, size: 410 × 500 × 60 mm, weight: 700 g, polyvinyl chloride resin foam) for the clinical assessment of the effect of sole tactile sensory interaction on postural stability, related to the CTSIB (Clinical Test of Sensory Interaction in Balance) [34]. The mattress provided a stimulus to the participant's sole without the movement of the ankle joint [32].

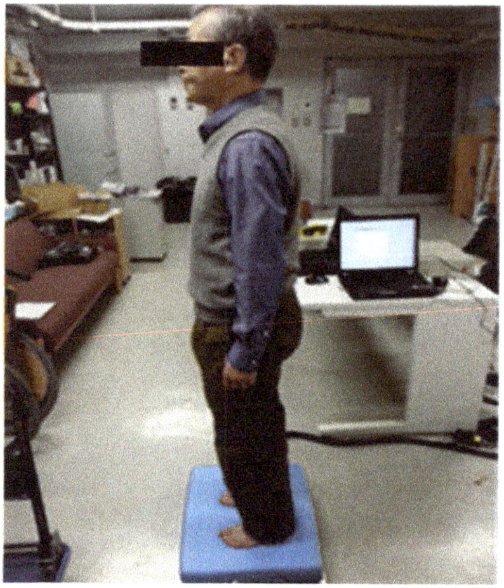

Figure 5. Image showing the evaluation scene of balance performance.

2.5. Analysis

The items for analysis from the trunk and sole sensory tests included the responses to stimulation of one and two sites. The items for statistical analysis obtained from the force plate included the data from four directions in the LoS test. The total LoS test value was also calculated based on the results of the left–right and right–anterior sways.

First, analysis of variance (ANOVA) was employed to identify significant differences between responses to stimulation of one and two sites, and to examine the main effects of the training group (control, trunk, and sole groups), number of rounds (1–3; Initial, intermediate, and final evaluations), positions to vibrate, and the interactions among these factors for these responses by the number of stimulated sites (0–2). Before the ANOVA, an aligned rank transformation (ART) [35,36] was performed on the scales, as the responses were non-normally distributed. The significance of the main effects was determined using post hoc multiple comparison methods, based on the least-squares means and Tukey's multiplicity adjustment [37,38]. Subsequently, we calculated the effect sizes, including the partial η^2 and Cohen's d, and determined the degree based on Cohen's effect size indices [39]. The level of significance was set at 5%.

Moreover, a robust multiple regression was performed with the dynamic sway data (five values from the LoS test: value for each of the four directions, including the anterior, posterior, left, and right values, and total value for the four directions) as dependent variables, and the experimental conditions and the rate of correct responses in sensory tests as the independent variables. We also calculated Pearson's correlation coefficients, and we checked the significance of these coefficients. The significance levels were set at 5% and 10%, respectively.

3. Results

3.1. Vibratory Sensation Evaluation

Figures 6–8 present the correct rates for guessing no stimulation, identifying when one vibration was presented, and identifying when two stimuli were presented, respectively. In these figures, the correct rate of vibration is plotted for each training group (control, sole, and trunk) and presentation location (sole and trunk) in relation to the number of rounds (one, two, and three). The thick black horizontal lines of these figures represent the median, while the red diamonds and error bars indicate the mean and standard error, respectively. In the absence of vibration, the mean and median percentages of correct responses were generally above 90%, regardless of the group allocation, stimulus location, or number of rounds, suggesting that few participants in the experiment experienced daily phantom vibrations. However, as the number of rounds increased, the percentage of such correct responses in the sole and trunk training groups increased, while in the third round, the percentage of correct responses in the sole and trunk presentations was 100% for both the sole and trunk groups, indicating that only the control group had a significant number of errors ($\chi^2(2) = 7.26$, $p = 0.027 < 0.05$. The adjusted Pearson's residual value for the control group were as follows: 2.69, $p = 0.043 < 0.05$).

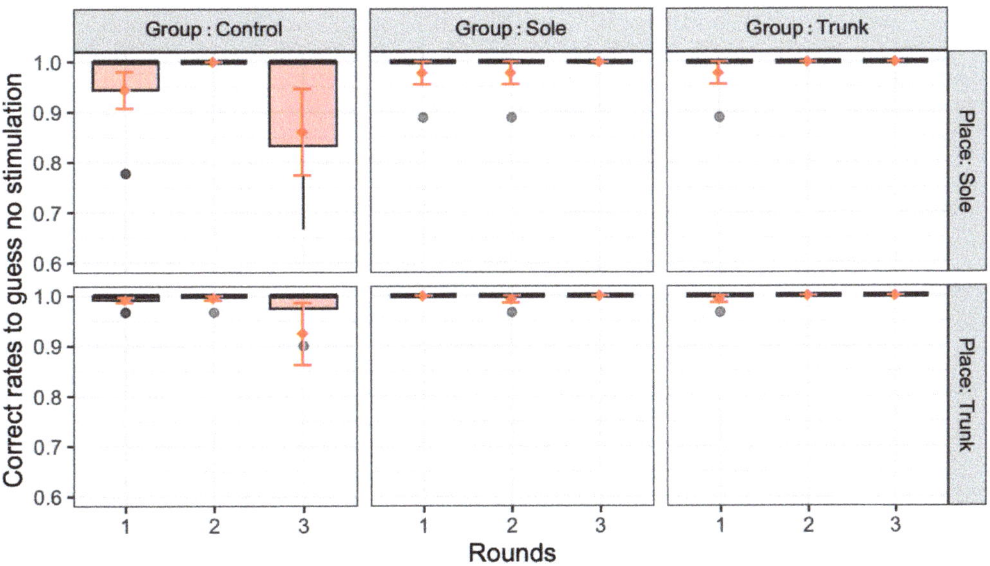

Figure 6. Correct rates for guessing no stimulation when there was no presented vibration. The thick black horizontal lines of these figures represent the median, while the red diamonds and error bars indicate the mean and standard error, respectively.

Regarding the one-stimulus condition, an ANOVA performed on the correct rates confirmed a significant main effect of the training group and vibration location ($p < 0.05$). The exact statistical value of these significant factors in the correct rates was as follows: training group: $F(1,2) = 15.8$, $p < 0.001$, partial $\eta^2 = 0.04$ (medium); vibration places: $F(1,1) = 270.8$, $p < 0.001$, partial $\eta^2 = 0.27$ (large). Furthermore, the interactions among these factors were significant, with the exact results as follows: training group and vibration place: $F(1,2) = 31.4$, $p < 0.001$, partial $\eta^2 = 0.08$ (medium). Although the significance level was not achieved, the following results are also noted: vibration place and number of rounds: $F(1,2) = 2.83$, $p = 0.060$, partial $\eta^2 = 0.008$ (negligible).

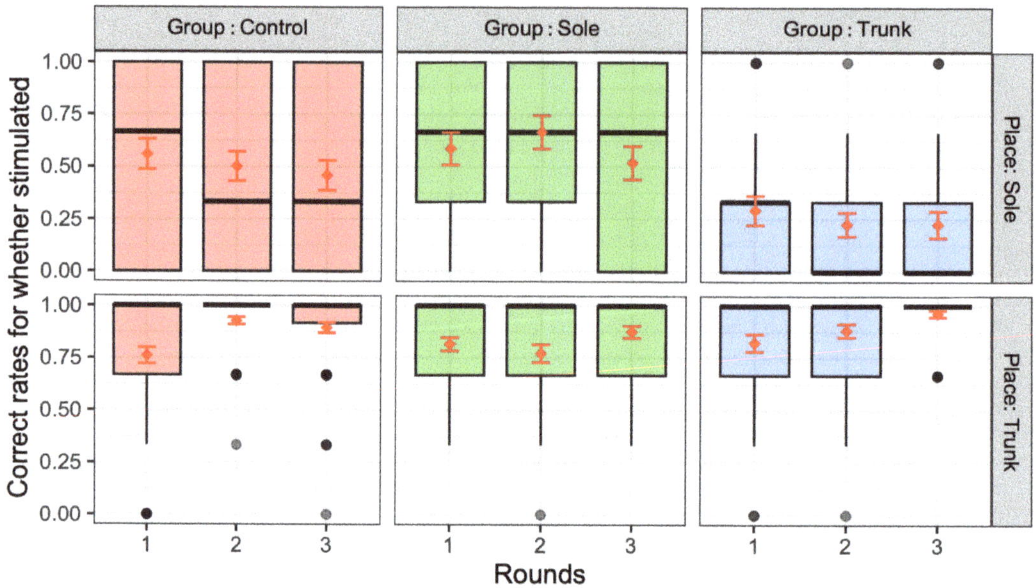

Figure 7. Correct rates for guessing a single vibration when a single vibration was presented to the participant. The thick black horizontal lines of these figures represent the median, while the red diamonds and error bars indicate the mean and standard error, respectively.

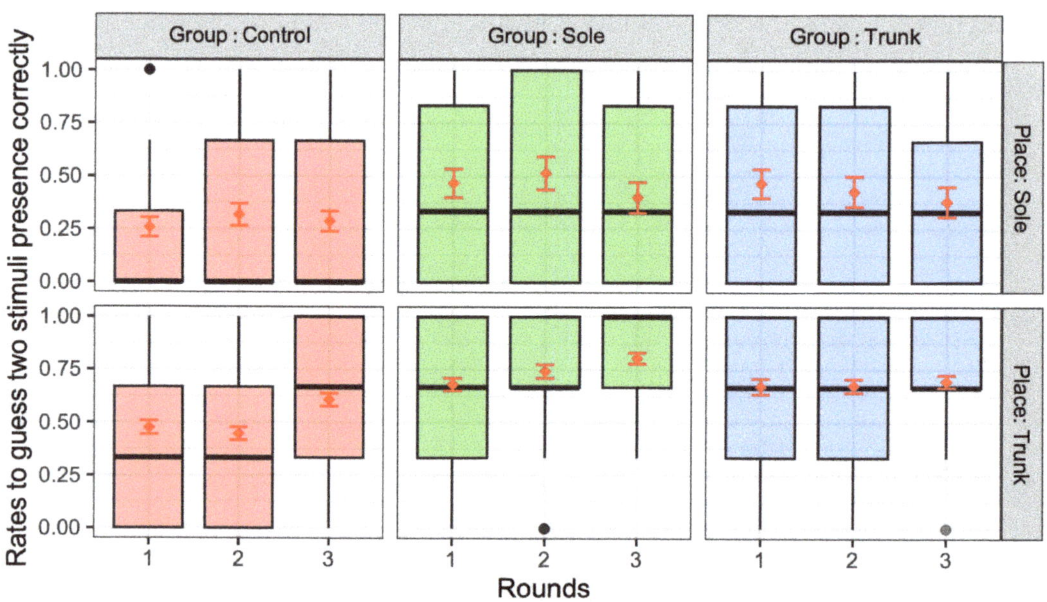

Figure 8. Correct rates for guessing two vibrations when two vibrations were presented to the sole and trunk. The thick black horizontal lines of these figures represent the median, while the red diamonds and error bars indicate the mean and standard error, respectively.

The correct rates for stimulation with one vibration was lower in the trunk training group than in the other groups, especially for the presentation of vibration to the sole (t(738) = 5.0, $p < 0.0001$, d = 0.51 (medium)), while the correct rate of vibration to the trunk increased significantly with the number of rounds (r = 0.27, t(133) = 3.14, p = 0.002). However, there was no significant difference between the sole and trunk training groups, even when the vibration was presented to the trunk.

Regarding the correct rates of guessing the presence of two stimuli, ANOVA identified significant main effects for the training group ($F(1,2) = 29.1$, $p < 0.001$, partial $\eta^2 = 0.048$, middle effect size) and vibration combinations ($F(1,9) = 35.4$, $p < 0.001$, partial $\eta^2 = 0.22$, large effect size). For the number of rounds, although the p-value approached but did not reach the conventional significance threshold ($F(1,2) = 2.39$, $p = 0.09$, partial $\eta^2 = 0.004$), the effect size suggests this factor had minimal practical impact on the results. Further, the interactions among these factors were significant, as follows: training group and vibration combinations: $F(1,18) = 2.0$, $p = 0.008$, partial $\eta^2 = 0.03$ (medium); vibration combinations and number of rounds: $F(1,18) = 1.88$, $p = 0.014 < 0.05$, partial $\eta^2 = 0.028$ (small).

The rate of correctly guessing the presence of the two stimuli tended to be higher in both the trunk and sole training groups compared with the control group ($p < 0.001$). Moreover, the correct rates changed with repetition, with the training group showing a significant increase in the correct rates for trunk vibrations. Figure 9 presents the correct rates for each combination of the two stimulation points in the sole and trunk, with an effect size d, as compared with the performance of the horizontal vibration on the trunk for convenience. For the sole, the percentage of correct responses was significantly higher when stimulation was applied to the proximal first metatarsal (P1M) and anywhere else vs. when stimulating the other two points of the sole. In particular, the correct response rate was significantly lower when the heel was stimulated than when the first proximal metatarsal was stimulated. The two-point discrimination results for the trunk were also significantly more accurate than those for the sole, except when the proximal first metatarsal and another point were stimulated. For convenience, Figure 10 presents the relative correct rates when two vibrations were presented on the trunk for each training group, with an effect size d, when compared to the control group. The correct response rates were significantly higher in the trunk and sole training groups than in the control group. Figure 11 presents the correct rates in the training sessions for convenience, with an effect size d, when compared to the results of round 1. The correct rates for round 3 were significantly higher than those for rounds 1 and 2.

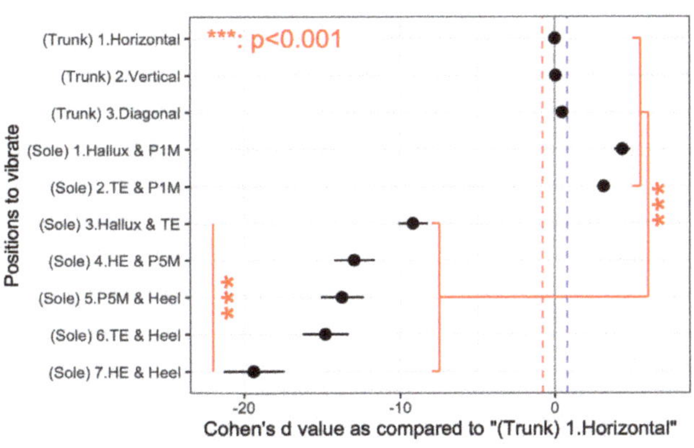

Figure 9. Effect size of the correct response rate for each of the two stimulus locations on the trunk and sole for participants to correctly guess the presence of the two stimuli. Effect sizes are relative to the (Trunk) 1. Horizontal condition. Significant differences were obtained through multiple comparisons. The red and blue dotted lines indicate values with large effect sizes.

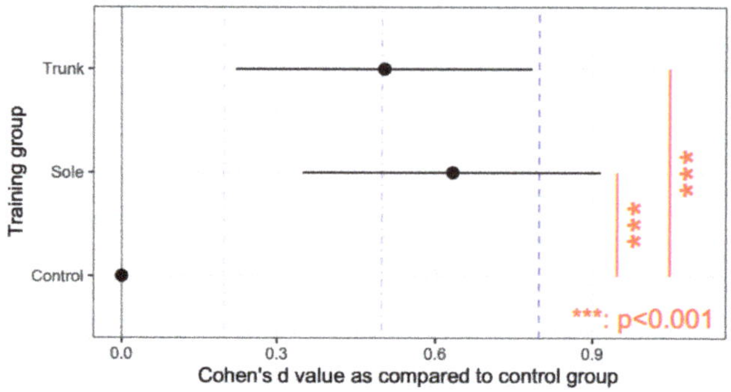

Figure 10. Effect size of the correct response rate for each of the two stimulus locations on the trunk and sole for participants to correctly guess the presence of the two stimuli. Effect sizes are relative to the control group. Significant differences were obtained by multiple comparisons. The blue dotted lines indicate values for which the effect size is about large (0.8), medium (0.5), or small (0.2).

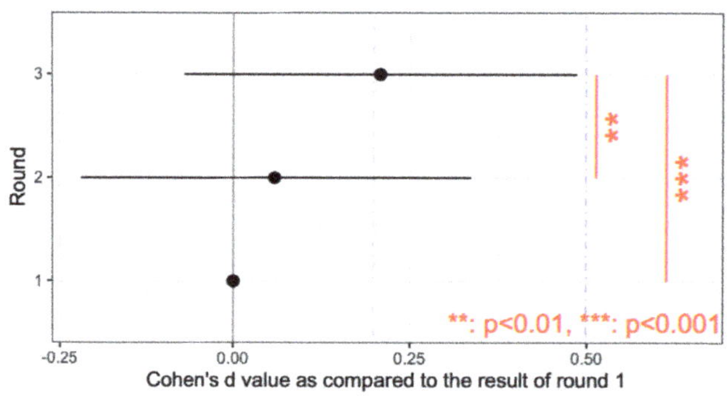

Figure 11. Effect size of the correct response rate for each of the two stimulus locations on the trunk and sole for participants to correctly guess the presence of the two stimuli. Effect sizes are relative to the results of round 1. Significant differences were obtained by multiple comparisons. The blue dotted lines indicate values for which the effect size is about medium (0.5), or small (0.2).

3.2. Evaluation of Standing Balance Performance with a Force Plate

Dynamic balance was evaluated using the mean maximum displacement values with the body inclined in the anterior, posterior, right and left directions (tilts) while standing. Figure 12 shows the tilt performance difference in the training groups from the first to fourth rounds and control groups in these directions with or without a mattress. Figure 13 shows the results of the total LoS test for the same groups with and without a mattress. In the initial evaluation, the maximum displacements in the control group were approximately 60 mm anterior tilt, 54 mm posterior tilt, 60 mm right tilt, and 57 mm left tilt. Conversely, the maximum displacement values in the trunk-training group were approximately 79 mm of anterior tilt, 78 mm of posterior tilt, 74 mm of right tilt, and 88 mm of left tilt. In the post-training evaluation, the maximum displacement values in the trunk-training group were approximately 80 mm anterior tilt, 85 mm posterior tilt, 83 mm right tilt, and 82 mm left tilt.

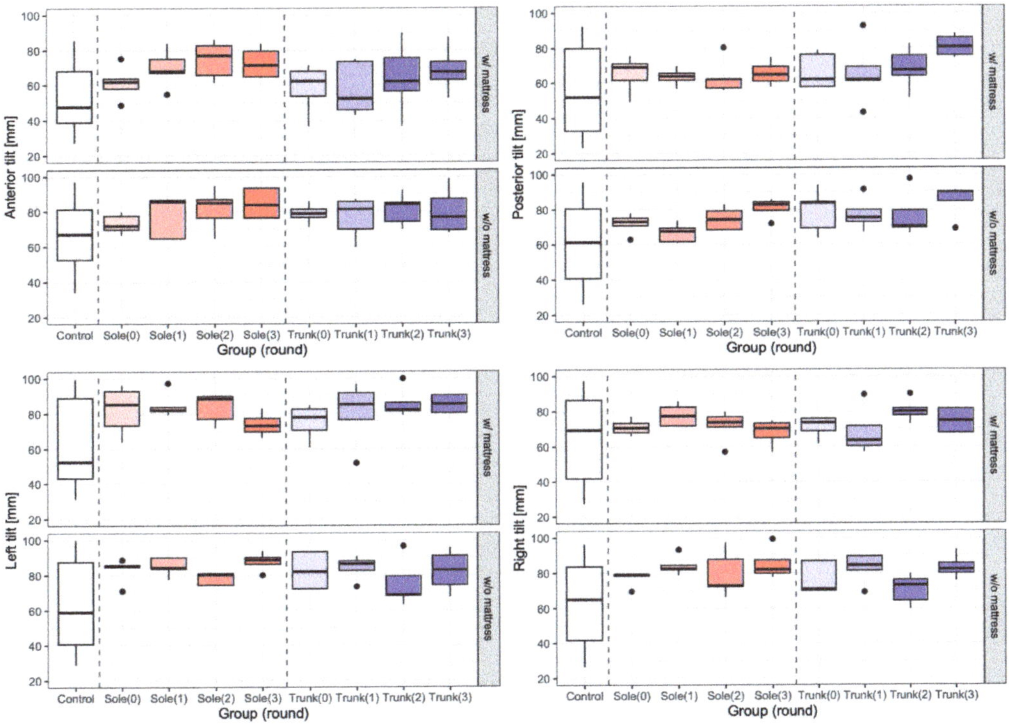

Figure 12. Dynamic balance performance with and without a mattress. Top left: anterior tilt, top right: posterior tilt, bottom left: left tilt, bottom right: right tilt. The top and bottom of each graph indicate the case with and without a mattress, respectively. Round 0 refers to the period before the intervention. The box plots in white, red and blue are the results for the control, sole training and trunk training groups, respectively.

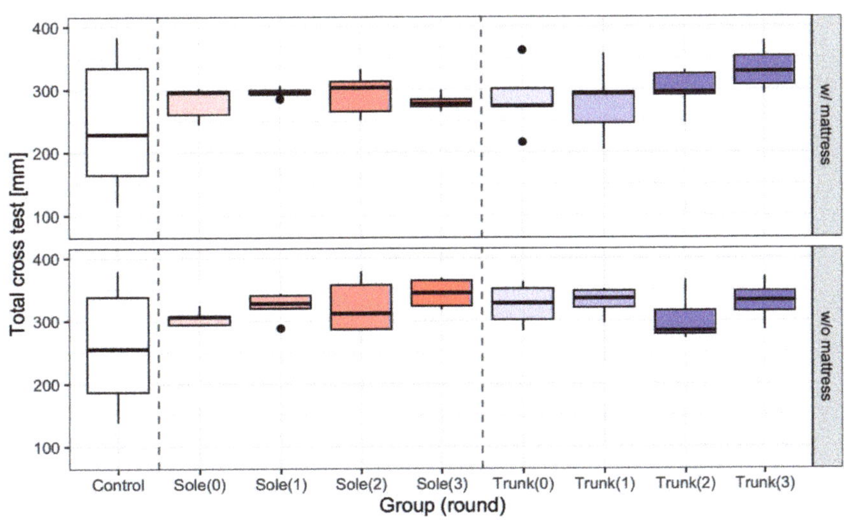

Figure 13. Performance of the total LoS test with and without a mattress. Round 0 refers to the period before the intervention. The box plots in white, red and blue are the results for the control, sole training and trunk training groups, respectively.

Table 3 presents the statistical results of the effects of the experimental conditions on dynamic balance performance. In general, significant differences were found in some balance metrics in the trunk and sole training groups against the control group. While significant differences were confirmed in the number of rounds and the use of the mattress in the anterior and posterior tilts as well as in the total tilt of LoS test, no significant differences in the number of rounds were confirmed in the left and right tilts. Furthermore, with regard to the correct response rate for vibration, the higher the discriminative ability in the trunk, the greater the tilts, but there was no significant relationship between the correct response rate for the sole and the tilts. Table 4 shows the correlation coefficient between correct rates of vibrations and LoS tilts. When the correct response rate was high for the two vibrations on the sole and trunk, a correlation was confirmed in which the tilt value became significantly larger. According to the value of the correlation coefficient, while the correct response rate of the two vibrations on the sole was significantly correlated, that of a single vibration on the sole would correlate negatively to the tilt values. However, as no significant difference was found in the correct rates for the sole in Table 3, the significant correlation on the sole might be less dominant than the sole training group itself.

Table 3. The p-values acquired by robust multiple regression analysis for rounds, mattress usage, correct rates to the two vibrations, places to vibrate, and training groups with dynamic balance performances (LoS test). The results are rounded to the fourth decimal place.

	Anterior Tilt		Posterior Tilt		Right Tilt		Left Tilt		Total Cross Test	
	p		p		p		p		p	
Rounds	<0.001	***	<0.001	***	0.130		0.415		0.029	*
Mattress usage	<0.001	***	<0.001	***	0.008	**	0.169		<0.001	***
Correct rates (sole)	0.626		0.324		0.896		0.599		0.550	
Correct rates (trunk)	0.024	*	0.003	**	0.004	**	0.005	**	0.015	**
Training group (sole)	<0.001	***	<0.001	***	0.007	**	0.007	***	<0.001	***
Training group (trunk)	<0.001	***	<0.001	***	0.001	**	0.001	***	<0.001	***

***: $p < 0.001$, **: $p < 0.01$, *: $p < 0.05$.

Table 4. The correlation coefficient between correct rates of vibrations (column) and LoS tilts (row). Orange and red bold text indicates significant coefficients ($p < 0.05$) with small and medium effect sizes by Cohen's criterion [39].

	Sole			Trunk		
	0 Vibration	1 Vibration	2 Vibrations	0 Vibration	1 Vibration	2 Vibrations
Anterior tilt	0.10	−0.06	**0.19**	0.16	−0.02	**0.41**
Posterior tilt	0.08	**−0.29**	0.16	0.08	0.05	**0.43**
Right tilt	0.10	**−0.19**	**0.27**	0.01	0.03	**0.45**
Left tilt	0.07	**−0.20**	**0.28**	0.08	−0.02	**0.48**
Total tilt	0.10	**−0.21**	**0.25**	0.09	0.01	**0.49**

Therefore, based on the results described in Figures 12 and 13, as well as Tables 3 and 4, vibration training for both the trunk and the sole positively impacts balance ability. The larger sway seen in the training groups versus controls reflects a better capability to shift the center of pressure towards stability limits while maintaining balance. This increased movement range signifies improved dynamic postural control rather than instability, as supported by previous research [31]. In dynamic balance tasks such as our LoS assessment, larger controlled movements usually suggest superior balance performance and increased movement confidence, contrary to static balance tasks, where reduced sway is generally preferred [40]. However, when examining the relationship between discrimination ability and balance ability, it was found that while vibration discrimination ability for the trunk could have a positive relationship with balance ability, the discrimination ability for the soles may not affect to balance ability.

When comparing the training groups, the anterior and posterior tilts and the total LoS test for both the trunk and sole training groups were larger than those of the control group for factors where significant differences were observed. In the anterior tilt, the sole exercise group showed significantly greater improvement than the trunk exercise group ($p = 0.013 < 0.05$, d = 0.27 (small)), whereas in the posterior tilt, the trunk exercise group showed significantly greater improvement than the sole exercise group ($p < 0.001$, d = 0.46 (medium)). There was no significant difference in the left and right tilts between the plantar and trunk groups ($p > 0.10$, d < 0.2 (negligible)).

Thus, the results indicated that after 10 weeks of training, there could be a significant improvement in dynamic balance performance in the sole and trunk training groups compared with the control group.

4. Discussion

The flexibility and stability of the foot arches are closely related to standing and walking balance [41]. In particular, a low medial longitudinal arch (MLA) can negatively affect balance by disrupting foot stability and the relationship between the foot and the floor [42–44]. Moreover, several studies have reported a relationship between arch pathologies and poor postural sway in young adults and seniors aged over 65 years [45]. Because the longitudinal arch is known to have a significant influence on balance, in the present study, we decided to present vibration stimulation methods focusing on the medial arch of the sole, which is particularly important.

Several researchers have proven the effectiveness of vibrator stimulation at improving dynamic balance [12,46,47]. For the plantar vibrator stimulation, Khalifeloo et al. [48] indicated that vibratory stimuli applied to the plantar region of patients' post-stroke could have beneficial effects on dynamic balance, as assessed by the timed "Up & Go" (TUG) test [49,50]. Önala et al. further showed the effectiveness of local vibration stimulation training applied to the plantar region of the foot with conventional rehabilitation on static and dynamic balance in stroke patients [51]. The results of the present study showed that the effects of 10 weeks of plantar vibration stimulation training may improve dynamic balance ability.

Regarding the influence of trunk vibration somatosensory stimulation on standing balance, Goldberg et al. reported that trunk repositioning errors (TREs) were reliable and valid measures of underlying balance impairment in older adults, indicating that TREs may ultimately be proven to be a marker of fall risk. Further, TREs indicated the assessment of trunk position sense difficulty [52]. In another study, Sonasath et al. reported that children with spastic diplegic C.P. with better lumbar position sense scored greater in static and dynamic balance [53]. To the best of our knowledge, studies investigating the effects of somatosensory stimulation on the trunk on balance are rare. In this study, similar to plantar vibration stimulation training, the results showed that trunk vibration stimulation training could be expected to have an effect on dynamic balance ability.

Overall, this study found no significant difference between the two groups in the vibration sensation training group for the sole and the trunk (Figure 10); however, the correct response rate with stimulation of the two sites was generally lower than that with stimulation of one site after training (Figures 7 and 8). This is similar to the finding that older adults tend to show decreased sensitivity to vibratory stimulation in threshold tests for vibratory stimulation delivered to their legs [12,14,54]. On the other hand, the correct response rate for vibration stimulation showed a significant increase as the number of training sessions increased (Figure 11). Therefore, it was suggested that vibration sensation training enhanced vibration sensation. Although no significant difference was observed in this study, the fact that the effect size was larger when the vibration stimulators were positioned diagonally than when they were arranged horizontally or vertically (Figure 9) is consistent with the results of previous studies that investigated tactile pressure sensation in the fingers [55,56].

According to the results of Tables 3 and 4, there was a significant positive correlation between the correct response rate for each of the two-point stimuli on the trunk and sole, and the limits of stability (LoS) test. However, for the sole, the positive response rate for single-point stimulation was negatively correlated with the ability to maintain dynamic postural stability. In other words, improving sensation through sensory training of the trunk and sole could be related to improving dynamic balance. However, improving sensation at a single point on the sole may have a greater effect on static dynamic balance than dynamic balance [6,11,15,56]. A one-point stimulus is a local stimulus and a two-point stimulus indicates the direction of the stimulus, providing a sense of spatial awareness related to dynamic balance. Further investigation is needed to explore how single- and two-point stimulations affect static and dynamic standing balances. These findings suggest that improving the tactile function of the trunk and the sole is important for posture control. Additionally, the results in Tables 3 and 4 also highlight the importance of discriminating between multiple vibrations. These findings suggest that improving the tactile function of the trunk and the sole is important for posture control, and the results in Table 4 also suggest that discriminating between multiple vibrations is particularly essential. Indeed, it has been reported that the simultaneous stimulation of two sites requires more complex processing than a single stimulation of one site, and hence, it is more difficult for older people to perceive [57,58].

Mechanoreceptors that react to the simultaneous stimulation of the two sites are likely to affect spatial resolution and postural changes. Improvement in sensing and reaction to stimulation of the two sites may, therefore, allow a person to perceive movements of the center of gravity and thus control posture, meaning that trunk sensory training may be important for postural control.

The results further indicated that plantar stimulation improved the dynamic balance ability in the direction of the anterior and posterior body sway. Parsons et al. [59] further indicated that plantar sensation on the affected side of patients with stroke was correlated with the Berg Balance Scale (BBS) [60] and the anteroposterior center of pressure variability in the eyes-closed standing position. Moreover, Wanderley et al. reported that the application of local vibration to the plantar region has beneficial effects on postural control along the anteroposterior axis [61]. These findings are consistent with our results.

In the present study, the results of the logistic regression analysis showed an association between the correct response rate with vertical stimulation of the two sites and the forward and backward displacement values in the LoS test; however, equations were only found for the total anteroposterior movement of the center of gravity, which is easy to understand as the movement of the trunk, and vertically paired stimulation of the trunk region, which had a good rate of correct responses. Several prior studies have reported that tactile sensations, such as touch–pressure sensation and vibratory sensations of the sole, are important in relation to standing balance and gait performance [62–64]. Several studies have also reported that the reactions to tactile sensation of the sole are dominant over reactions to visual and vestibular sensations as reactions for postural control [65,66]. From this, it could be concluded that tactile sensations in the soles and trunk are particularly important for avoiding falls while standing or walking. The high correlation between the tactile sensation of the trunk and the dynamic center of gravity data in the present study indicates the importance of sole and trunk sensory in preventing falls.

Several scholarly articles address the physiological mechanisms through which vibration sensory stimulation training influences human physical movement. Vibratory sensory stimulation impacts motor control by activating sensory receptors and integrating information within the somatosensory and association cortices. This study posits that vibration applied to the trunk or soles may enhance postural muscle activity in older adults experiencing age-related sensory decline; however, the underlying neural mechanisms require further investigation [67]. This study examined whether subsensory vibratory noise generated by a piezoelectric insole could enhance sensation, balance, and gait among older individuals. The findings indicated improvements in balance and gait, suggesting that applying stochastic resonance to the foot's sensory systems may contribute to fall prevention. In contrast to our study, previous research employed short-term stimulation (lasting less than two weeks), specifically targeting only the medial plantar arch [68]. Neck muscle vibration (NMV) and trunk proprioception significantly influence body perception and postural control. NMV induces an illusion of muscle stretching, thereby shifting the center of pressure (COP), while trunk vibration modifies gait trajectory. Both observations imply that vibratory stimulation can effectively modulate COP, showcasing its utility as a tool for postural training [69]. Sensory training aimed at both the trunk and soles can enhance standing balance, although their individual contributions remain ambiguous. Further research should investigate the effects of trunk and plantar sensations on postural control across various movements, such as standing, walking, and different phases of gait, to optimize sensory training tailored to each posture.

In clinical implications, vibratory stimulation is inherently safe, poses no risk of side effects, and is cost-effective, making it highly practical. The results of this study have clarified that sensory training of the soles of the feet or the trunk is connected to improved dynamic standing balance ability. Accordingly, when the standing balance ability of older adults is decreased or lost, we believe that it is important to actively evaluate and train the senses of the trunk and the soles of the feet, in addition to the conventional balance training practiced in clinical settings. Furthermore, the type of shoe insole and trunk orthosis with vibratory stimulators are considered valuable as portable sensory training devices that can facilitate the sensation of the soles of the feet and the trunk. By utilizing a vibration device or a balance training app based on IMU (Inertial measurement unit), motion analysis can be conducted in a game-like manner, which can boost user motivation and create a more effective training method under appropriate medical professional guidance.

Limitations

Although the LoS data were used as an index of dynamic balance ability in this study, adjustments may be necessary when comparing groups of different heights. To further clarify the relationship between dynamic balance ability and sensory training, it is essential to measure trunk and lower extremity joint movements and muscle activity using various motion analysis methods to analyze the relationship factors with higher accuracy. Additionally, it is important to consider measuring brain activity to support the impact of sensory training on standing balance ability. When collecting data on older adults' characteristics, it is essential to acknowledge that differences in age, slight variations in sensory thresholds, and personal physical activity abilities may also influence responses to vibratory stimulation. This will include examination of the superiority of the effects on standing balance of a trunk training group and a sole training group, examination of the effects on standing balance of long-term sensory training of 12–14 weeks or more with a larger sample size, examination of sex differences, and examination of the specifications of the vibratory device, including miniaturization and vibratory stimulation at different frequencies.

The sample size in this study may have been insufficient. Concerning the result of the χ^2 test presented in Section 3.1, which indicated that the control group committed significantly more errors than both the sole and trunk training groups as the number of rounds increased, the power analysis conducted using the *pwr* (ver. 1.3.0) and *pwrss* (ver. 0.3.1) packages in R [70,71] revealed a value of 0.67, which falls short of the threshold of 0.8. However, a post hoc power analysis of the ANOVA results presented in the same section, conducted using the *Superpower* package (ver. 0.2.0) of the R software (ver. 4.2.2) [72], indicated that the statistical power exceeded 0.8 for all the factors and interactions that demonstrated significance. When we analyzed the post hoc power of the significant results from the multiple comparisons using the *PMCMRplus* package (ver. 1.9.10) in R software [73], we found that the power exceeded 0.8 whenever a significant difference was observed. Furthermore, concerning the outcomes of the robust regression illustrated in Figure 3, the power analysis based on R^2 utilizing the aforementioned *pwr* and *pwrss* packages [70,71] revealed that all tilt parameters exhibited a power greater than 0.8. This observation also indicates that internal validity was upheld to some extent, despite the limitations imposed by the sample size. Using the same power analysis packages, we also conducted a post hoc power analysis on the correlations with a medium effect size presented in Table 4 and found that the statistical power exceeded 0.8, even for the small samples in this study. In instances where a small correlation coefficient is observed, if the absolute value does not surpass 0.25, the statistical power remains below 0.8. Nonetheless, despite the significance and sufficient statistical power yielded by these results, limitations persist regarding the demonstration of consistent internal validity and the establishment of a clear causal relationship. Therefore, additional studies are imperative to thoroughly investigate both internal and external validities, as well as precise causality, involving a larger participant pool. At that time, it will be crucial to examine the various dynamic and static balance metrics in relation to diverse participant characteristics, such as age, gender, and personality traits, within an expanded group of older adults encompassing a range of influencing factors.

5. Conclusions

In the present study, we investigated the effects of vibratory stimulation training on standing balance using a new vibratory sensation test device. The participants were all elderly individuals aged 65 years or older, who were divided into two training groups and a control group for comparison and analysis. Trunk or sole region vibratory sensation training was carried out for 10 weeks. Balance was measured as dynamic balance, while vibratory sensation was evaluated as the rate of correct responses. Overall, the trunk and the sole training group showed an improvement in the correct response rate over time, as well as an improvement in dynamic balance performance. A significant relationship was found between vibratory sensation and dynamic balance performance, both of which are linked to the causes of falls. The results of a series of analyses indicated that the intervention in this study led to improvements in the correct response rate for vibrations and balance performance. These improvements, combined with the effects of the intervention itself, led to improvements in dynamic balance performance, indicating that they could be used as interventions to reduce falls in older adults. To validate and expand upon our findings, future work should examine the superiority of the effects of trunk and sole training on standing balance and the effects of long-term sensory training for 12–14 weeks or more on standing balance using a larger sample size.

Author Contributions: Conceptualization, T.T.; methodology, T.T.; validation, T.M.; formal analysis, Y.M. and T.M.; investigation, Y.M.; data curation, T.T. and T.M.; writing—original draft preparation, T.T. and T.M.; writing—review and editing, T.T.; visualization, Y.M.; project administration, T.T.; funding acquisition, T.T. All authors have read and agreed to the published version of the manuscript.

Funding: This work was supported by Japan Society for the Promotion of Science (JSPS), KAKENHI, Grant Number JP20K20494, and JP21H04580.

Institutional Review Board Statement: This study was conducted with the approval of the Institutional Review Board of The University of Tokyo (approval review no. 21-230, 21-231). Approval date: 21 September 2021.

Informed Consent Statement: Informed consent was obtained from all participants involved in the study.

Data Availability Statement: The datasets analyzed during this study are available from the corresponding author upon reasonable request.

Conflicts of Interest: The authors declare no conflicts of interest.

References

1. American Geriatrics Society; British Geriatrics Society; American Academy of Orthopaedic Surgeons Panel on Falls Prevention. Guideline for the prevention of falls in older persons. *J. Am. Geriatr. Soc.* **2001**, *49*, 664–672. [CrossRef]
2. Blake, A.J.; Morgan, K.; Bendall, M.J.; Dallosso, H.; Ebrahim, S.B.; Arie, T.H.; Fentem, P.H.; Bassey, E.J. Falls by elderly people at home: Prevalence and associated factors. *Age Ageing* **1988**, *17*, 365–372. [CrossRef] [PubMed]
3. Yoshida, H.; Hunkyung, K. Frequency of falls and their prevention. *Clin. Calcium* **2006**, *16*, 1444–1450. [PubMed]
4. Birmingham, T. Test-retest reliability of lower extremity functional instability measures. *Clin. J. Sport Med.* **2000**, *10*, 264–268. [CrossRef]
5. Brouwer, B.; Culham, E.G.; Liston, R.A.; Grant, T. Normal variability of postural measures: Implications for the reliability of relative balance performance outcomes. *Scand. J. Rehabil. Med.* **1998**, *30*, 131–137. [CrossRef]
6. Maeda, Y.; Tanaka, T.; Miyasaka, T.; Shimizu, K. A Preliminary Study of Static and Dynamic Standing Balance and Risk of Falling in an Independent Elderly Population with a Particular Focus on the Limit of Stability Test. *J. Phys. Ther. Sci.* **2011**, *23*, 803–806. [CrossRef]
7. Duncan, P.W.; Weiner, D.K.; Chandler, J.; Studenski, S. Functional Reach: A New Clinical Measure of Balance. *J. Gerontol.* **1990**, *45*, M192–M197. [CrossRef]
8. Dibble, L.E.; Lopez-Lennon, C.; Lake, W.; Hoffmeister, C.; Gappmaier, E. Utility of disease-specific measures and clinical balance tests in prediction of falls in persons with multiple sclerosis. *J. Neurol. Phys. Ther.* **2013**, *37*, 99–104. [CrossRef]
9. Poncumhak, P.; Srithawong, A.; Duangsanjun, W.; Amput, P. Comparison of the Ability of Static and Dynamic Balance Tests to Determine the Risk of Falls among Older Community-Dwelling Individuals. *J. Funct. Morphol. Kinesiol.* **2023**, *8*, 43. [CrossRef]
10. Bronstein, A.M.; Brandt, T.; Woollacott, M.; Nutt, J.G. *Clinical Disorders of Balance, Posture and Gait*, 2nd ed.; A Hodder Arnold Publication: Cary, NC, USA, 2004.
11. Tanaka, T.; Noriyasu, S.; Ino, S.; Ifukube, T.; Nakata, M. Objective method to determine the contribution of the great toe to standing balance and preliminary observations of age-related effects. *IEEE Trans. Rehabil. Eng.* **1996**, *4*, 84–90. [CrossRef]
12. Tanaka, T.; Shirogane, S.; Izumi, T.; Ino, S.; Ifukube, T. The Effect of Brief Moving Vibratory Stimulation on the Feet for Postural Control in a Comparison Study. *Phys. Occup. Ther. Geriatr.* **2005**, *24*, 1–23. [CrossRef]
13. Inglis, J.T.; Horak, F.B.; Shupert, C.L.; Jones-Rycewicz, C. The importance of somatosensory information in triggering and scaling automatic postural responses in humans. *Exp. Brain Res.* **1994**, *101*, 159–164. [CrossRef] [PubMed]
14. Kenshalo, D.R. Somesthetic sensitivity in young and elderly humans. *J. Gerontol.* **1986**, *41*, 732–742. [CrossRef]
15. Ballardini, G.; Florio, V.; Canessa, A.; Carlini, G.; Morasso, P.; Casadio, M. Vibrotactile Feedback for Improving Standing Balance. *Front. Bioeng. Biotechnol.* **2020**, *8*, 94. [CrossRef]
16. Xu, J.; Bao, T.; Lee, U.H.; Kinnaird, C.; Carender, W.; Huang, Y.; Sienko, K.H.; Shull, P.B. Configurable, wearable sensing and vibrotactile feedback system for real-time postural balance and gait training: Proof-of-concept. *J. Neuroeng. Rehabil.* **2017**, *14*, 102. [CrossRef]
17. LeVeau, B.F. *Williams and Lissner's Biomechanics of Human Motion*, 3rd ed.; WB Saunders: Philadelphia, PA, USA, 1992; pp. 12–14.
18. Jijimol, G.; Fayaz, R.K.; Vijesh, P.V. Correlation of trunk impairment with balance in patients with chronic stroke. *NeuroRehabilitation* **2013**, *32*, 323–325. [CrossRef]
19. Johansson, G.; Jarnlo, G. Balance training in 70-year-old women. *Physiother. Theory Pract.* **1991**, *7*, 121–125. [CrossRef]

20. Dean, C.M.; Channon, E.F.; Hall, J.M. Sitting training early after stroke improves sitting ability and quality and carries over to standing up but not to walking: A randomized trial. *Aust. J. Physiother.* **2007**, *53*, 97–102. [CrossRef]
21. Hopewell, S.; Adedire, O.; Copsey, B.J.; Boniface, G.J.; Sherrington, C.; Clemson, L.; Close, J.C.; Lamb, S.E. Multifactorial and multiple component interventions for preventing falls in older people living in the community. *Cochrane Database Syst. Rev.* **2018**, *23*, 7. [CrossRef]
22. Buchner, D.M.; Cress, M.E.; De Lateur, B.J.; Esselman, P.C.; Margherita, A.J.; Price, R.; Wagner, E.H. The effect of strength and endurance training on gait, balance, fall risk, and health services use in community-living older adults. *J. Gerontol. Ser. A Biol. Sci. Med. Sci.* **1997**, *52*, M218–M224. [CrossRef]
23. Lord, S.R.; Ward, J.A.; Williams, P.; Strudwick, M. The effect of a 12-month exercise trial on balance, strength, and falls in older women: A randomized controlled trial. *J. Am. Geriatr. Soc.* **1995**, *43*, 1198–1206. [CrossRef] [PubMed]
24. Zhang, S.L.; Liu, D.; Yu, D.Z.; Zhu, Y.T.; Xu, W.C.; Tian, E.; Guo, Z.Q.; Shi, H.B.; Yin, S.K.; Kong, W.J. Multisensory Exercise Improves Balance in People with Balance Disorders: A Systematic Review. *Curr. Med. Sci.* **2021**, *41*, 635–648. [CrossRef] [PubMed]
25. Allison, L.K.; Kiemel, T.; Jeka, J.J. Sensory-Challenge Balance Exercises Improve Multisensory Reweighting in Fall-Prone Older Adults. *J. Neurol. Phys. Ther.* **2018**, *42*, 84–93. [CrossRef]
26. Sienko, K.H.; Balkwill, M.D.; Oddsson, L.I.E.; Wall, C. Effects of multi-directional vibrotactile feedback on vestibular-deficient postural performance during continuous multi-directional support surface perturbations. *J. Vestib. Res.* **2013**, *23*, 33–43. [CrossRef]
27. Ma, C.Z.; Wong, D.W.; Lam, W.K.; Wan, A.H.; Lee, W.C. Balance improvement effects of biofeedback systems with state-of-the-art wearable sensors: A systematic review. *Sensors* **2016**, *16*, 434. [CrossRef]
28. Orr, R. The effect of whole body vibration exposure on balance and functional mobility in older adults: A systematic review and meta-analysis. *Maturitas* **2015**, *80*, 342–358. [CrossRef]
29. Peters, R.M.; McKeown, M.D.; Carpenter, M.G.; Inglis, J.T. Losing touch: Age-related changes in plantar skin sensitivity, lower limb cutaneous reflex strength, and postural stability in older adults. *J. Neurophysiol.* **2016**, *116*, 1848–1858. [CrossRef]
30. Allum, J.H.; Carpenter, M.G.; Honegger, F.; Adkin, A.L.; Bloem, B.R. Age-dependent variations in the directional sensitivity of balance corrections and compensatory arm movements in man. *J. Physiol.* **2002**, *542*, 643–663. [CrossRef]
31. Juras, G.; Słomkal, K.; Fredyk, A.; Sobota, G.; Bacik, B. Evaluation of the Limits of Stability (LOS) Balance Test. *J. Hum. Kinet.* **2008**, *19*, 39–52. [CrossRef]
32. Shumway-Cook, A.; Horak, F.B. Assessing the influence of sensory interaction on balance. *Phys. Ther.* **1986**, *66*, 1548–1550. [CrossRef]
33. Hu, M.H.; Woollacott, M.H. Multisensory training of standing balance in older adults: I. Postural stability and one-leg stance balance. *J. Gerontol.* **1994**, *49*, M52–M61. [CrossRef] [PubMed]
34. Hirase, T.; Inokuchi, S.; Matsusaka, N.; Okita, M. Effects of a Balance Training Program Using a Foam Rubber Pad in Community-Based Older Adults. A Randomized Controlled Trial. *J. Geriatr. Phys. Ther.* **2015**, *38*, 62–70. [CrossRef] [PubMed]
35. Wobbrock, J.O.; Findlater, L.; Gergle, D.; Higgins, J.J. The aligned rank transform was used for non-parametric factorial analyses using only anova. In Proceedings of the SIGCHI Conference on Human Factors in Computing Systems, Vancouver, BC, Canada, 7–12 May 2011; pp. 143–146.
36. Elkin, L.A.; Kay, M.; Higgins, J.J.; Wobbrock, J.O. Rank transform procedure for multifactor contrast tests. In Proceedings of the 34th Annual ACM Symposium on User Interface Software and Technology, Virtual, 10–13 October 2021; pp. 754–768.
37. Lenth, R.V. Least-squares means: R package lsmeans. *J. Stat. Softw.* **2016**, *69*, 1–33. [CrossRef]
38. Lenth, R.; Singmann, H.; Love, J.; Buerkner, P.; Herve, M. Emmeans: Estimated Marginal Means, aka Least-Squares Means. R Package Version 1.10.7. 2018. Available online: https://cran.r-project.org/web/packages/emmeans/emmeans.pdf (accessed on 13 March 2025).
39. Cohen, J. A power primer. *Psychol. Bull.* **1992**, *112*, 155. [CrossRef]
40. Horak, F.B. Postural orientation and equilibrium: What do we need to know about neural control of balance to prevent falls? *Age Ageing* **2006**, *35* (Suppl. S2), ii7–ii11. [CrossRef]
41. Wright, W.G.; Ivanenko, Y.P.; Gurfinkel, V.S. Foot anatomy specialization for postural sensation and control. *J. Neurophysiol.* **2012**, *107*, 1513–1521. [CrossRef]
42. Tsai, L.-C.; Yu, B.; Mercer, V.S.; Gross, M.T. Comparison of different structural foot types for measures of standing postural control. *J. Orthop. Sports Phys. Ther.* **2006**, *36*, 942–953. [CrossRef]
43. Al Abdulwahab, S.S.; Kachanathu, S.J. The effect of various degrees of foot posture on standing balance in a healthy adult population. *Somatosens. Mot. Res.* **2015**, *32*, 172–176. [CrossRef]
44. Anzai, E.; Nakajima, K.; Iwakami, Y.; Sato, M.; Ino, S.; Ifukube, T.; Yamashita, K.; Ohta, Y. Effects of foot arch structure on postural stability. *Clin. Res. Foot Ankle* **2014**, *2*, 132.
45. Saghazadeh, M.; Tsunoda, K.; Tomohiro, O. Foot arch height and rigidity index associated with balance and postural sway in elderly women using a 3D foot scanner. *Foot Ankle Online J.* **2014**, *7*, 10-3827.

46. Lee, S.W.; Cho, K.H.; Lee, W.H. Effect of a local vibration stimulus training programme on postural sway and gait in chronic stroke patients: A randomized controlled trial. *Clin. Rehabil.* **2013**, *27*, 921–931. [CrossRef] [PubMed]
47. Priplata, A.A.; Niemi, J.B.; Harry, J.D.; Lipsitz, L.A.; Collins, J.J. Vibrating insoles and balance control in elderly people. *Lancet* **2003**, *362*, 1123–1124. [CrossRef] [PubMed]
48. Khalifeloo, M.; Naghdi, S.; Ansari, N.N.; Akbari, M.; Jalaie, S.; Jannat, D.; Hasson, S. A study on the immediate effects of plantar vibration on balance dysfunction in patients with stroke. *J. Exerc. Rehabil.* **2018**, *14*, 259–266. [CrossRef]
49. Podsiadlo, D.; Richardson, S. The Time "Up & Go": A Test of Basic Functional Mobility for Frail Elderly Persons. *J. Am. Geriatr. Soc.* **1991**, *39*, 142–148.
50. Shumway Cook, A.; Brauer, S.; Woolacott, M. Predicting the Probability for Falls in Community Dwelling Older Adults Using the Timed Up & Go Test. *Phys. Ther.* **2000**, *80*, 896–903.
51. Önala, B.; Sertelb, M.; Karacaca, G. Effect of plantar vibration on static and dynamic balance instroke patients: A randomised controlled study. *Physiotherapy* **2022**, *116*, 1–8. [CrossRef]
52. Goldberg, A.; Hernandez, M.E.; Alexander, N.B. Trunk repositioning errors are increased in balance-impaired older adults. *J. Gerontol. Ser. A Biol. Sci. Med. Sci.* **2005**, *60*, 1310–1314. [CrossRef]
53. Sonasath, M.K.; Shah, D.S. Effect of Lumbar Position Sense on Lumbar Muscle Strength, Static versus Dynamic Balance and Functional Status in Children with Spastic Diplegic Cerebral Palsy: A Cross-Sectional Study. *Int. J. Health Sci. Res.* **2024**, *14*, 20–27. [CrossRef]
54. Whanger, A.; Wang, H.S. Clinical correlates of the vibratory sense in elderly psychiatric patients. *J. Gerontol.* **1974**, *29*, 39–45. [CrossRef]
55. Johansson, R.S.; Vallbo, A.B. Tactile sensory coding in the glabrous skin of the human hand. *Trends Neurosci.* **1983**, *6*, 27–32. [CrossRef]
56. Ino, S.; Shimizu, S.; Hosoe, F.; Izumi, T.; Takahashi, M.; Ifukube, T. A Basic Study on Tactile Display for Tele-presence. In Proceedings of the IEEE International Workshop on Robot and Human Communication, RO-MAN'92, Tokyo, Japan, 1–3 September 1992; pp. 58–62.
57. Franco, P.G.; Santos, K.B.; Rodacki, A.L. Joint positioning sense, perceived force level and two-point discrimination tests of young and active elderly adults. *Braz. J. Phys. Ther.* **2015**, *19*, 304–310. [CrossRef]
58. Maurer, C.; Mergner, T.; Bolha, B.; Hlavacka, F. Human balance control during cutaneous stimulation of the plantar soles. *Neurosci. Lett.* **2001**, *302*, 45–48. [CrossRef] [PubMed]
59. Parsons, S.L.; Mansfield, A.; Inness, E.L.; Patterson, K.K. The relationship of plantar cutaneous sensation and standing balance post-stroke. *Top. Stroke Rehabil.* **2016**, *23*, 326–332. [CrossRef] [PubMed]
60. Berg, K.; Wood-Dauphinee, S.; Williams, J.I.; Gayton, D. Measuring balance in the elderly: Preliminary development of an instrument. *Physiother. Can.* **1989**, *41*, 304–311. [CrossRef]
61. Wanderley, F.S.; Alburquerque-Sendin, F.; Parizotto, N.A.; Rebelatto, J.R. Effect of plantar vibration stimuli on the balance of older women: A randomized controlled trial. *Arch. Phys. Med. Rehabil.* **2011**, *92*, 199–206. [CrossRef]
62. Menz, H.B.; Lord, S.R.; St George, R.; Fitzpatrick, R.C. Walking stability and sensorymotor function in older people with diabetic peripheral neuropathy. *Arch. Phys. Med. Rehabil.* **2004**, *85*, 245–252. [CrossRef]
63. Lord, S.R.; Clark, R.D.; Webster, I.W. Postural stability and associated physiological factors in a population of aged persons. *J. Gerontol.* **1991**, *46*, M69–M76. [CrossRef]
64. Kavounoudias, A.; Roll, R.; Roll, J.-P. Foot sole and ankle muscle inputs contribute jointly to human erect posture regulation. *J. Physiol.* **2001**, *532*, 869–878. [CrossRef]
65. Dietz, V.; Trippel, M.; Horstmann, G.A. Significance of proprioceptive and vestibulo-spinal reflexes in the control of stance and gait. In *Adaptability of Human Gait*; Patla, A.E., Ed.; Elsevier: Amsterdam, The Netherlands, 1991; pp. 17–52.
66. Massion, J.; Wollacott, M. Normal balance and postural control. In *Clinical Aspects of Balance and Gait Disorders*; Bronstein, A.M., Brandit, T., Woollacott, M., Eds.; Edward Arnold: London, UK, 1996.
67. Shumway-Cook, A.; Woollacott, M.H. *Motor Control: Translating Research into Clinical Practice*, 3rd ed.; Lippincott Williams & Wilkins: Philadelphia, PA, USA, 2007; pp. 52–62.
68. Lipsitz, L.A.; Lough, M.; Niemi, J.; Travison, T.; Howlett, H.; Manor, B. A shoe insole delivering subsensory vibratory noise improves balance and gait in healthy elderly people. *Arch. Phys. Med. Rehabil.* **2015**, *96*, 432–439. [CrossRef]
69. Hirosawa, M.; Takehara, I.; Moriyama, Y.; Amimoto, K. Effects of unilateral neck muscle vibration on standing postural orientation and spatial perception in healthy subjects based on stimulus duration and simultaneous stimulation of trunk muscles. *PLoS ONE* **2023**, *18*, e0281012. [CrossRef] [PubMed]
70. Champely, S.; Ekstrom, C.; Dalgaard, P.; Gill, J.; Weibelzahl, S.; Anandkumar, A.; Ford, C.; Volcic, R.; De Rosario, H. pwr: Basic Functions for Power Analysis. 2017. Available online: https://cran.r-project.org/web/packages/pwr/ (accessed on 6 March 2025).

71. Bulus, M. Pwrss: Statistical Power and Sample Size Calculation Tools. Available online: https://CRAN.R-project.org/package=pwrss (accessed on 6 March 2025).
72. Lakens, D.; Caldwell, A.R. Simulation-based power analysis for factorial analysis of variance designs. *Adv. Methods Pract. Psychol. Sci.* **2021**, *4*, 2515245920951503. [CrossRef]
73. Pohlert, T. PMCMRplus: Calculate Pairwise Multiple Comparisons of Mean Rank Sums Extended. R Package Version 1.9.10. 2023. Available online: https://CRAN.R-project.org/package=PMCMRplus (accessed on 6 March 2025).

Journal of
Functional Morphology and Kinesiology

MDPI

Article

Effects of Functional Partial Body Weight Support Treadmill Training on Mobility in Children with Ataxia: A Randomized Controlled Trial

Alexandra Lepoura [1,*], Sofia Lampropoulou [2], Antonis Galanos [3], Marianna Papadopoulou [1], Georgios Gkrimas [4], Magda Tziomaki [4] and Vasiliki Sakellari [1,*]

1 Physiotherapy Department, School of Health and Care Sciences, University of West Attica, Agiou Spidonos 28, 2243 Athens, Greece; mpapad@uniwa.gr
2 Department of Physiotherapy, School of Health Rehabilitation Science, University of Patras, 26504 Rion, Greece; lampropoulou@upatras.gr
3 Laboratory for Research of the Musculoskeletal System (LRMS), School of Medicine, National and Kapodistrian University of Athens, University Campus, 15784 Athens, Greece; galanostat@yahoo.gr
4 Gait & Motion Analysis Center, ELEPAP, Kononos 16, 11634 Athens, Greece; gait_lab@elepap.gr (G.G.); mtziomaki@gmail.com (M.T.)
* Correspondence: alepoura@uniwa.gr (A.L.); vsakellari@uniwa.gr (V.S.); Tel.: +30-69-4862-0233 (A.L.)

Abstract: Background/Objectives: Ataxia is quite common in pediatric neuromotor disorders and has a highly heterogeneous etiology. Mobility difficulties and functional limitations reflect the lack of coordination in this population. The aim of this study is to assess the effectiveness of an intensive program of Functional Partial Body Weight Support Treadmill Training (FPBWSTT) on the mobility and functionality of children with ataxia. **Methods:** Through a stratified randomized control trial, a sample of 18 children with progressive and non-progressive ataxia and GMFCS II-IV (mean age: 14 years; standard deviation: 2.5) was assessed prior to the intervention, post-intervention, and 2 months after its end. Motor and functional skills were assessed with the Gross Motor Function Measure (GMFM, items D-E), the Pediatric Balance Scale (PBS), a 10 m walk test (10 MWT), a 6 min walk test (6 MWT), the Scale for Assessment and Rating Ataxia (SARA), the TimedUp and Go (TUG) test, spatiotemporal gait parameters, and kinetic and kinematic variables of the pelvis and lower limb. **Results:** Statistically significant interactions and changes in favor of the FPBWSTT were found in all functional assessments and spatiotemporal gait parameters ($p < 0.05$), the majority of which were maintained for two months. There was no statistical interaction or change in kinematic parameters ($p > 0.05$), while kinetic variables were insufficiently collected and were not statistically analyzed. **Conclusions:** The FPBWSTT is more effective on the mobility and functionality of children with ataxia who are 8–18 years old, compared to typical physiotherapy. Kinematic variables may not be sensitive indicators of change over a short period of time and/or in this population.

Keywords: functional; treadmill training; partial body weight support; children; ataxia

1. Introduction

Ataxia in childhood is a clinical manifestation of neuromotor disorders, the occurrence of which is estimated at about 26/100,000 children in Europe and probably reflects a minimum prevalence worldwide [1]. In many countries, including Greece, official data on the prevalence of ataxia in the pediatric population are lacking, while both assessment and intervention strategies seem to have been poorly studied worldwide [2].

The pathogenesis of childhood ataxia is characterized by great heterogeneity, with progressive and non-progressive cerebellar ataxia being its two main types [3]. The causes of this movement disorder can be acquired, such as cerebellar tumors; congenital, such as cerebral palsy; or genetic, such as Friedrich's ataxia [3]. European data show that the highest incidence of ataxia in children is overall ataxia of genetic origin (14.61/100,000 births), while ataxia as a result of CP is the most studied in Europe and the most frequent among non-progressive disorders (10.65/100,000 births) [1]. In accordance with European data, a recent Greek cross-cultural adaptation [4] of the Scale for Assessment and Rating Ataxia (SARA) [5] found a rate of 54.4% for ataxic cerebral palsy and a rate of 62.5% for Friedrich ataxia in the non-progressive and progressive ataxia categories, respectively.

The symptoms of a taxi are ferto a set of difficulties that manifest in each type and etiology of ataxia, with varying degrees of severity and limitations in daily activities [6]. Lack of balance and coordination are the primary difficulties, evident in the quality and quantity of daily activities where children interact. Ataxic gait, dysmetria, dysdiadochokinesia, tremor, nystagmus, and dysarthria are some of the key clinical features underlying the symptomatology of cerebellar ataxia, regardless of its etiology [7–9]. According to Hartley et al. [2], investigating the assessment and treatment of children with various types of ataxia, it appeared that over forty different outcome measures were used in the twenty studies included in their systematic review. The majority of these studies focused on balance, gait, and gross motor function, identifying gait performance as a basic physiotherapy goal. The few data existing from children with ataxia report reduced cadence, step, and stride length; increased step width; variability in gait measures; and abnormalities in motor and kinematic characteristics [10–13]. These factors may serve as sensitive indicators of the progression of ataxia but also indicate the "instability" of ataxic gait pattern within the heterogeneous population investigated [10–13]. However, it seems that changes in gait performance and parameters in the pediatric population with ataxia after physiotherapy interventions have been poorly studied, mainly within short-term frames [2].

Treadmill interventions with and without partial body weight support are suggested as a means of faster gait acquisition, gross motor and gait parameters' improvement in pediatric populations with various neuromotor disorders. However, the application of different protocols in different neuromotor populations, coupled with the small sample sizes, fail to demonstrate a clear and effective guideline [2,14–17]. An important factor of the therapeutic effectiveness is the dosage of training, which varies according to the intensity (e.g., treadmill speed, incline) or duration [17], prompting the need to standardize and test protocols appropriately designed for specific pediatric populations. The strategy of increasing speed during gait training has been well documented with positive results, but speed alternations, as suggested by Bjornson et al. [18], for children with CP, are so far a rather "challenging" approach, worthy of investigation, especially in ataxia. The cerebellum, the main dysfunctional structure resulting in ataxia, has a regulatory role in gait speed control, and its activation during such challenging gait training [19] may be a promising therapeutic intervention. Another suggested therapeutic strategy recorded in adults with neuromotor deficits [20,21] and pediatric populations [22,23] seems to be dual-task training, which defines a functional and demanding approach, especially when combined with gait, capable of promoting neuroplasticity [24].

Through this study, we aim to investigate the effects of integrating speed-alternation treadmill training with dual-task functional activities on improving gait performance and gross motor function in children with ataxia. We anticipate that this study will provide further clinical, practical, and research insights, as well as a better understanding for future therapeutic purposes.

2. Materials and Methods

A stratified, randomized, controlled trial of 4-week Functional Partial Body Weight Support Treadmill Training (FPBWSTT), with a 2-month follow-up period, was applied to children with ataxia (progressive and non-progressive), aged 8–18 years and Gross Motor Function Classification System (GMFCS) II-IV. The clinical trial was registered to ISRCTN (ISRCTN54463720), following ethical approval from the University of West Attica (study protocol: 14η/26 April 2021) and 'ATTIKON' General University Hospital of Athens (study protocol: Γ ΠΑΙΔ, ΕΒΔ 149/20 March 2020). Participant recruitment started in June 2021 and was finally completed in the middle of December 2022, with the last data collected in the end of March 2023.

The protocol of this study with all methodological information was applied as was published in March 2022 [25]. The consort checklist is further provided as a Supplementary Materials.

2.1. Group Allocation

Inclusion and exclusion criteria for participant recruitment was administered as originally planned in the study protocol [25]. Participants were randomly allocated to the intervention group (FPBWSTT group) or control group, using a stratification method, based on the type of ataxia disorder. Two strata were used to stratify the sample: progressive and non-progressive ataxia type [26]. An independent researcher from data collection was responsible for creating the allocation process, which was kept hidden from the rest of the research team. Children from both groups continued to receive their typical therapy (physiotherapy and any other therapies they received, such as occupational therapy, speech therapy, etc.). The FBPWSTT group additionally followed the 4-week intervention program (FPBWSTT).

2.2. Intervention and Settings

The FPBWSTT was designed based on the implementation of a treadmill gait protocol with speed change intervals [18] combined with dual-task functional activities, according to applications in different population groups [20,21,27–29]. The implementation of functional motor activities in children with neuromotor disorders, as well as their progressivity, has been shown to be a potentially effective therapeutic strategy [30,31]. These activities were implemented in a cyclical rotation, as described in detail in the study protocol [25]. This approach creates a satisfactory repetition of challenges, during gait, to enhance performance [32]. The 4-week physiotherapy intervention has been studied both in children with cerebral palsy [18] and in children with ataxia [12], and this period seems to be a duration with beneficial therapeutic effects. A partial body weight support of <40% of each participant was applied through the use of LiteGait. This limit of body weight support has been suggested by the literature in order to improve gait performance in different types of gait disorder populations [14,33–35].

Twenty (20) sessions over 4 weeks (5 days/week) constituted the intensive FPBWSTT program. The session was divided into two phases. Phase 1 consisted of 20 min gait training on the treadmill, with no handlebars, and speed intervals of 30 s between low and high speed. Both low and high speeds were individualized and modulated at 75–80% of each child's respective ground speeds according to the 10 MWT. The high speed was progressively increased per session up to 5% of the defined maximum speed achieved from the previous day (Figure 1). Phase 2 consisted of 15 min functional dual-task training. In this phase, functional activities were applied during the individualized fixed low-pace treadmill gait. In each session, 3 of a total of 6 activities were applied in a cyclical rotation, with each one lasting up to 5 min (Figure 1). In every session, each child's performance was recorded. The physiotherapist encouraged the gradual improvement in motor performance in each activity with verbal and visual guidance. Participants wore their shoes throughout the intensive program, along with any insoles they might have used. At the completion of the two phases, a total of 35 min of gait (20 min with speed intervals and 15 min with dual-task functional activities) was completed and displayed on the treadmill monitor. The total time from preparation to completion and release of the child from the LiteGait system ranged from 45 min to 1 h "with breaks".

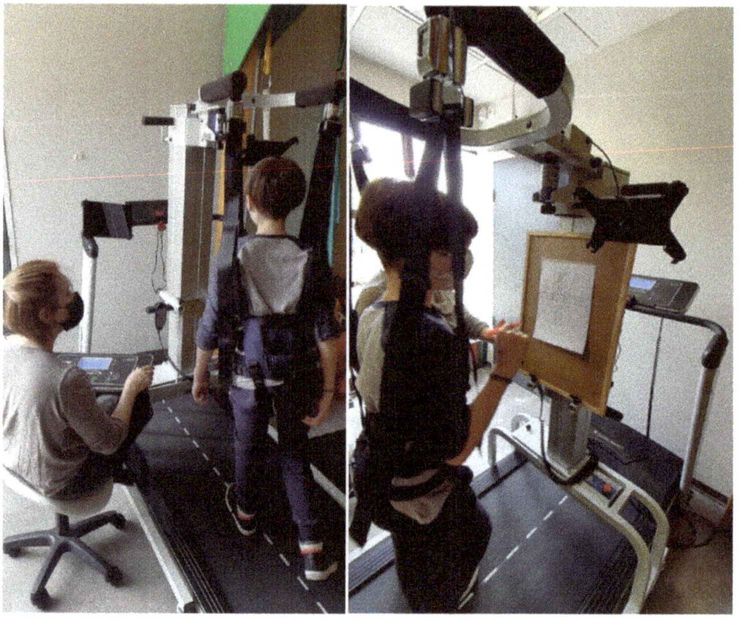

Figure 1. Application of the FPBWSTT. The left image shows gait training with speed intervals (phase 1), and the right image shows the application of the dual-activity of "target demonstration"(phase 2).

The FPBWSTT, as well as the assessment of all participants' spatiotemporal gait characteristics, was performed using a LiteGait LG 200 P (Mobility Research, Tempe, AZ, USA) partial body weight support system, accompanied by a Gait Keeper (Gait-Keeper S22, Mobility Research, Tempe, AZ, USA) electric treadmill system with a low-gait start speed (0.1 km/h). Two tablets were used for monitoring, recording, and collecting data from LiteGait.

For the 3D gait analysis, two force plates, specially designed platforms (AMTIs), placed in the middle section of a 10 m path were used to obtain the kinetic data. For the kinematic data, 16 self-adhesive reflective markers were appropriately placed at anatomical points of the pelvis and lower limbs. These data were acquired from 10 Vicon cameras (6MXT10 and 4 Verov2.2) at 100 Hz and 2 Basler digital video cameras (Pentaxlenses, Basler IND CCD Pentax TV Lens 8.5 mm 1:15, Tokyo, Japan) at 50 Hz.

2.3. Typical Therapy

Participants in both groups continued to receive their regular therapeutic program, consisting of physiotherapy and any other form of therapy the child needed, such as occupational therapy, speech therapy, etc. Typical physiotherapy (co-counting therapeutic swimming or equine therapy) did not exceed a total of 3 days per week, as otherwise it could be considered an intensive physiotherapy program [36,37]. The typical physiotherapy included 45 min sessions 1–2 times per week with functional exercises aimed at improving standing and gait skills. These included exercises on the mat to strengthen the trunk and lower limbs, therapeutic Pilates exercise, standing exercises, maintaining an upright position with balance boards, transitions to and from the standing position, walking on the ground and/or on a treadmill, and climbing up and down stairs.

2.4. Measurement Outcomes

Demographic and anthropometric data, including the functional level of each child through the use of the Gross Motor Function Classification System (GMFCS) and data obtained by the Child quality of Life Questionnaire for children report were collected once in the baseline assessment [38,39]. Primary and secondary outcomes were assessed three times over a period of approximately 3 months. A first baseline assessment was performed prior to the 4-week intervention period (baseline), a 4-week post-assessment was conducted by the end of the 4-week intervention period (4-week), and a final 2-month post-assessment was conducted 2 months by the end of the 4-week intervention period (2 months) (Figure 2).

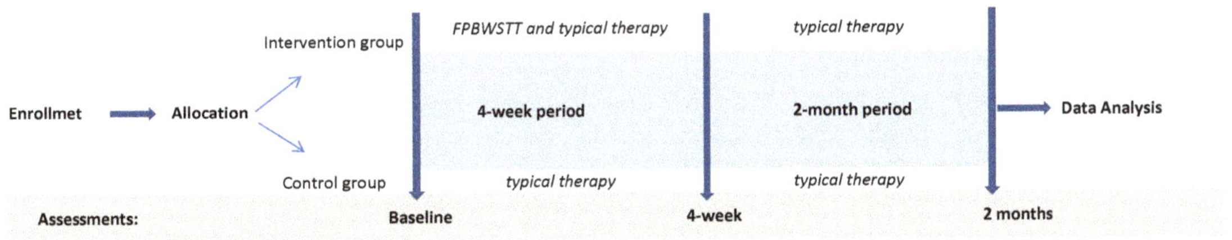

Figure 2. Flow of the events for the participants of this study.

Primary Outcomes:

- The Gross Motor Function Measure (GMFM-88) dimension D/E (GMFM-D /GMFM-E), were expressed as percentage scores (%) for the assessment of the motor performance and functional ability in standing, walking, running, and jumping [40].

Secondary Outcomes:

- The Pediatric Balance Scale (PBS), with scores in a range of 0–56 (the higher score indicates better balance), was used for the assessment of functional balance skills [41].
- The 10-meter walk test (10 MWT) for the assessment of self-selected slow-(10 MWT-SLOW) and high-speed (10 MWT-FAST) gaits over ground and determination of individualized training speeds on the treadmill were expressed as meters/second (m/s) [18,42,43].
- The Timed Up and Go (TUG) test for the assessment of dynamic balance control was expressed in seconds (s) [44].
- The 6-minute walk test (6 MWT) for the assessment of physical condition and endurance was expressed in meters (m) [45].

- The Scale for Assessment and Rating Ataxia (SARA), applied in the Greek version (SARAgr), was used for the assessment of ataxia features, with scores in a range of 0–40 (a higher score indicates more severe ataxia) [4].
- Three-dimensional kinematic and kinetic analysis of lower limbs through motion and gait analysis was applied, with the electronic recording of kinematics elements for the pelvis, hip, knee, and foot of both lower limbs in the three planes of motion (sagittal, frontal, and transverse). Since laterality severity does not occur in ataxia, each participant's dominant ankle power absorption and generation, expressed as Watt/kg, was collected for the kinetic variable. Similarly, the dominant lower limb's mean gait deviations index (MGDI) during 1. pelvis movement in all three planes of motion; 2. hip, knee, and ankle movement in the sagittal plane; and 3. ankle movement in the transverse plane (foot progression) were collected and expressed as normally disturbed data, categorized as Normal Standard Deviations (NSDs) through Gait Deviation Index (GDI) analysis [46]. Data recording and collection were obtained by the Gait and Motion Analysis Lab of ELEPAP in Athens.
- Analysis of spatiotemporal gait features was performed through 2 min recordings on the treadmill with partial body weight support at a personalized slow walking speed (75% of each participant's self-selected walking speed based on the 10 MWT over ground). GaitSens software (version 2.0), incorporated in the LiteGait equipment, was used for recording and collecting the gait parameters. The dominant lower limb's step length, stride length, and width length were expressed in terms of meters (cm), while step and stride time were expressed in seconds (s).

2.5. Assessment Procedure and Raters

Assessments were conducted according to the suggested guidelines of the outcome measure creators, following the same conditions, the same equipment across all participants, and across all time points. All assessments were conducted barefoot, except for the 10 MWT, 6 MWT, and 2 min gait recording on LiteGait, in which participants wore their shoes, as these were not possible or safe to be assessed barefoot. The procedure to assess the spatiotemporal gait parameters on the treadmill was performed with minimal partial body weight support (0–15%) at the individualized low walking speed (75% of the walking speed chosen by each participant based on 10 MWT on the ground). Equipment placement on LiteGait was the same as in the intervention procedure. All the assessments besides the 3D gait analysis took place in the same private pediatric faculty, from the same physiotherapy team, which was not blind to each child's allocation group.

For the 3D gait analysis, a total of 16 self-adhesive reflective markers were initially placed on participants at key anatomical points, according to the standard Plug-in-Gait biomechanical analysis model (Vicon, Oxford, UK) for the pelvis and lower limbs in order to collect kinematic data. Participants were instructed to walk on the 10 m path, completing a total of five barefoot walking trials in sequence, at their self-selected speeds, independently or with the help of a parent or physiotherapist, according to each child's GMFCS level. Upon completion of five left and five right gait cycles, valid motor data were determined from the force platform, on which each leg of each participant had to be placed and on which each leg "landed" wholly and individually on the force plate. The recording and collection of the above kinematic and kinetic data (Figure 3) were performed by the Athens ELEPAP Gait and Motion Analysis Laboratory by a blind physiotherapy team.

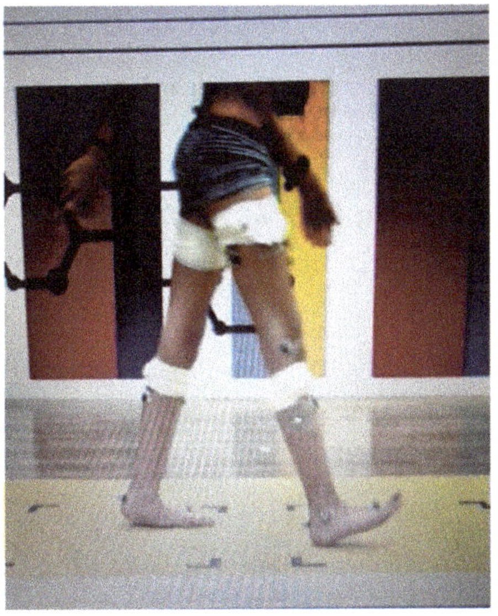

Figure 3. Gait procedure in a 10 m walking path during the 3D gait analysis in ELEPAP, Athens.

2.6. Statistical Analysis

The proposed sample size estimation could not be verified with the completion of 5 children per group, as was initially scheduled [25], due to the large heterogeneity among the participants at that time period. Despite the fact that an interim statistical analysis was not planned in the design of the protocol, in March 2023, with available data from a total of 18 children with ataxia, calculation of the primary end point of the GMFM-D was performed. This indicated statistically significant differences, which safely led to the adjustment of the sample size and therefore the termination of further sample search [47]. The variables were described using the mean and standard deviation or the median and interquartile range (in cases of violation of normality). The Kolmogorov–Smirnov test was used to check the normal distribution of the data. A comparison for homogeneity between the intervention groups in relation to the demographic and clinical indicators was performed using the independent samples t-test and the Chi-square test.

A two-way mixed ANOVA model was used, considering "intervention" (between groups) and "time" (within group) as factors for the analysis of the variables, applying the Bonferroni correction for all pairwise comparisons either between the intervention groups or between the time assessments.

Sensitivity analysis of the variables concerning the homogeneity of the groups at baseline (baseline–balance) was performed using two methods:

- The percentage change from baseline at all time points, where we compared the percentage changes between the intervention groups using the independent samples t-test or the Mann–Whitney test if the data did not follow a normal distribution.
- The absolute change from baseline at all time points, where we compared the absolute change in the variables (dependent variable) between the intervention groups (factor) and the baseline assessment (covariate) using the Analysis of Covariance (ANCOVA) model.

All statistical analyses were performed using the SPSS statistical package, version 21.00 (IBM Corporation, Somers, NY, USA). All tests were two-sided. A p-value < 0.05 was considered statistically significant.

3. Results

3.1. Participant Characteristics

Thirty-five (35) children with ataxia were assessed according to the eligibility criteria. A total of 21 children were randomized to either the intervention [Functional Partial Body Weight Support Treadmill Training (FPBWSTT)] or the control group, as shown in Figure 4. The data from 18 children were finally collected and statistically analyzed, from which only 9 children completed the 3D gait analysis in all three assessment periods, due to time-restricted periods from the 3D gait lab. Those data were processed for statistical analysis. The two groups were similar at baseline, in all clinical and demographic features, as well as in their perception of quality-of-life issues, as shown in Table 1.

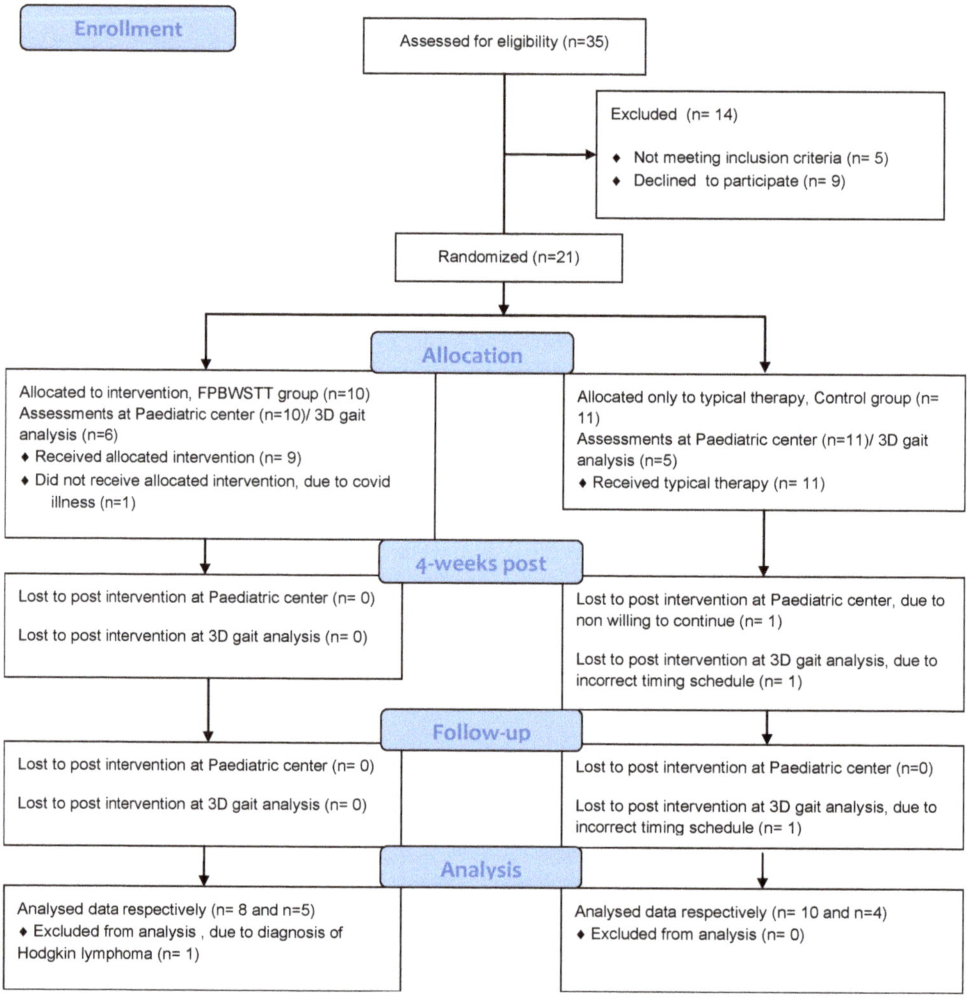

Figure 4. Flow chart of the study according to the Consolidated Standards of Reporting Trials "CONSORT" guidelines; pediatric center: private faculty for the evaluation of all the assessments; 3D: three-dimensional gait analysis at ELEPAP, Athens.

Table 1. Comparison of demographic, clinical, and quality-of-life characteristics between groups.

Characteristics	FPBWSTT Group	Control Group	p-Value
Age (years), mean ± SD	14.69 ± 2.05	13.45 ± 2.73	0.304
Sex, male/female	7 (87.5%)/1 (12.5%)	7 (70%)/3 (30%)	0.588
Weight (kg), mean ± SD	41.56 ± 8.79	46.55 ± 14.53	0.407
Height (cm), mean ± SD	157.38 ± 11.17	151.90 ± 14.67	0.397
BMI, mean ± SD	16.86 ± 2.20	19.72 ± 3.56	0.058
Type of ataxia, (non-P/P)	7 (87.5%)/1 (12.5%)	9 (90%)/1 (10%)	1.000
GMFCS, (II/III/IV)	6 (75%)/1 (12.5%)/1 (12.5%)	7 (70%)/2 (20%)/1 (10%)	0.909
Laterality, (right/left)	8 (100%)/0 (0%)	9 (90%)/1 (10%)	1.000
Quality of life Questionnaire			
Friends/Family, mean ± SD	7.18 ± 0.92	6.81 ± 0.82	0.375
Participation, mean ± SD	6.06 ± 2.31	5.65 ± 1.79	0.675
Communication, mean ± SD	6.58 ± 1.28	6.00 ± 1.50	0.395
Use of limbs, mean ± SD	5.99 ± 1.78	6.23 ± 1.62	0.683
Self-care, median ± IR	7.00 ± 0.0	7.00 ± 0.0	0.537
Equipment, mean ± SD	4.21 ± 1.38	4.21 ± 0.76	1.00
Pain-discomfort, mean ± SD	2.98 ± 0,77	2.98 ± 0.93	0.991
Sense of happiness, median ± IR	7.00 ± 1.0	7.00 ± 0.5	0.573
Assistance with questionnaire completion, mean ± SD	2.38 ± 1.06	2.40 ± 1.07	0.961

Abbreviations: SD, standard deviation; IR, interquartile range; BMI, Body Mass Index; non-P, non-progressive; P, progressive; GMFCS: Gross Motor Function Classification System. Note: Values are presented numerically, unless otherwise stated. There are no statistically significant differences between the groups at baseline ($p > 0.05$).Quality of Life Questionnaire: Scores are based on a Likert scale, from 1 (bad) to 9 (very good), except for the last question where the options range from 1 (no) to 4 (yes, very). Group Composition: **FPBWSTT Group** includes children with cerebral palsy ataxia (n = 5) [subsequent genetic testing revealed a variant of CACNA1A in 1 case], neuroblastoma (n = 1; 2 years post-surgical resection], CACNA1A-related ataxia (n = 1; previous CP diagnosis) and Friedreich Ataxia (n = 1). **Control Group** comprises children with cerebral palsy ataxia (n = 4), neuroblastoma (n = 1; 3.5 years post-surgical resection), CACNA1A-related ataxia (n = 1), ataxia of unknown etiology (n = 1), Gillespie syndrome (n = 1), TBI-related ataxia (n = 1; 6 years post-injury), and Menkes-like ataxia (n = 1).

3.2. Primary Outcomes: Domains D and E of the GMFM-88 (%)

The FPBWSTT group was statistically significant improved in GMFM domains D (standing) and E (gait) at 4 weeks by a mean of 6.45% (95% CI 3.34–9.57, $p < 0.001$) for standing and by a mean of 4.68% (95% CI 1.66–7.70, $p = 0.005$) for gait, compared to the control group. These improvements were also maintained at 2 months, by a mean of 5.56% (95% CI 1.46–9.67, $p = 0.011$) and by a mean of 8.51% (95% CI 2.91–14.11, $p = 0.005$), compared to the control group, respectively. Gross motor functionality of standing and gait changed significantly through time for the FPBWSTT group ($p < 0.005$), but no significant changes were found for the control group ($p > 0.05$). This is reinforced by the significant interaction of the groups and time for both variables ($p = 0.002$), as shown in Figure 5.

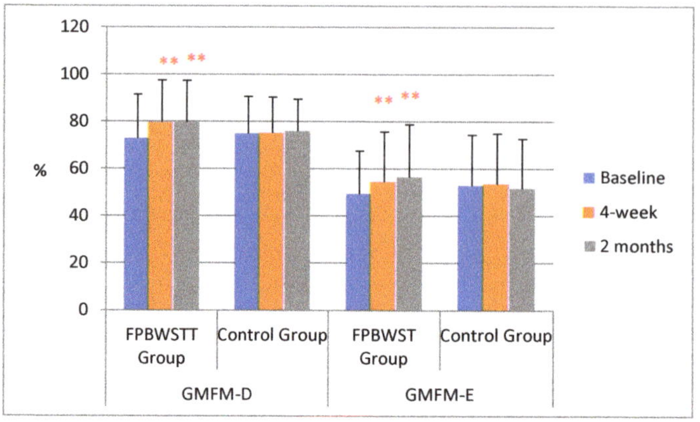

Figure 5. Mean values and standard deviation of gross motor function in standing (GMFM-D) and gait (GMFM-E) of the two groups at baseline, 4 weeks, and 2 months. Asterisks (**) represent statistically significant values, with $p \leq 0.005$.

3.3. Secondary Outcomes

Analyses of the data of secondary outcome measures are presented in Table 2,showing that in most of them, the FPBWSTT group had statistically significant improvement ($p < 0.05$) at 4 weeks, compared to the control group. The intervention group maintained their improvements in the PBS, 6 MWT, and spatiotemporal gait parameters at 2 months, as shown in Table 2 and Figure 6. There were baseline differences between the groups, both in stride and step length, with greater values obtained in the control group (Table 3). Interestingly, the slow self-paced 10 MWT did not show statistically significant improvement at 4 weeks (mean: 0.07 m/s, 95% CI −0.04/0.18, $p > 0.05$) and at 2 months (mean:0.05 m/s, 95% CI −0.05/0.15, $p = 0.307$), for the FPBWSTT group. This was in stark contrast to the fast self-selected gait pace at 4 weeks, in which the intervention group showed statistically significant improvement, by a mean of 0.19 m/s (95% CI 0.00–0.38, $p = 0.046$).

Table 2. Sensitivity analysis using ANCOVA model (baseline vs. 4-week and 2-month outcomes).

Secondary Outcome	4-Week Mean Difference (95% CI)	p-Value	2-Month Mean Difference (95% CI)	p-Value
PBS	3.73 (1.13–6.33)	0.008	3.85 (−0.14 to 7.71)	0.05
TUG (s)	2.19 (0.7–3.67)	0.007	1.29 (−0.53 to 3.10)	0.151
10 MWT-SLOW (m/s)	0.07 (0.04–0.18)	0.193	0.05 (0.05–0.15)	0.307
10 MWT-FAST (m/s)	0.19 (0–0.38)	0.046	0.04 (−0.12 to 0.21)	0.620
6 MWT (m)	56.09 (29.22–82.96)	<0.005	36.92 (7.34–66.50)	0.018
SARAgr	1.22 (0.44–2.01)	0.005	1.00 (−0.31 to 2.34)	0.125
Step Length (cm)	8.84 (1.67–16.01)	0.019	5.36 (−3.64 to 14.35)	0.224
Stride Length (cm)	8.29 (−3.98 to 20.57)	0.170	12 (−5.52 to 29.54)	0.165
Step Time (s)	0.38 (0.01–0.74)	0.043	0.45 (0.01–0.90)	0.048
Stride Time (s)	0.45 (0.16–0.75)	0.005	0.77 (0.05–1.49)	0.038
Step Width (cm)	6.74 (4.20–9.29)	<0.005	7.41 (4.18–10.64)	<0.005

Abbreviations: CI, confidence interval; PBS, Pediatric Balance Scale; TUG, Timed Up and Go; 10 MWT, 10 meter walk test; 6 MWT, 6 minute walk test; SARAgr, Scale for Assessing and Rating Ataxia (Greek version). Red highlights the statistically significant p-values.

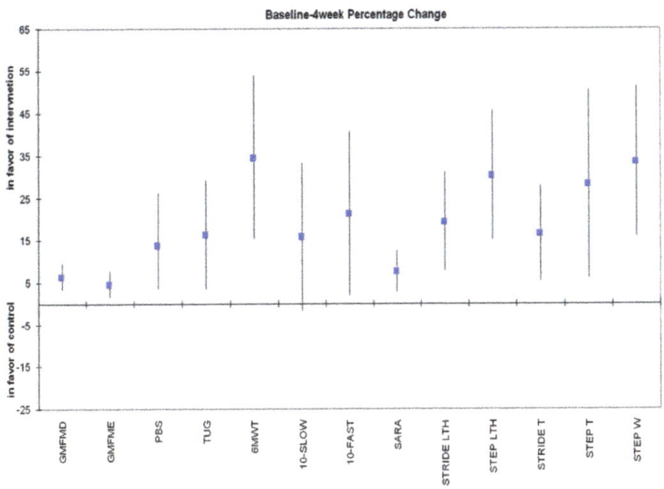

Figure 6. Percentage change from baseline to 4 weeks of all variables in which all 18 children were assessed. All changes are statistically significant ($p < 0.05$), in favor of the experimental group, except for 10 MWT-Slow, which is marginally statistically significant ($p = 0.072$).

Table 3. Mixed two-way ANOVA for the step length and stride length variables.

Groups	Step Length (cm)			Stride Length (cm)		
	Baseline	4-Week	2 Months	Baseline	4-Week	2 Months
	Mean ± SD	Mean ± SD	Mean ± SD	Mean ± SD	Mean ± SD	Mean ± SD
FPBWSTT	22.85 ± 7.56	28.19 ± 8.69 *	27.49 ± 8.65	47.72 ± 12.74	54.79 ± 14.69	58.16 ± 18.66
Control	38.01 ± 7.04	35.99 ± 9.63	32.88 ± 7.00	72.29 ± 17.77	68.51 ± 18.27	64.57 ± 16.63
Comparison between groups by time	$p < 0.005$	$p = 0.094$	$p = 0.163$	$p = 0.005$	$p = 0.104$	$p = 0.453$
Interaction between group and time	F(2.32) = 6.94, $p < 0.005$			F(2.32) = 6.34, $p = 0.005$		

Abbreviations: SD, standard deviation. Asterisk (*) indicates $p < 0.05$ vs. baseline. Red highlights the statistically significant p-values.

The percentage change of primary and secondary outcomes after 4 weeks and 2 months of all participants is presented, respectively, in Figures 6 and 7.

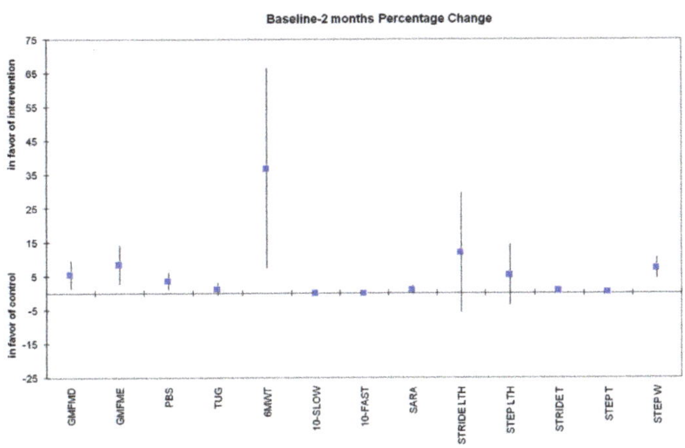

Figure 7. Percentage change from baseline to 2 months of all variables in which all 18 children were assessed. Most changes were still statistically significant ($p < 0.05$), in favor of the experimental group, except for TUG, 10 MWT-Slow, 10 MWT-Fast, and SARAgr.

Secondary Variables from 3D Gait Analysis

Three-dimensional gait analysis was obtained only in a total of 9 children (FPBWSTT group $n = 5$; control group $n = 4$). Kinetic variables were inadequately collected, due to the insufficient placing of the entire foot or due to the coexistence of both feet on the platform during gait.

The values of the kinematic variable of the pelvis in the sagittal plane were highly heterogeneous with extreme values. Additionally, given the small sample size, the statistical analysis of this variable was excluded, as no valid result could be attributed [48]. The kinematic variables that were analyzed were the ones obtained from 1.pelvis movement in the frontal and transverse planes of motion; 2. hip, knee and ankle movement in the sagittal plane; and 3. ankle movement in the transverse plane (foot progression). Those findings indicated no statistically significant differences between the groups and no statistically significant changes for either of the groups, as shown in Table 4.

Table 4. Sensitivity analysis of kinematic variables, using ANCOVA model (baseline vs. 4-week and 2-month outcomes).

Kinematic Variables	4-Week Mean Difference (95% CI)	p-Value	2-Month Mean Difference (95% CI)	p-Value
Pelvis Frontal Plane (NSDs)	−0.11 (−0.76 to 0.74)	0.972	0.57 (−0.42 to 1.57)	0.210
Pelvis Transverse Plane (NSDs)	−0.08 (−1.45 to 1.29)	0.888	−0.22 (−1.41 to 0.97)	0.671
Hip Sagittal Plane (NSDs)	−0.21 (−0.98 to 0.54)	0.512	−0.54 (−0.45 to 1.53)	0.232
Knee Sagittal Plane (NSDs)	−0.42 (−1.68 to 0.85)	0.450	−0.06 (−1.41 to 1.29)	0.919
Ankle Sagittal Plane (NSDs)	−0.21 (−0.70 to 0.28)	0.337	0.18 (−0.42 to 0.78)	0.482
Ankle Transverse Plane (NSDs)	−0.09 (−01.05 to 0.88)	0.829	−0.42 (−1.69 to 0.86)	0.452

Abbreviations: CI, confidence interval; NSDs, normal standard deviations.

4. Discussion

The results of the clinical study, alongside compliance to the protocol and the absence of adverse effects, indicate that the FPBWSTT can be a highly effective intensive program for children8–18 years old with moderate functional severity of ataxia, more than typical physical therapy. The significant improvements in gross motor function in the areas of standing and walking were accompanied with similar changes in ataxia symptoms, functional balance skills, gait speed, dynamic balance control, physical condition and endurance, and spatiotemporal gait parameters, in favor of the FPBWSTT group. The majority of these were sustained two months after the end of the intensive program. The collection and statistical analysis of the kinematic variables of the 3D gait analysis did not reveal significant differences between groups, and neither significantly changed in any of the two groups between the different time measurements. The sample that completed the 3D gait analysis was too small (only nine children), which limits the statistical power for these specific measures and may affect the robustness of the conclusions drawn from these data. However, these findings may indicate that such measurements may not be sensitive enough for detecting functional changes in the specific population and/or at such a short time frame.

Children in both groups had similar clinical and demographic features. Confounding factors that could affect the outcome, as well as the interpretation of the results, were taken into account. This was obtained through the admission and exclusion criteria of the participants, as well as their recruitment, based on stratification of the type of disorder. Each group had one participant with progressive type of ataxia and GMFCS IV, while the remaining participants belonged to the non-progressive ataxia category, between

GMFCS II-III. Children who had undergone surgical resection of the posterior fossa tumor (neuroblastoma), as well as the child with ataxia as a result of traumatic brain injury, all far exceeded the time frame for spontaneous recovery of balance ability, determined to be up to one year [49].

According to the results in gross motor function, particularly in standing and walking after the end of the of the present study, the children who completed the FPBWSTT significantly improved intensive program, which were maintained at follow-up. At the same time, statistically significant differences emerged between the two groups in the changes from the initial measurement, both after the end of the 4-week period and after the 2-month period. The domains of standing (domain D) and walking (domain E) in gross motor function, according to the GMFM, are the most representative domains of motor difficulties in children and youth with CP [50,51], as well as in children with ataxia [2,12].

The findings of the present study are even more encouraging than the reference range of 0.8–5.2% and 2.3–6.5% suggested by Storm et al. [52] as a Minimum Clinically Important Difference (MCID) for the improvement of GMFM-D in children with cerebral palsy and TBI, respectively, after one month of robotic gait training. Accordingly, the reference range of clinically significant difference for GMFM-E varies from 0.3 to 4.9% for children with CP and 2.8–6.5% for children with TBI. Specifically, in the study there was a total of 182 children, aged 4–18 years with movement disorders as a result of CP and TBI, who followed 20 sessions of 45 minutes of gait training and typical physical therapy each (total 90 min session) over a 4-week period [52].

In the present study, the change in gross motor function in standing position after the end of 4 weeks was 6.81% for FPBWSTT group and only 0.35% for the control group, while the change in gross motor function in gait was 5.30% for FPBWSTT and only 0.62% for the control group. Those findings are in accordance with the pilot study of Peri et al. [12], which investigated the effects of a 4-week gait training program in 11 children with ataxia due to TBI, additionally reinforcing the clinical significance of gross motor function change in standing and gait domains in such a short time frame. An interesting point found in the present study and confirmed through the research of Peri et al. [12] is that both programs focused on gait training produced greater changes in standing gross mobility than in gait. In other words, what is evident is that even if there are no exercises focused on static and dynamic standing skills, gait training contributes significantly to the enhancement of gross motor function in standing.

The exact same trend in change, similar to GMFM-D, was found for the PBS, with a clinically significant change, based on the proposed reference range after a 6-month period for children up to 6.5 years old with CP [53]. The same study showed a strong correlation between the total score of GMFM-66 and PBS. Based on our findings, GMFM-D and PBS share common characteristics with a trend change consistent with basic principles of neuroplasticity [33], as practicing a motor activity promotes a type of transfer to the acquisition and improvement of similar activities to the one being trained. It appears that gait training, as a functional activity, and the way in which speed alternations and dual-task functional activities were combined, were able to promote simultaneous or subsequent changes, through a network of neural circuits for other functional activities, in addition to those of gait. Motor training alone is capable of activating angiogenic mechanisms in the motor cortex and cerebellum and promoting the growth and survival of neurons in many brain regions [54,55]. The activity of gait involves activation of somatosensory and motor areas of the whole body, and the application of FPBWSTT through both speed and dual-task challenges appears to be sufficiently able to promote the appropriate synaptic connections and form a fertile environment to support structural brain changes related to standing functional activities.

A statistically and clinically significant difference was also found for gross motor function in gait (GMFM-E), with an interesting, continuous improvement observed 2 months after the end of the FPBWSTT. This finding could be due to a possible increase in the relevant daily activities of the children who completed the FPBWSTT as a "habit" formed as a result of the intensive gait program. As supported by theories and research on motor learning, neuroplasticity is an ongoing process, rather than a single event [54].The consolidation of a motor behavior involves time and repetition that often depend on the time period after the end of the motor training [54], which could explain the continuous increase in GMFM-E, 2 months after the end of the training. Unfortunately, this remains an assumption, based on theoretical knowledge that can not be directly correlated with other studies, which investigated short-term and post intervention results or the total GMFM score of all domains [2].

The change in ataxic symptoms was only significant just after the end of the 4-week program for the FPBWSTT group, without reaching the minimum clinically important difference reported in adult studies [56,57] and in the pediatric population [12,58]. It is possible that further clinical reduction in the SARA score can be achieved by a more targeted therapeutic approach on functional activities, related to the ataxic signs and increased time practice, as the cerebellum, the main responsible structure causing ataxia, requires sufficient temporal processing [55].

Improvements in dynamic balance control following various applications of therapeutic protocols have been reported in children with ataxia with reference to fall risk reduction and functional mobility skill improvement [2]. However, the heterogeneity of study protocols in the measurement of TUG and the need for chronological age correlation with a standard reference value [59] restrict the clinical interpretation of TUG's change seen in the present study. Nevertheless, the improvement and significant change found for the FPBWSTT compared to the control group at 4 weeks indicates developing functional independence in children [60]. This is reinforced by the improvements in the self-selected pace and the significant change in10 MWT-fast, which further points out the ability of adjusting and regulating gait speed—an extremely difficult task for people with cerebellum deficits [19]. Besides the above, the increase in gait speed found for the FPBWSTT is even more apparent in the way that 6 MWT changed. Even though 6 MWT measures physical condition and endurance, it has been widely used informally for walking speed calculation in children with CP [61], while a strong correlation with 10 MWT has been supported in adults with neurological deficits [62]. Based on the increased 46, 25 m by the end of the FPBWSTT, a study similar in population, duration, and type of intervention [12] identified an improvement of 48 m, post 4-week gait training. These findings may verify an important reference range for the functional improvements of children with ataxia, after 4-week, 20-sessiongait training.

Children who underwent the FPBWSTT significantly reduced their step width at all time periods, showing statistically significant changes, compared to children who underwent a standard program. Despite the fact that the children of the FPBWSTT group had significantly shorter stride and stride lengths compared to the control group at baseline, there was a statistically significant increase in their stride and step length after 4 weeks, in contrast to children of the control group who even demonstrated a decline in those gait variables. However, from the absolute changes, only that of the step length at 4 weeks was statistically significantly improved. The increase in stride length continued further, even 2 months after the end of FBPWSTT, while step length showed a slight decrease. This may be due to an increased variability of steps with non-symmetrical bilateral steps at the given time point. In a systematic review by Buckley et al. [10], regarding gait characteristics in adults with ataxia, increased variability of stride length, but not of step length, was reported at low speeds compared to higher speeds. Given the above, this finding could be due to the difficulty of adapting gait to a walking speed lower than what has now been achieved, as the speed of evaluation of all spatiotemporal characteristics in all three time periods was the same (75–80% of low self-selected baseline ground speed).

The overall spatiotemporal gait changes are of particular importance, as they highlight an adapting ability and the possibility of adopting a new gait strategy within the same gait speed. Increased step and stride time characterize ataxic gait, compared to typical values of adults and children [10,12]. According to the present findings, what theoretically appears as worsening actually reveals adaptation of a gait pattern in order to maintain the same pace. It seems that temporal gait variables act as a compensatory index to maintain walking pace when spatial parameters (step and stride length) are increased as a result of the FPBWSTT program. This adaptation skill is a well-established indicator of improved motor functionality [63].

4.1. Kinematic Changes

According to current data, joint mobility in children with ataxia has been assessed in relation to the maximum trajectory range achieved during gait, expressed in degrees, compared to a healthy population [12,13] and immediately after gait training [12]. The assessment of the maximum range of motion at a joint and whether this is close to standard reference values is not necessarily an indication of improvement, as it is unknown whether this range of motion is utilized at the appropriate time during gait. The use of the MGDI seems to reflect the deviation between the pathological and typical gait, as it is calculated in such way as to estimate and compare the absolute value of each momentary deviation with the corresponding value of normal data [64].To our knowledge, the present study is the first in this population to assess changes in mean joint mobility deviations throughout the gait cycle, as derived from standard gait analysis values, relative to a control group and in the long term.

During 3D gait analysis of the nine children, there was an inability to collect kinetic variables due to incorrect and insufficient placement of the foot on the force-recording platform. Additionally, there was great heterogeneity with extreme values in the kinematic variables of the pelvis in the sagittal plane, an observation confirmed in adults with ataxia [65,66]. The instability of the trunk and pelvis in all directions of movement and especially in the sagittal plane, seems to be particularly pronounced in adults with ataxia, perhaps due to an effort to maintain an energy-efficient gait [65,66]. In a similar study by Peri et al. [12], changes in pelvic kinematics, measured by maximal range of motion after 4-week gait training showed greater values in deviation from the normal reference ones and increased standard deviation, following a different course of change, than the otherwise functional improvements of the participants. It seems that pelvis kinematics' deterioration or even variability may be part of an effort for trunk stability in a newly adopted gait strategy.

All other kinematic variables did not show a specific change trend in any of the two groups, which differs from the findings reported by Peri et al. [12]. The latter argue that changes in knee and ankle mobility, close to standard values, may be indicators of the effectiveness of a therapeutic program. The pilot study of Peri et al. [12] applied 20 sessions of typical physiotherapy alongside with the 20 sessions of gait training, which aimed to improve balance skills and correct the movement pattern. On the other hand, in the present study, neither the typical physiotherapy nor FPBWSTT, specifically focused on "correction" or facilitation techniques, aimed to improve joint mobility. Changes in some kinematic variables could be expected over a longer time period, perhaps as an indication of a "consolidated" gait, without clarifying whether these changes will align with the reference standard values. What needs further clarification is whether these variables are associated with functional improvements in this population and whether physiotherapy should aim for "correction" of those.

4.2. Limitations

From the study design, a limitation is the lack of blind data collection by the assessors of the outcome measures, conducted at the private pediatric center, as they were also FPBWSTT therapists. The only blind assessors were the ones from the 3D gait analysis. This can be appropriately anticipated in future research, and the risk of bias arising can be therefore reduced.

The 2-month follow-up may not fully capture the long-term impact of the intervention, so future studies should involve a longer follow-up period to better evaluate the treatment effects over time.

5. Conclusions

In conclusion, our study provides robust evidence that FPBWSTT is a feasible and effective intervention for improving mobility and functionality in children with ataxia. Specifically, children in the FPBWSTT group exhibited a statistically significant improvement in gross motor function, with a 6.45% increase in standing performance (GMFM-D, $p < 0.001$) and a 4.68% increase in gait performance (GMFM-E, $p = 0.005$) after the 4-week intervention. These improvements were maintained at the 2-month follow-up, as demonstrated by significant differences between the intervention and control groups ($p < 0.05$). In addition, significant enhancements in dynamic balance and endurance, as measured by the Pediatric Balance Scale and the 6-Minute Walk Test, further support the efficacy of the FPBWSTT program and its maintained benefits over a period of 2 months. Interestingly, significant changes in some gait parameters indicate the adapting ability and the possibility of adopting a new gait strategy with the completion of the FPBWSTT. Although the kinematic variables did not show significant changes—likely due to a limited sample size—the observed functional improvements are both statistically and clinically meaningful. These results underscore the real-world applicability of FPBWSTT in pediatric rehabilitation settings, suggesting that this intervention can substantially enhance daily functional activities and overall quality of life for children with moderate ataxia.

Supplementary Materials: The following supporting information can be downloaded at https://www.mdpi.com/article/10.3390/jfmk10020123/s1.

Author Contributions: Conceptualization: A.L., S.L. and V.S.; methodology: A.L., S.L., V.S., M.P. and A.G.; software: A.L., G.G. and A.G.; validation: V.S.; formal analysis: A.L. and A.G.; investigation: A.L., G.G. and M.T.; resources: A.L.; data curation: A.L., A.G. and V.S.; writing—original draft preparation: A.L.; writing—review and editing: A.L., S.L., M.P. and V.S.; visualization: A.L.; supervision: V.S.; project administration: A.L. All authors have read and agreed to the published version of the manuscript.

Funding: This research received no external funding.

Institutional Review Board Statement: This study was conducted according to the guidelines of the Declaration of Helsinki and approved by the Ethics Committee of the University of West Attica (study's protocol: 14η/26 April 2021) and the Review Board of 'ATTIKON' General University Hospital of Athens (study's protocol: Γ ΠΑΙΔ, ΕΒΔ 149/20 March 2020).

Informed Consent Statement: Written informed consent was obtained from all participants involved in this study. Parents and children above the age of 16 years old were asked to sign the consent form.

Data Availability Statement: The data presented in this study are available on request from the corresponding authors.

Acknowledgments: We are deeply grateful to all the children and their families who spent some of their time participating in this research study during the difficult period of the COVID-19 pandemic. We would also like to thank all our colleagues for their help in the sample search and especially those from the pediatric faculty "Motivation and Movement: Child's Functional Therapy" for their valuable contribution and support of the research process.

Conflicts of Interest: The authors declare no conflicts of interest.

References

1. Musselman, K.E.; Stoyanov, C.T.; Marasigan, R.; Jenkins, M.E.; Konczak, J.; Morton, S.M.; Bastian, A.J. Prevalence of ataxia in children: A systematic review. *Neurology* **2014**, *82*, 80–89. [CrossRef] [PubMed]
2. Hartley, H.; Cassidy, E.; Bunn, L.; Kumar, R.; Pizer, B.; Lane, S.; Carter, B. Exercise and Physical Therapy Interventions for Children with Ataxia: A Systematic Review. *Cerebellum* **2019**, *18*, 951–968. [CrossRef] [PubMed]
3. Pavone, P.; Praticò, A.D.; Pavone, V.; Lubrano, R.; Falsaperla, R.; Rizzo, R.; Ruggieri, M. Ataxia in children: Early recognition and clinical evaluation. *Ital. J. Pediatr.* **2017**, *43*, 6. [CrossRef] [PubMed]
4. Lepoura, A.; Lampropoulou, S.; Galanos, A.; Papadopoulou, M.; Sakellari, V. Scale for Assessment and Rating Ataxia (SARA) in Children with Ataxia: Greek Cultural Adaptation and Psychometric Properties. *Open Access J. Neurol. Neurosurg.* **2023**, *18*, e555976.
5. Schmitz-Hübsch, T.; du Montcel, S.T.; Baliko, L.; Berciano, J.; Boesch, S.; Depondt, C.; Giunti, P.; Globas, C.; Infante, J.; Kang, J.S.; et al. Scale for the assessment and rating of ataxia: Development of a new clinical scale. *Neurology* **2006**, *66*, 1717–1720.
6. Pinto, W.B.; Pedroso, J.L.; Souza, P.V.; Albuquerque, M.V.; Barsottini, O.G. Non-progressive cerebellar ataxia and previous undetermined acute cerebellar injury: A mysterious clinical condition. *Arq. Neuropsiquiatr.* **2015**, *73*, 823–827. [CrossRef]
7. Panzeri, D.; Bettinelli, M.S.; Biffi, E.; Rossi, F.; Pellegrini, C.; Orsini, N.; Recchiuti, V.; Massimino, M.; Poggi, G. Application of the Scale for the Assessment and Rating of Ataxia (SARA) in pediatric oncology patients: A multicenter study. *Pediatr. Hematol. Oncol.* **2020**, *37*, 687–695. [CrossRef]
8. Sullivan, R.; Yau, W.Y.; O'Connor, E.; Houlden, H. Spinocerebellar ataxia: An update. *J. Neurol.* **2019**, *266*, 533–544.
9. Steinlin, M. Non-progressive congenital ataxias. *Brain Dev.* **1998**, *20*, 199–208.
10. Buckley, E.; Mazzà, C.; McNeill, A. A systematic review of the gait characteristics associated with Cerebellar Ataxia. *Gait Posture* **2018**, *60*, 154–163.
11. Milne, S.C.; Hocking, D.R.; Georgiou-Karistianis, N.; Murphy, A.; Delatycki, M.B.; Corben, L.A. Sensitivity of spatiotemporal gait parameters in measuring disease severity in Friedreich ataxia. *Cerebellum* **2014**, *13*, 677–688. [CrossRef]
12. Peri, E.; Panzeri, D.; Beretta, E.; Reni, G.; Strazzer, S.; Biffi, E. Motor Improvement in Adolescents Affected by Ataxia Secondary to Acquired Brain Injury: A Pilot Study. *Biomed. Res. Int.* **2019**, *2019*, 8967138. [CrossRef]
13. Vasco, G.; Gazzellini, S.; Petrarca, M.; Lispi, M.L.; Pisano, A.; Zazza, M.; Della Bella, G.; Castelli, E.; Bertini, E. Functional and Gait Assessment in Children and Adolescents Affected by Friedreich's Ataxia: A One-Year Longitudinal Study. *PLoS ONE* **2016**, *11*, e0162463. [CrossRef]
14. Damiano, D.L.; DeJong, S.L. A systematic review of the effectiveness of treadmill training and body weight support in pediatric rehabilitation. *J. Neurol. Phys. Ther.* **2009**, *33*, 27–44. [CrossRef]
15. Molina-Rueda, F.; Aguila-Maturana, A.M.; Molina-Rueda, M.J.; Miangolarra-Page, J.C. Pasarelarodante con o sin sistema de suspension del peso corporal enninos con paralisis cerebral infantil: Revision sistematica y metaanalisis [Treadmill training with or without partial body weight support in children with cerebral palsy: Systematic review and meta-analysis]. *Rev. Neurol.* **2010**, *51*, 135–145.
16. Qian, G.; Cai, X.; Xu, K.; Tian, H.; Meng, Q.; Ossowski, Z.; Liang, J. Which gait training intervention can most effectively improve gait ability in patients with cerebral palsy? A systematic review and network meta-analysis. *Front. Neurol.* **2023**, *13*, 1005485. [CrossRef]
17. Valentin-Gudiol, M.; Bagur-Calafat, C.; Girabent-Farrés, M.; Hadders-Algra, M.; Mattern-Baxter, K.; Angulo-Barroso, R. Treadmill interventions with partial body weight support in children under six years of age at risk of neuromotor delay: A report of a Cochrane systematic review and meta-analysis. *Eur. J. Phys. Rehabil. Med.* **2013**, *49*, 67–91.
18. Bjornson, K.F.; Moreau, N.; Bodkin, A.W. Short-burst interval treadmill training walking capacity and performance in cerebral palsy: A pilot study. *Dev. Neurorehabil.* **2019**, *22*, 126–133. [CrossRef]
19. Hamacher, D.; Herold, F.; Wiegel, P.; Hamacher, D.; Schega, L. Brain activity during walking: A systematic review. *Neurosci. Biobehav. Rev.* **2015**, *57*, 310–327. [CrossRef]

Journal of
Functional Morphology and Kinesiology

MDPI

Article

May Patients with Chronic Stroke Benefit from Robotic Gait Training with an End-Effector? A Case-Control Study

Mirjam Bonanno [1,†], Paolo De Pasquale [1,*,†], Antonino Lombardo Facciale [1], Biagio Dauccio [1], Rosaria De Luca [1], Angelo Quartarone [1,2] and Rocco Salvatore Calabrò [1]

1 IRCCS Centro Neurolesi Bonino-Pulejo, 98124 Messina, Italy; mirjam.bonanno@irccsme.it (M.B.); antonino.lombardo@irccsme.it (A.L.F.); biagio.dauccio@irccsme.it (B.D.); rosaria.deluca@irccsme.it (R.D.L.); angelo.quartarone@irccsme.it (A.Q.); roccos.calabro@irccsme.it (R.S.C.)

2 Department of Biomedical and Dental Sciences and Morphofunctional Imaging, University of Messina, 98125 Messina, Italy

* Correspondence: paolo.depasquale@irccsme.it

† These authors contributed equally to the work.

Abstract: Background: Gait and balance alterations in post-stroke patients are one of the most disabling symptoms that can persist in chronic stages of the disease. In this context, rehabilitation has the fundamental role of promoting functional recovery, mitigating gait and balance deficits, and preventing falling risk. Robotic end-effector devices, like the G-EO system (e.g., G-EO system, Reha Technology, Olten, Switzerland), can be a useful device to promote gait recovery in patients with chronic stroke. **Materials and Methods:** Twelve chronic stroke patients were enrolled and evaluated at baseline (T0) and at post-treatment (T1). These patients received forty sessions of robotic gait training (RGT) with the G-EO system (experimental group, EG), for eight weeks consecutively, in addition to standard rehabilitation therapy. The data of these subjects were compared with those coming from a sample of twelve individuals (control group, CG) matched for clinical and demographic features who underwent the same amount of conventional gait training (CGT), in addition to standard rehabilitation therapy. **Results:** All patients completed the trial, and none reported any side effects either during or following the training. The EG showed significant improvements in balance (p = 0.012) and gait (p = 0.004) functions measured with the Tinetti Scale (TS) after RGT. Both groups (EG and CG) showed significant improvement in functional independence (FIM, p < 0.001). The Fugl-Meyer Assessment—Lower Extremity (FMA-LE) showed significant improvements in motor function (p = 0.001, p = 0.031) and passive range of motion (p = 0.031) in EG. In EG, gait and balance improvements were influenced by session, age, gender, time since injury (TSI), cadence, and velocity (p < 0.05), while CG showed fewer significant effects, mainly for age, TSI, and session. EG showed significantly greater improvements than CG in balance (p = 0.003) and gait (p = 0.05) based on the TS. **Conclusions:** RGT with end-effectors, like the G-EO system, can be a valuable complementary treatment in neurorehabilitation, even for chronic stroke patients. Our findings suggest that RGT may improve gait, balance, and lower limb motor functions, enhancing motor control and coordination.

Keywords: robotic gait training; neurorehabilitation; gait and balance; end-effector; lower limb; chronic stroke

1. Introduction

Gait and balance alterations in post-stroke patients are some of the most disabling symptoms that can persist in the chronic stages of the disease [1–3]. Generally, post-stroke patients can manifest abnormal gait patterns characterized by temporal and spatial asymmetry between steps [4]. This asymmetry during gait could result in postural instability and a lack of coordination to both self-induced and external balance perturbations [5]. According to some authors [2,3], stroke-related gait deficits, leading to fall risk, comprise reduced propulsion at push-off, decreased hip and knee flexion during the swing phase, and reduced stability during the stance phase. All these gait features can represent the cause of falling in this patient population, leading to further medical complications. It is noteworthy that post-stroke patients represent a heterogeneous group due to variations in the location and extent of brain damage. As a result, they may exhibit diverse step length patterns in both the paretic and non-paretic limbs. These variations are often linked to compensatory adjustments involving the pelvis and the unaffected side of the body [6].

In this context, physiotherapy is fundamental to promoting functional recovery, mitigating gait and balance deficits, and preventing fall risk [7,8]. Both conventional rehabilitation approaches and innovative technologies have proved their effectiveness in post-stroke patients [7,8]. However, limited evidence exists in the context of chronic stroke patients [9,10], in which it is commonly thought that neuroplastic processes and the subsequent functional recovery are already exhausted.

Among the innovative approaches, robotic rehabilitation devices play a crucial role, enabling intensive, repetitive, and task-oriented training to stimulate neuroplastic processes, even in chronic stages [10,11]. Robotic devices are generally categorized into two main types based on their biomechanical interaction with patients: exoskeletons and end-effectors [8].

End-effectors, such as the G-EO system (Reha Technology, Olten, Switzerland), are equipped with a single distal control, providing a propulsive motion of the legs thanks to two footplates that replicate the motion of stance and swing phases during gait training [12]. This design contrasts with exoskeletons, wearable powered orthoses that guide joint movements more proximally (e.g., Ekso-GT, Indego, or Lokomat) [12,13]. While exoskeletons, especially the Lokomat, have demonstrated effectiveness in promoting functional recovery and brain connectivity changes in chronic post-stroke patients [10], evidence supporting the efficacy of end-effector devices, particularly the G-EO system, remains limited [14] in this population. Most available studies have focused on acute and subacute stages [15–17], leaving a gap in the literature regarding their use in chronic stroke.

Given this background, this study aims to evaluate the effects of robotic end-effector gait rehabilitation training (RGT) in patients with chronic stroke and compare the functional outcomes with a matched control group receiving conventional gait training (CGT). To achieve this, we clinically assessed both rehabilitation approaches at baseline and post-treatment. A linear mixed effects (LME) model was employed to analyze the influence of demographic, clinical, and rehabilitation variables on the outcomes in both groups.

2. Materials and Methods

Twelve chronic post-stroke patients, attending the Robotic and Behavioral Neurorehabilitation Unit of the IRCCS Centro Neurolesi "Bonino-Pulejo" between January 2021 and August 2021, were evaluated for inclusion in this study.

Inclusion criteria were (i) hemiplegia/hemiparesis due to a first-ever stroke; (ii) at least one year after stroke; (iii) supervision-dependent ambulation (Functional Ambulation Classification—FAC $\geq$ 3); (iv) patients aged between 18 and 75 years. Patients were excluded if they presented the following criteria: (i) age > 75 years; (ii) diagnosis of concurrent psychiatric conditions or other significant medical comorbidities that could interfere with the RGT; (iii) presence of deficits (e.g., cognitive, visual, or auditory) that could limit the comprehension and/or execution of the proposed exercise; (iv) comorbidities that prevented upright posture and walking (e.g., hypotension); (v) refused consent or were unable to provide informed consent; (vi) recent bone fractures. In addition, we excluded patients if they had contraindications to the use of the technological instrumentation, such as a weight > 150 kg and open lesions or bandages in contact with the harness.

The enrolled patients were evaluated at baseline (T0) and after the experimental training (T1), consisting of forty sessions of RGT (experimental group—EG) for eight consecutive weeks.

The data of these subjects were compared with those coming from a sample of 12 individuals (control group, CG) matched for clinical and demographic features who underwent the same amount of CGT with no robotic assistance, in addition to standard rehabilitation therapy.

All experiments were conducted according to the ethical policies and procedures approved by the local ethics committee (IRCCSME-45/2020 approved on 14/12/2020). All participants gave their written informed consent.

The clinical–demographic characteristics of both groups are summarized in Table 1.

Table 1. Demographic and clinical characteristics of both groups (experimental—RGT and control—conventional rehabilitation training).

Characteristic	All	EG	CG	p-Value	Test
Patients	24 (100%)	12 (50%)	12 (50%)		
Age	51.13 ± 13.72	47 ± 12.54	55.25 ± 14.12	0.14	t-test
Education (years)	12.92 ± 2.96	12.92 ± 2.64	12.92 ± 3.37	0.82	U
Sex					
Male	16 (66.67%)	8 (66.67%)	8 (66.67%)	1	Fisher
Female	8 (33.33%)	4 (33.33%)	4 (33.33%)	1	Fisher
Time since injury (years)	2.25 ± 1.62	2.33 ± 1.78	2.17 ± 1.53	1	U
Etiology					
Ischemic	13 (54.17%)	7 (58.33%)	6 (50%)	0.68	χ^2
Hemorrhagic	11 (45.83%)	5 (41.67%)	6 (50%)	0.68	χ^2
Most affected side					
Left	11 (45.83%)	5 (41.67%)	6 (50%)	0.68	χ^2
Right	13 (54.17%)	7 (58.33%)	6 (50%)	0.68	χ^2

Legend: Fisher (Fisher's exact test); χ^2 (chi-squared test); U (Mann–Whitney U test).

2.1. Procedures

All the included patients were submitted for the same amount of training. However, they diverged in the type of rehabilitation approaches. The EG (n. 12) underwent RGT with the G-EO system, while the CG (n. 12) received CGT. Both groups followed the same rehabilitation protocol (as per the total amount of training), consisting of five sessions per week over eight weeks (by our established clinical research and standard care protocols). Each session included approximately one hour of gait training, followed by 45 min of conventional physiotherapy. Importantly, while the duration and structure of the sessions were identical, the type of gait training differed between groups: the EG used the G-EO system, whereas the CG received conventional overground gait training. In addition to gait training, both groups also received conventional physiotherapy, including stretching exercises, passive and active-assisted limb mobilization, and therapeutic exercises aimed at improving range of motion and overall muscle strength, lasting approximately 45 min per session (see Table 2 for more details).

Table 2. Summary of the characteristics linked to RGT and CGT protocols.

Rehabilitation Intervention Elements	CGT	RGT
Setting	Conventional physiotherapy gym	G-EO system robotic device
Duration of gait training	1 h	1 h
Gait training	10′ postural alignment with the aid of the physiotherapist 20′ gait training exercises: walking over obstacles of different sizes, tandem and slalom walking 10′ weight-shifting, core muscle strengthening, monopodal and bipodal balance exercises, 10′ ascending and descending stairs 10′ cool down and return to sitting position	10′ postural alignment with G-EO system 30′ gait training on the G-EO system, focusing on proper weight distribution between the two legs 10′ ascending and descending stairs with G-EO 10′ cool down and return to sitting position
Ascending and descending stairs	Yes With the supervision and manual guidance of the physiotherapist	Yes With the supervision of the physiotherapist and the guidance provided by the robotic device
Guidance	Manual guidance provided by the physiotherapist	BWS and robotic guidance—when needed, the physiotherapist provided supervision and/or hands-on support to the paretic knee of the patients
Audio–visual Feedback	Verbal feedback provided by the physiotherapist	Visual feedback provided by the monitor of the G-EO system and verbal feedback provided by the physiotherapist, as needed
Fatigue management	Yes Visible signs of fatigue (e.g., changes in gait quality or shortness of breath)	Yes Visible signs of fatigue (e.g., changes in gait quality or shortness of breath)
Rehabilitation parameters	No	Yes Step cadence and velocity
Conventional physiotherapy	Yes 45′ of stretching exercises, passive and active-assisted limb mobilization, and therapeutic exercises	Yes 45′ of stretching exercises, passive and active-assisted limb mobilization, and therapeutic exercises

All patients underwent a clinical visit and neurological evaluation at T0 and T1. However, only the patients who underwent RGT were also evaluated with the Fugl-Meyer—Lower Extremity assessment to understand the effects of robotics on body segmental outcomes, as well as specific parameters coming from the device.

2.2. Outcome Measures

Motor and functional clinical assessment scales/tests were administered by a skilled physiotherapist (ALF) at T0 and T1, and the subsequent analyses were performed by a biomedical engineer (PDP). In particular, the physiotherapist, who was blinded to the training allocation of the patient, administered a complete motor battery, including (i) the 10 Meters Walking Test (10MWT) [18] to assess walking speed in meters per second over a short distance; (ii) the Tinetti Scale (TS) [19], made up of 16 items, with 7 items assessing gait (with scores ranging from 0 to 12) and 9 items evaluating balance (with scores ranging from 0 to 16); (iii) the Modified Ashworth Scale (MAS) [20] was used to assess spasticity in lower limbs (hip, knee, and ankle), and it ranges from 0 (no increase in muscle tone) to 4 (rigid limb movement). Intermediate scores indicate varying degrees of increased muscle tone, from slight resistance (1, 1+) to marked stiffness (2, 3); (iv) the Functional Independence Measure (FIM) [21] was utilized to assess overall functioning across 18 items divided into six subscales—self-care, sphincter control, transfer, locomotion, communication, and social cognition ability. A higher score indicates less disability for basic daily functions.

After the allocation assignment, EG patients were also evaluated with the Fugl-Meyer—Lower Extremity (FMA-LE) assessment [22], which assesses reflexes and motor functioning at the hip, knee, and ankle (part E ranging from 0 to 28), coordination (part F ranging from 0 to 6), sensory functioning (part H ranging from 0 to 12), joint range of motion (part JI ranging from 0 to 20), and joint pain (part JII ranging from 0 to 20). In addition, specific rehabilitation parameters, regarding RGT, were extracted from the G-EO system, such as mean values of step cadence (steps/min) and walking speed (m/s).

2.3. G-EO System

The G-EO system [23] is an advanced robotic end-effector designed specifically for lower limb rehabilitation. This innovative device is equipped with footplates, or pedals, that guide the movement of the lower limbs along fully programmable trajectories. These footplates are designed to facilitate a range of natural motion patterns, moving from the bottom to the top in a manner that closely mimics real-life walking. The system allows for precise adjustment of key parameters, including step length (from 0 to 55 cm), step height (up to 400 mm), footplate angles (up to 90 degrees), movement velocity (up to 2.3 km/h), and acceleration peaks (up to 10 m/s^2). These customizable settings enable tailored rehabilitation programs that meet individual patient needs.

Unlike traditional systems that rely on the hips and knees for leg movement, the G-EO system focuses on ankle actuation, which is critical for simulating accurate walking mechanics. The patient's feet are securely fastened to the footplates using straps, ensuring proper alignment and safety during therapy sessions. This setup enables the device to replicate forward and backward walking motions, as well as stair-climbing activities, including both ascending and descending movements.

To enhance patient safety and support, the system features handrails on both sides, providing stability during therapy. Additionally, it incorporates a Body Weight Support (BWS) system, which reduces the load on the patient's lower limbs and allows for controlled weight-bearing exercises. This combination of features makes the G-EO system a highly versatile and effective tool for gait rehabilitation, offering a comprehensive approach to improving mobility and function in patients with lower limb impairments. The gait training session can be monitored through two displays providing visual feedback for therapists and patients. Moreover, this robotic device allows clinicians to supervise therapy progress over time through a detailed report, in which mean values of step length and cadence, walking speed, number of steps, and stairs are reported. In this way, therapists and clinicians can personalize each gait training session according to patients' parameters. During the rehabilitation sessions conducted on the G-EO system, patients began walking at an initial comfortable pace. This velocity was incrementally increased by 0.1 m/s based on the motor capacity and the state of fatigability of the patients. Once this threshold was achieved, the main phase of the session began. This progressive approach was implemented daily, with adjustments made based on the patient's performance and safety. Additionally, the therapists were allowed to modify step length parameters to tailor the RGT session to each patient. The primary goal was to increase gait parameters such as step length and velocity within safe and effective ranges. If a patient demonstrated the ability to sustain these parameters, those parameters were retained for the session. If not, the training proceeded at the previously established parameters from the prior session. The intensity of the training was individualized to prevent overexertion, with patients being closely monitored by clinicians. In instances of noticeable fatigue, the walking speed was decreased to a more comfortable pace, ensuring the patient could continue training effectively without risking overfatigue or injury. In general, all the RGT sessions were supervised by the physiotherapist, providing support to the paretic knee of the patient as needed.

Initially, BWS was set at 80% discharge for both floor walking and stair climbing, gradually decreasing by 10% each week until reaching 10% or the highest tolerated BWS; however, individual adjustments were implemented as needed based on patient tolerance and fatigue to ensure a safe and effective progression. Refer to Figure 1 for a visual representation.

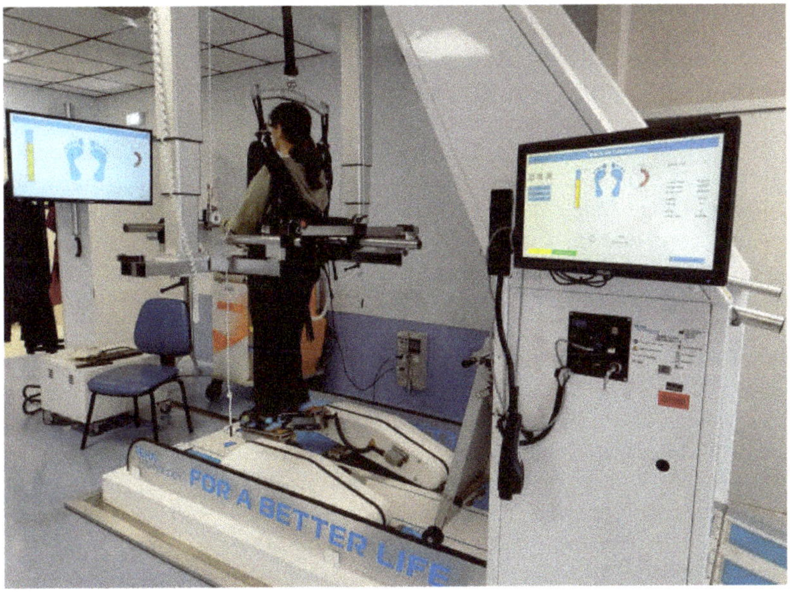

Figure 1. Post-stroke patient performing gait training on the G-EO system. The figure shows a patient performing an RGT session on the G-EO system. The monitor in front of the patient, as well as the second monitor of the therapist, provides visual real-time feedback on the patient's performance, including footplate pressure feedback, active therapy duration, repetitions, and distance covered.

2.4. Conventional Gait Training

Conventional gait training (CGT) sessions lasted one hour, followed by 45 min of conventional physiotherapy, in line with the protocol used for the EG (see Table 2).

In particular, the CGT included various exercises such as weight-shifting, core muscle strengthening, monopodal and bipodal balance exercises, and gait training involving obstacles, tandem, and slalom walking.

Like the EG, the intensity of training in the CG was individually tailored to prevent fatigue, with close monitoring of patients. Additionally, throughout all sessions, post-stroke patients received manual guidance and supervision from physiotherapists to minimize the risk of falls.

2.5. Statistical Analysis

The sample participants' sociodemographic and clinical parameters were analyzed, and differences between the experimental and control groups were assessed. Descriptive statistics were expressed as mean $\pm$ standard deviation for continuous variables and as frequencies (percentages) for categorical variables. Age, years of education, and years since injury were treated as continuous variables, while gender, etiology, and most affected side were analyzed as categorical variables. Normality for continuous variables was tested using the Shapiro–Wilk test (MATLAB R2022a, Natick, MA, USA, function swtest). Because the age distribution in both groups was normal, a parametric *t*-test (MATLAB function ttest) was used to evaluate group differences for age. In contrast, due to non-normal distributions of years of education and years since injury, group differences for these variables were assessed with the Mann–Whitney U test (MATLAB function ranksum). For the categorical variables, contingency tables were constructed; Fisher's exact test (MATLAB function fishertest) was applied when expected frequencies were low, whereas a chi-squared test (MATLAB function chi2cdf) was used otherwise.

Clinical data collected before and after treatment were compared within both groups. First, normality was evaluated using the Shapiro–Wilk test, and because not all distributions were normal, non-parametric methods were employed. Within-group changes were assessed with the Wilcoxon signed-rank test on paired pre-treatment (T0) and post-treatment (T1) data. To evaluate differences in treatment effects between groups, we computed the change (delta) for each subject (post-treatment value minus pre-treatment value) and compared these delta values between the experimental and control groups using the Mann–Whitney U test (i.e., a rank-sum test on the pre–post differences). Baseline equivalence was further confirmed by comparing the T0 values of the experimental group with those of the control group using the same non-parametric approach.

The dependency of clinical evaluations on demographic factors and patients' clinical status was tested using linear mixed effects models (LMEs) [24] via MATLAB's fitlme function. Separate models were constructed for the experimental and control groups, with participants included as a random effect to account for inter-individual variability. The age (A), gender (G), time since injury (I), and session (S) were treated as fixed effect factors. The experimental factors G and S were treated with categorical (dummy) variables, as they could take categorical outcomes: G = 0 for male, G = 1 for female, S = 0 for T0, S = 1 for T1. RGT parameters, which were selected by the therapist as step cadence (C) and velocity (V) during therapy, were included in the EG model based on their established relevance as indicators of gait function and rehabilitation outcomes after stroke [25–27]. Moreover, the interactions between sessions and each variable were evaluated. The normality of the residuals, which supports the model choice, was verified using a Lilliefors test applied to the residuals.

$$Y = g(u_0 + \alpha_0 A + \beta_0 G + \gamma_0 I + \delta_0 S + \theta_0 SA + \iota_0 SG + \kappa_0 SI + \epsilon) \quad (1)$$

$$Y = g(u_0 + \alpha_0 A + \beta_0 G + \gamma_0 I + \delta_0 S + \zeta_0 C + \eta_0 V + \theta_0 SA + \iota_0 SG + \kappa_0 SI + \lambda_0 SC + \mu_0 SV + \epsilon) \quad (2)$$

Equations. In Equations (1) and (2), u_0 represents the individual intercept and accounts for interindividual differences. The coefficients α_0, β_0, γ_0, δ_0, ζ_0, η_0, θ_0, ι_0, κ_0, λ_0, and μ_0 represent fixed effects; thus, the modulation of the response variable by the main factors A, G, I, S, C, V, and their interactions, ϵ, is the error-term.

In both Equations (1) and (2), g represents the identity link function. Control data were fitted using Equation (1), while experimental data were fitted with Equation (2), which considers rehabilitation training input parameters. In both cases, model parameters were estimated using maximum likelihood.

The significance of each fixed-effect term in the models was tested using the Wald Test [24], which evaluates the contribution of each fixed effect based on its coefficients and associated covariance structure. Given the number of clinical outcome measures and fixed effects analyzed, the risk of inflated type I errors due to multiple comparisons was addressed by applying a False Discovery Rate (FDR) correction using the Benjamini–Hochberg procedure [28].

The FDR correction was applied to the *p*-values obtained from the Wald tests at the term level, separately within each outcome-specific model. This correction method was applied independently for each clinical outcome, reflecting the independent testing of distinct functional domains.

Both uncorrected and FDR-corrected *p*-values are provided in the Supplementary Materials (Tables S1 and S2). Statistical significance was based on FDR-corrected *p*-values; effects not surviving correction but with *p*-values close to the threshold were interpreted cautiously as indicative of trends.

3. Results

At the baseline, there were no significant differences in the demographic and clinical features between the groups, as shown in Table 1. All patients completed the trial, and none reported any side effects during or after the training.

We found that the TS evaluating balance and gait was significantly improved after (T1) the RGT in the EG ($p = 0.012$, $p = 0.004$). Regarding the 10MWT, we found a statistically significant improvement in the CG ($p = 0.014$), while the EG showed an increased score, without achieving statistical significance. Moreover, we found that independence in daily activities (FIM) in both groups ($p < 0.001$), as shown in Table 3.

Table 3. Statistical comparisons (*p*-values) between T0 and T1 for each group and between EG and CG at T0 and T1 (EG vs. CT).

Scale/Test	EG T0–T1	CG T0–T1	EG vs. CG T0–T0	EG vs. CG Δ (T1–T0)
10MWT	0.069	**0.014**	0.295	0.255
Tinetti–Balance	**0.012**	0.277	0.6	**0.003**
Tinetti–Gait	**0.004**	0.25	0.06	**0.05**
MAS	0.078	0.453	0.17	0.342
FIM	**<0.001**	**<0.001**	0.977	0.183

Legend: 10WMT (10 m Walking Test), MAS (Modified Ashworth Scale), FIM (Functional Independence Measure); Δ (T1–T0): difference of "after treatment–before treatment". Significant *p*-values are reported in bold.

On the other hand, the FMA scores also improved, especially in the motor function (items E-F) (E, $p = 0.001$, F, $p = 0.031$, E-F, $p = 0.001$) and in the passive range of motion (JI, $p = 0.031$), as shown in Figure 2.

At the baseline, there were no significant differences in the clinical scales/tests scores between the two groups, as shown in Table 3. Regarding the statistical comparison between the two groups, we found statistically significant differences between EG and CG only in the TS for balance and gait ($p = 0.003$; $p = 0.05$), as shown in Table 3.

In particular, the EG showed a greater improvement in the TS for both balance and gait, compared to the CG, as shown in Figure 3.

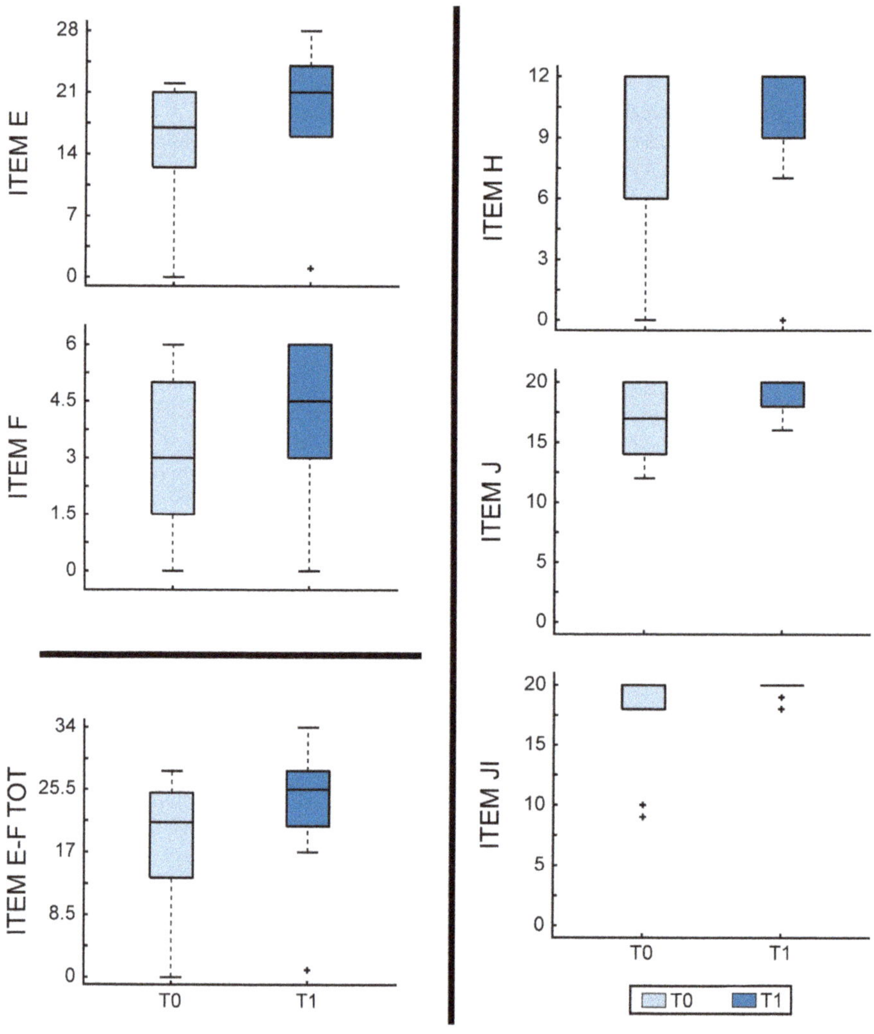

Figure 2. Fugl-Meyer Assessment—Lower extremity (FMA-LE) scores evaluated before and after RGT in the EG. The figure shows boxplots for each item of FMA-LE comparing before (T0—light blue) and after (T1—dark blue) RGT. Item E = lower extremity; Item F = coordination/speed; Item total E-F = motor function; Item H = sensation; Item JI = passive joint motion; Item JII = joint pain. The outliers are plotted using the + marker symbol.

The analysis, conducted using an LME model and evaluated via the Wald Test, was performed to detect treatment-associated changes while simultaneously assessing the influence of various factors (age, gender, TSI, and session) on clinical outcomes. Additionally, for the experimental group, treatment-specific parameters, such as velocity and cadence, which were adjusted by the therapist session by session, were integrated into the model. This comprehensive approach enabled us to identify the parameters that most significantly influenced the success of the intervention, thereby providing valuable insights into the determinants of treatment efficacy. In this study, we have reported only the statistically significant effects detected by the model.

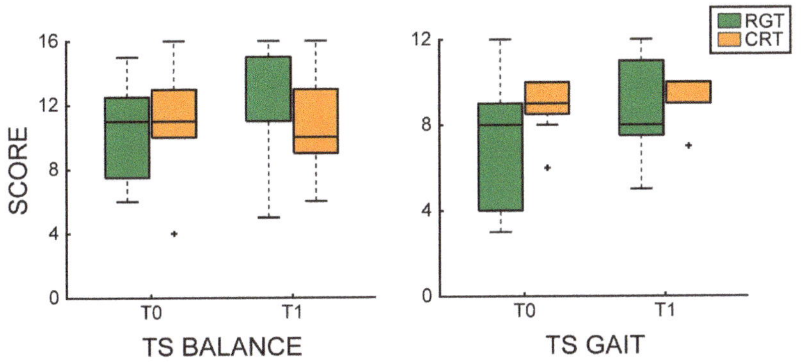

Figure 3. Tinetti Scale (TS) evaluating balance and gait functions. The left panel shows the TS balance boxplot comparing before (T0) and after (T1) RGT (green) and CGT (orange). The right panel shows the TS gait boxplot comparing before (T0) and after (T1) RGT (green) and CGT (orange). The outliers are plotted using the + marker symbol.

In the TS evaluating balance in the EG (R^2 = 0.98), significant effects were found for velocity (p = 0.049), gender × session (p = 0.049), TSI × session (p = 0.016), cadence × session (p = 0.016), and velocity × session (p = 0.016). Also, for the TS evaluating gait in the EG (R^2 = 0.98), significant effects were detected for session ($p < 0.001$), velocity ($p < 0.001$), gender × session ($p < 0.001$), and velocity × session ($p < 0.001$). In the control group (R^2 = 0.83), significant interactions were found for age × session (p = 0.019) and TSI × session (p = 0.024). For the MAS Scale in the EG (R^2 = 0.97), significant effects were observed for gender (p = 0.020), while a trend toward a significant effect of TSI (p = 0.074) was observed. Regarding the FIM Scale in the EG (R^2 = 0.98), we found that significant effects were observed for gender (p = 0.001), TSI ($p < 0.001$), cadence ($p < 0.001$), velocity (p =0.024), age × session (p = 0.024), gender × session ($p < 0.001$), and cadence × session ($p < 0.001$). On the other hand, in the CG (R^2 = 0.96), we found only the following significant effects: session (p = 0.023), TSI (p = 0.023), while a trend toward a significant effect of the interaction gender × session (p = 0.065) was observed. For FMA Item H in the EG (R^2 = 1), significant effects were detected for TSI (p = 0.019), velocity ($p < 0.001$), age × session ($p < 0.001$), and TSI × session ($p < 0.001$). For Item JI in the experimental group (R^2 = 0.97), significant effects were found for session ($p < 0.001$), TSI (p = 0.013), age × session ($p < 0.001$), gender × session ($p < 0.001$), TSI × session (p = 0.012), and a trend toward a significant effect of the interaction velocity × session (p = 0.079) was observed. For Item JII in the experimental group (R^2 = 0.93), significant effects were observed for TSI ($p < 0.001$), cadence (p = 0.017), and TSI × session ($p < 0.001$).

Although the effect on the 10MWT evaluation in the EG (R^2 = 0.99) did not reach statistical significance after FDR correction, a trend toward significance was observed for the following interactions: gender × session (p = 0.073), TSI × session (p = 0.089), and cadence × session (p = 0.073).

4. Discussion

In this case-control study, we aimed to investigate the effects of rehabilitation with the G-EO system, a robotic end-effector, on lower limb function in chronic post-stroke patients, compared to a CG that received CGT. At baseline, no significant differences were observed between groups in demographic and clinical characteristics. However, following the intervention, the EG demonstrated significant improvements in balance and gait performance (TS evaluating gait and balance, see Figure 3), as well as significant differences compared to the CG. These results may indicate that RGT enhanced postural control and dynamic stability, likely due to its ability to provide task-specific and repetitive movement patterns, which might facilitate neuromuscular adaptation (as demonstrated by previous studies [29,30]). In line with our findings, Kim et al. [31] found that RGT with an end-effector, combined with conventional physiotherapy, was associated with an improvement in balance scores, in comparison with CGT alone. According to the literature [2,5,32,33], lower limb alterations (e.g., muscle stiffness, spasticity, sensory loss) in post-stroke patients can be associated with a reduced efficiency in gait and balance, leading to an increased risk of falls in this patient population. In this context, neurorehabilitation strategies aim to achieve better neuromuscular control of lower limbs to promote a higher level of independence [34]. Innovative technologies, like robotic devices, have the advantage of carrying out personalized and task-oriented training that can motivate the patients, leading to longer therapy sessions [8]. Specifically, end-effector robotic devices are stationary devices with a distal movable part requiring active participation. In particular, the end-effectors are suitable tools that can be adapted to different shapes and sizes. Our results are likely influenced by the suitability of end-effector devices for patients who had residual locomotor functions, indicating a sufficient activation of proximal joints and muscles. It is noteworthy that the G-EO system provides repetitive, intensive, and task-oriented training that can enhance motor learning by engaging both efferent motor pathways and afferent sensory pathways throughout the training process [35]. Repetitive movements guided by the robotic device can play a crucial role in the re-acquisition of motor functions, promoting muscle memory and improving motor coordination [35]. It has been demonstrated that repetitive motor tasks facilitate neuroplasticity and brain reorganization in stroke patients, resulting in enhanced motor recovery after stroke [36]. In addition, the G-EO system promotes proximal muscle activity. In this sense, some authors found that proximal lower limb control plays a key role in improving gait speed and walking performance after stroke [36]. In this regard, we found that the RGT session with the G-EO system influenced the 10MWT scores in the EG. However, we did not find statistically significant differences between CG and EG in gait speed, maybe due to the small sample. Moreover, other authors studied the effects of RGT in chronic stroke patients with Lokomat, an exoskeleton, suggesting that FMA scores were significantly different in comparison with the conventional rehabilitation group. However, no significant differences in other clinical scales or tests were found in both groups. According to our results, RGT with the G-EO system improved FMA-LE scores, especially lower limb movements (FMA-LE part E), coordination (FMA-LE part F), and joint passive range of motion (FMA-LE part JI). This aspect could be explained by the fact that repetitive movements, provided by the robotic device, can serve as a fundamental element in the acquisition of motor skills [37], improving motor coordination and precision over time. A key outcome of this study was the improvement in functional independence (FIM) in both groups. This suggests that while both RGT and conventional therapy contribute to functional recovery, RGT with the G-EO system may offer additional benefits, allowing for the simulation of real-world experiences, such as ascending and descending stairs. In this way, by incorporating different stimuli and environmental conditions, therapy sessions become more dynamic and reflect the challenges encountered in everyday life [38], explaining our improvements in FIM scores.

The LME analysis showed that RGT treatment parameters (e.g., velocity and cadence) had significant effects across different assessment scales, indicating that adjustments made during the intervention have a dynamic impact on motor function recovery. In addition, as the LME analysis revealed that patients' demographic and clinical characteristics influenced various assessment scales, these findings underscore the importance of adopting a personalized rehabilitation approach that considers both baseline characteristics and adaptive treatment strategies to optimize motor recovery. Moreover, some clinical scales, such as FMA, showed significant interactions between sessions and various fixed effects. For instance, we found a significant session × age interaction (FMA, items H and JI), suggesting that the magnitude or pattern of motor recovery differs across age groups, with younger patients potentially exhibiting a more pronounced improvement than older patients.

This aspect is particularly important, as in the acute and subacute phases of stroke, it appears that there is no significant difference in motor and cognitive recovery between younger and older patients. Several studies, including the one by Kugler et al. [39], have demonstrated that age is a poor predictor of functional recovery during these early stages. However, in the chronic phase of stroke, age seems to play a more substantial role. Yoo et al. [40] found that functional recovery between 6- and 30-months post-stroke differed significantly between patients younger than 70 years and those aged 70 years or older.

Moreover, we found a statistically significant effect of velocity and an interaction between velocity and session on gait and balance outcomes (TS), as well as the effect of the interaction between cadence and session on balance outcome (TS for balance). According to Tomida et al. [41], increasing walking speed on a treadmill can significantly increase cadence in post-stroke patients. Generally, in healthy individuals, increasing gait speed requires taking longer steps, which necessitates moving the leg forward more quickly [42]. On the other hand, in post-stroke patients, enhancing propulsive force and facilitating a rapid forward swing of the lower limbs, achieved through an increased push-off moment via ankle plantar flexion during the late stance phase, augmented pull-off via hip flexion in the initial swing phase, and greater angular velocity, are key factors in improving walking speed [41].

Walking with end-effectors allows high degrees of freedom motions, which may provide a more realistic gait [43]. This aspect could have increased the passive range of motion scores in FMA-LE (FMA item JI), suggesting that the G-EO promoted an effective recovery instead of relying solely on behavioral compensation mechanisms. Furthermore, the significant effects and potential trends identified in passive range of motion (FMA item JI) and joint pain (FMA item JII) highlight the complex interplay between intrinsic patient characteristics and the optimization of tailored treatment parameters.

Unlike conventional rehabilitation training, the RGT with the G-EO offers visual feedback for patients and therapists. In this way, patients could have exploited the visual cues on the screen to increase their motivation during the training session. According to Nascimento et al. [44], walking training accompanied by cues for cadence can be an effective rehabilitation strategy to positively affect cadence, speed, and step length. On the other hand, the 10MWT showed a significant improvement in the CG, while the EG exhibited an increased score without reaching statistical significance. This finding suggests that CGT may still be more effective for certain aspects of mobility.

Similar findings were reported by Goffredo et al. [45], where the 10MWT did not show significant improvement in the RGT group treated either with an end-effector or with an exoskeleton, while the CGT group achieved statistical significance in this test. Likewise, in the study by Aprile et al. [14], the 10MWT did not yield any significant differences between T0 and T1 in either the RGT or CGT groups.

However, in our study, the LME analysis revealed a potential trend of the following interactions: age × session, gender × session, TSI × session, and cadence × session in the EG, related to the 10MWT, indicating that considering both demographic and clinical patients characteristics as well as RGT training parameters can positively affect the outcomes over time.

Among the interactions identified in the 10MWT evaluation for the EG, the cadence × session is particularly noteworthy. This finding potentially indicates that changes in cadence throughout the treatment could be significantly associated with improvements in walking performance [44]. Given that cadence represents the rhythm and pace of steps [46], a critical element of effective gait, the significant interaction suggests that adjustments made to cadence during each session contributed meaningfully to overall performance gains [47]. Specifically, the dynamic modulation of cadence, which was tailored by the therapist on a session-by-session basis, appears to have played a crucial role in enhancing neuromuscular coordination and gait efficiency. As the treatment progressed, the evolving relationship between cadence and session highlighted its potential as both a therapeutic target and a sensitive indicator of treatment responsiveness. In essence, these results underscore the importance of personalized adjustments in cadence to optimize rehabilitation outcomes, suggesting that fine-tuning this parameter could be key to achieving more effective gait training in patients undergoing robotic-assisted interventions [48,49].

Regarding muscle tone and motor control, both the EG and CG exhibited lower MAS scores post-treatment compared to baseline, indicating a reduction in spasticity. However, while the overall improvement in MAS scores was not statistically significant in the CG, the EG demonstrated statistically significant effects of gender and a trend toward a significant effect of TSI.

These findings suggest that, although both interventions led to a decrease in muscle tone, RGT may have a more pronounced impact on reducing spasticity in certain subgroups of patients [15]. In particular, the effect of gender and TSI can modulate the response of the MAS to robotic-assisted therapy, underscoring the potential for a more patient-specific rehabilitation approach.

According to a previous study in the multiple sclerosis population [35], the RGT with the G-EO system showed that MAS scores were significantly improved compared to the CGT. It has been suggested that RGT, by stimulating neuroplastic processes, may help regulate corticospinal excitability mechanisms involved in spasticity [8,35]. Spasticity is characterized by an increase in velocity-dependent tonic stretch reflexes, often associated with exaggerated tendon jerks [50]. From this perspective, the repetitive movements performed at a tolerated speed, according to the patients' needs, during RGT could mitigate spasticity by engaging spinal locomotor centers and influencing corticospinal pathway activity.

Our study has some limitations that should be acknowledged. First, the main limitation is related to the lack of randomization. Randomized trials (RCTs) allow for an unbiased assessment of treatment effects and ensure that, on average, treatment groups are balanced across all covariates. Secondly, the small sample prevents us from generalizing our findings. In this context, future larger sample RCTs on RGT in chronic post-stroke patients should be designed to minimize selection bias. Increasing the sample size would enhance the statistical power to confirm the positive trend of our study. Furthermore, we employed a demographic matching approach in our case-control design, which offers more limited control over potential confounding factors. Unlike simple demographic matching, propensity score matching accounts for multiple covariates simultaneously to achieve a more comprehensive balance between groups. In our study, the two groups were mostly balanced, although the TS gait at baseline was close to reaching statistical significance. Therefore, future studies should aim for greater homogeneity between groups to improve comparability and reduce potential confounding effects.

Future research should incorporate quantitative gait analysis methods, such as motion capture systems, force plates, and electromyography, to provide deeper insights into the effects and underlying mechanisms of motor recovery during RGT in chronic stroke patients. It is also important to implement clinical and quantitative evaluations not only in the short term but also in the long term through appropriate follow-up assessments. Lastly, we cannot exclude the possibility that the RGT group experienced a psychological placebo effect as compared to the non-robotic group, potentially influencing the results. However, unlike pharmacological or neuromodulation studies, where sham treatments can be implemented to control placebo effects, rehabilitation research faces inherent limitations: patients are fully aware of the type of intervention they receive, making it difficult to eliminate such biases.

Our study was intended to be preliminary evidence focusing on the feasibility and potential effectiveness of RGT with an end-effector in post-stroke patients compared to conventional gait training to provide basic information on determining the appropriateness of candidates that could benefit from this kind of treatment.

5. Conclusions

In conclusion, our results suggest that RGT with end-effectors, such as the G-EO system, may serve as an adjunctive and complementary treatment in neurorehabilitation, even for patients with chronic stroke, where recovery is typically considered to have plateaued. According to our findings, the G-EO system improved gait and balance functions compared to CGT. Furthermore, RGT promoted improvements in lower limb motor functions, indicating enhanced motor control and coordination, which are both key factors in fall prevention.

Supplementary Materials: The following supporting information can be downloaded at https://www.mdpi.com/article/10.3390/jfmk10020161/s1, Table S1: Results of linear mixed effects models for the experimental group (RGT): corrected and uncorrected *p*-values and significance for each clinical outcome. The table reports the results of linear mixed effects models (LMEs) for each clinical outcome in the experimental group. For each model, *p*-values obtained from Wald tests at the term level and their corresponding false discovery rate (FDR)-corrected values are presented, along with the assigned significance symbols. Statistical significance is indicated as *** $p < 0.001$, ** $p < 0.01$, * $p < 0.05$ after FDR correction, † indicates results significant before but not after correction, ns denotes non-significant effects; Table S2: Results of linear mixed effects models for the control group (CGT): corrected and uncorrected *p*-values and significance for each clinical outcome. The table reports the results of linear mixed effects models (LMEs) for each clinical outcome in the experimental group. For each model, *p*-values obtained from Wald tests at the term level and their corresponding false discovery rate (FDR)-corrected values are presented, along with the assigned significance symbols. Statistical significance is indicated as *** $p < 0.001$, ** $p < 0.01$, * $p < 0.05$ after FDR correction, † indicates results significant before but not after correction, ns denotes non-significant effects.

Author Contributions: Conceptualization, M.B., P.D.P., and R.S.C.; methodology, A.L.F. and P.D.P.; software, P.D.P.; validation, all authors; formal analysis, P.D.P.; investigation, M.B., B.D., and A.L.F.; resources, A.Q. and R.S.C.; data curation, P.D.P. and A.L.F.; writing—original draft preparation, M.B., P.D.P., and R.D.L.; writing—review and editing, R.S.C.; visualization, all authors; supervision, R.S.C., A.Q., and R.D.L.; project administration, A.Q. and R.S.C.; funding acquisition, A.Q. All authors have read and agreed to the published version of the manuscript.

Funding: This research was supported by Current Research Funds 2025, Ministry of Health, Italy.

Institutional Review Board Statement: The study was conducted in accordance with the Declaration of Helsinki and approved by the local Ethics Committee, IRCCS Centro Neurolesi Bonino Pulejo (IRCCSME-45-2020, 12 December 2020).

Informed Consent Statement: Written and informed consent was obtained from all subjects involved in the study.

Data Availability Statement: The data presented in this study are available on request from the corresponding author. The data are not publicly available due to the privacy of research participants.

Conflicts of Interest: The authors declare no conflicts of interest.

Abbreviations

The following abbreviations are used in this manuscript:

10MWT	10 Meters Walking Test
BWS	Body Weight Support
CG	Control Group
CGT	Conventional Gait Training
EG	Experimental Group
FAC	Functional Ambulation Classification
FDR	False Discovery Rate
FIM	Functional Independence Measure
FMA-LE	Fugl-Meyer Assessment—Lower Extremity
LME	Linear Mixed Effects
MAS	Modified Ashworth Scale
RGT	Robotic Gait Training
T0	Baseline Timepoint
T1	Post-Treatment Timepoint
TS	Tinetti Scale
TSI	Time Since Injury

References

1. Mohan, D.M.; Khandoker, A.H.; Wasti, S.A.; Ismail Ibrahim Ismail Alali, S.; Jelinek, H.F.; Khalaf, K. Assessment Methods of Post-Stroke Gait: A Scoping Review of Technology-Driven Approaches to Gait Characterization and Analysis. *Front. Neurol.* **2021**, *12*, 650024. [CrossRef]
2. Mizuta, N.; Hasui, N.; Kai, T.; Inui, Y.; Sato, M.; Ohnishi, S.; Taguchi, J.; Nakatani, T. Characteristics of Limb Kinematics in the Gait Disorders of Post-Stroke Patients. *Sci. Rep.* **2024**, *14*, 3082. [CrossRef]
3. Bonanno, M.; De Nunzio, A.M.; Quartarone, A.; Militi, A.; Petralito, F.; Calabrò, R.S. Gait Analysis in Neurorehabilitation: From Research to Clinical Practice. *Bioengineering* **2023**, *10*, 785. [CrossRef]
4. Wang, Y.; Mukaino, M.; Ohtsuka, K.; Otaka, Y.; Tanikawa, H.; Matsuda, F.; Tsuchiyama, K.; Yamada, J.; Saitoh, E. Gait Characteristics of Post-Stroke Hemiparetic Patients with Different Walking Speeds. *Int. J. Rehabil. Res.* **2020**, *43*, 69–75. [CrossRef]
5. Weerdesteyn, V.; de Niet, M.; van Duijnhoven, H.J.R.; Geurts, A.C.H. Falls in Individuals with Stroke. *J. Rehabil. Res. Dev.* **2008**, *45*, 1195–1213. [CrossRef]
6. Lee, K.B.; Kim, J.S.; Hong, B.Y.; Sul, B.; Song, S.; Sung, W.J.; Hwang, B.Y.; Lim, S.H. Brain Lesions Affecting Gait Recovery in Stroke Patients. *Brain Behav.* **2017**, *7*, e00868. [CrossRef]
7. Pollock, A.; Baer, G.; Campbell, P.; Choo, P.L.; Forster, A.; Morris, J.; Pomeroy, V.M.; Langhorne, P. Physical Rehabilitation Approaches for the Recovery of Function and Mobility Following Stroke. *Cochrane Database Syst. Rev.* **2014**, *2014*, CD001920. [CrossRef]
8. Calabrò, R.S.; Sorrentino, G.; Cassio, A.; Mazzoli, D.; Andrenelli, E.; Bizzarini, E.; Campanini, I.; Carmignano, S.M.; Cerulli, S.; Chisari, C.; et al. Robotic-Assisted Gait Rehabilitation Following Stroke: A Systematic Review of Current Guidelines and Practical Clinical Recommendations. *Eur. J. Phys. Rehabil. Med.* **2021**, *57*, 460–471. [CrossRef]
9. Ward, N.S.; Brown, M.M.; Thompson, A.J.; Frackowiak, R.S.J. Neural Correlates of Motor Recovery after Stroke: A Longitudinal fMRI Study. *Brain* **2003**, *126*, 2476–2496. [CrossRef]
10. Manuli, A.; Maggio, M.G.; Latella, D.; Cannavò, A.; Balletta, T.; De Luca, R.; Naro, A.; Calabrò, R.S. Can Robotic Gait Rehabilitation plus Virtual Reality Affect Cognitive and Behavioural Outcomes in Patients with Chronic Stroke? A Randomized Controlled Trial Involving Three Different Protocols. *J. Stroke Cerebrovasc. Dis.* **2020**, *29*, 104994. [CrossRef]
11. Calabrò, R.S.; Naro, A.; Russo, M.; Leo, A.; De Luca, R.; Balletta, T.; Buda, A.; La Rosa, G.; Bramanti, A.; Bramanti, P. The Role of Virtual Reality in Improving Motor Performance as Revealed by EEG: A Randomized Clinical Trial. *J. Neuroeng. Rehabil.* **2017**, *14*, 53. [CrossRef]
12. Bonanno, M.; Pioggia, G.; Santamato, A.; Calabrò, R.S. Robotics in Neurorehabilitation: From Research to Clinical Practice. In *Translational Neurorehabilitation: Brain, Behavior and Technology*; Calabrò, R.S., Ed.; Springer International Publishing: Cham, Switzerland, 2024; pp. 165–174. ISBN 978-3-031-63604-2.
13. Agarwal, P.; Deshpande, A.D. Exoskeletons: State-of-the-Art, Design Challenges, and Future Directions. In *Human Performance Optimization: The Science and Ethics of Enhancing Human Capabilities*; Matthews, M.D., Schnyer, D.M., Eds.; Oxford University Press: Oxford, UK, 2019; ISBN 978-0-19-045513-2.

14. Aprile, I.; Iacovelli, C.; Padua, L.; Galafate, D.; Criscuolo, S.; Gabbani, D.; Cruciani, A.; Germanotta, M.; Di Sipio, E.; De Pisi, F.; et al. Efficacy of Robotic-Assisted Gait Training in Chronic Stroke Patients: Preliminary Results of an Italian Bi-Centre Study. *NeuroRehabilitation* **2017**, *41*, 775–782. [CrossRef]
15. Aprile, I.; Iacovelli, C.; Goffredo, M.; Cruciani, A.; Galli, M.; Simbolotti, C.; Pecchioli, C.; Padua, L.; Galafate, D.; Pournajaf, S.; et al. Efficacy of End-Effector Robot-Assisted Gait Training in Subacute Stroke Patients: Clinical and Gait Outcomes from a Pilot Bi-Centre Study. *NeuroRehabilitation* **2019**, *45*, 201–212. [CrossRef]
16. Kim, J.; Kim, D.Y.; Chun, M.H.; Kim, S.W.; Jeon, H.R.; Hwang, C.H.; Choi, J.K.; Bae, S. Effects of Robot-(Morning Walk®) Assisted Gait Training for Patients after Stroke: A Randomized Controlled Trial. *Clin. Rehabil.* **2019**, *33*, 516–523. [CrossRef]
17. Lee, J.; Kim, D.Y.; Lee, S.H.; Kim, J.H.; Kim, D.Y.; Lim, K.-B.; Yoo, J. End-Effector Lower Limb Robot-Assisted Gait Training Effects in Subacute Stroke Patients: A Randomized Controlled Pilot Trial. *Medicine* **2023**, *102*, e35568. [CrossRef]
18. Cheng, D.K.-Y.; Dagenais, M.; Alsbury-Nealy, K.; Legasto, J.M.; Scodras, S.; Aravind, G.; Takhar, P.; Nekolaichuk, E.; Salbach, N.M. Distance-Limited Walk Tests Post-Stroke: A Systematic Review of Measurement Properties. *NeuroRehabilitation* **2021**, *48*, 413–439. [CrossRef]
19. Tinetti, M.E. Performance-oriented assessment of mobility problems in elderly patients. *J. Am. Geriatrics Soc.* **1986**, *34*, 119–126. [CrossRef]
20. Harb, A.; Kishner, S. Modified Ashworth Scale. In *StatPearls*; StatPearls Publishing: Treasure Island, FL, USA, 2025.
21. Biester, R.C. Chapter 12—Outcome Scales and Neuropsychological Outcome. In *Monitoring in Neurocritical Care*; Le Roux, P.D., Levine, J.M., Kofke, W.A., Eds.; W.B. Saunders: Philadelphia, PA, USA, 2013; pp. 107–113.e2. ISBN 978-1-4377-0167-8.
22. Hernández, E.D.; Forero, S.M.; Galeano, C.P.; Barbosa, N.E.; Sunnerhagen, K.S.; Alt Murphy, M. Intra- and Inter-Rater Reliability of Fugl-Meyer Assessment of Lower Extremity Early after Stroke. *Braz. J. Phys. Ther.* **2021**, *25*, 709–718. [CrossRef]
23. G-EO1 (n.d.). Reha Technology. Available online: https://www.rehatechnology.com/en/g-eo1/ (accessed on 11 February 2025).
24. McCulloch, C.E.; Searle, S.R. *Generalized, Linear, and Mixed Models*, 1st ed.; Wiley Series in Probability and Statistics; Wiley: Hoboken, NJ, USA, 2000; ISBN 978-0-471-19364-7.
25. Balasubramanian, C.K.; Bowden, M.G.; Neptune, R.R.; Kautz, S.A. Relationship Between Step Length Asymmetry and Walking Performance in Subjects With Chronic Hemiparesis. *Arch. Phys. Med. Rehabil.* **2007**, *88*, 43–49. [CrossRef]
26. Patterson, K.K.; Gage, W.H.; Brooks, D.; Black, S.E.; McIlroy, W.E. Changes in Gait Symmetry and Velocity After Stroke: A Cross-Sectional Study From Weeks to Years After Stroke. *Neurorehabil. Neural Repair.* **2010**, *24*, 783–790. [CrossRef]
27. Ada, L.; Dean, C.M.; Lindley, R.; Lloyd, G. Improving Community Ambulation after Stroke: The AMBULATE Trial. *BMC Neurol.* **2009**, *9*, 8. [CrossRef]
28. Benjamini, Y.; Hochberg, Y. Controlling the False Discovery Rate: A Practical and Powerful Approach to Multiple Testing. *J. R. Stat. Soc. Ser. B Stat. Methodol.* **1995**, *57*, 289–300. [CrossRef]
29. Calabrò, R.S.; Naro, A.; Russo, M.; Bramanti, P.; Carioti, L.; Balletta, T.; Buda, A.; Manuli, A.; Filoni, S.; Bramanti, A. Shaping Neuroplasticity by Using Powered Exoskeletons in Patients with Stroke: A Randomized Clinical Trial. *J. Neuroeng. Rehabil.* **2018**, *15*, 35. [CrossRef]
30. Androwis, G.J.; Pilkar, R.; Ramanujam, A.; Nolan, K.J. Electromyography Assessment During Gait in a Robotic Exoskeleton for Acute Stroke. *Front. Neurol.* **2018**, *9*, 630. [CrossRef]
31. Kim, H.; Park, G.; Shin, J.-H.; You, J.H. Neuroplastic Effects of End-Effector Robotic Gait Training for Hemiparetic Stroke: A Randomised Controlled Trial. *Sci. Rep.* **2020**, *10*, 12461. [CrossRef]
32. Darak, V.; Karthikbabu, S. Lower Limb Motor Function and Hip Muscle Weakness in Stroke Survivors and Their Relationship with Pelvic Tilt, Weight-Bearing Asymmetry, and Gait Speed: A Cross-Sectional Study. *Curr. J. Neurol.* **2020**, *19*, 1–7. [CrossRef]
33. Tyson, S.F.; Crow, J.L.; Connell, L.; Winward, C.; Hillier, S. Sensory Impairments of the Lower Limb after Stroke: A Pooled Analysis of Individual Patient Data. *Top. Stroke Rehabil.* **2013**, *20*, 441–449. [CrossRef]
34. Maier, M.; Ballester, B.R.; Verschure, P.F.M.J. Principles of Neurorehabilitation After Stroke Based on Motor Learning and Brain Plasticity Mechanisms. *Front. Syst. Neurosci.* **2019**, *13*, 74. [CrossRef]
35. Bonanno, M.; Maggio, M.G.; Ciatto, L.; De Luca, R.; Quartarone, A.; Alibrandi, A.; Calabrò, R.S. Can Robotic Gait Training with End Effectors Improve Lower-Limb Functions in Patients Affected by Multiple Sclerosis? Results from a Retrospective Case–Control Study. *J. Clin. Med.* **2024**, *13*, 1545. [CrossRef]
36. Mao, Y.-R.; Lo, W.L.; Lin, Q.; Li, L.; Xiao, X.; Raghavan, P.; Huang, D.-F. The Effect of Body Weight Support Treadmill Training on Gait Recovery, Proximal Lower Limb Motor Pattern, and Balance in Patients with Subacute Stroke. *Biomed. Res. Int.* **2015**, *2015*, 175719. [CrossRef]
37. Dayan, E.; Cohen, L.G. Neuroplasticity Subserving Motor Skill Learning. *Neuron* **2011**, *72*, 443–454. [CrossRef] [PubMed]
38. Banyai, A.D.; Brișan, C. Robotics in Physical Rehabilitation: Systematic Review. *Healthcare* **2024**, *12*, 1720. [CrossRef]
39. Kugler, C.; Altenhöner, T.; Lochner, P.; Ferbert, A. Hessian Stroke Data Bank Study Group ASH Does Age Influence Early Recovery from Ischemic Stroke? A Study from the Hessian Stroke Data Bank. *J. Neurol.* **2003**, *250*, 676–681. [CrossRef]

40. Yoo, J.W.; Hong, B.Y.; Jo, L.; Kim, J.-S.; Park, J.G.; Shin, B.K.; Lim, S.H. Effects of Age on Long-Term Functional Recovery in Patients with Stroke. *Medicina* **2020**, *56*, 451. [CrossRef] [PubMed]
41. Tomida, K.; Ohtsuka, K.; Teranishi, T.; Ogawa, H.; Takai, M.; Suzuki, A.; Kawakami, K.; Sonoda, S. Effects of Change in Walking Speed on Time-Distance Parameters in Post-Stroke Hemiplegic Gait. *Fujita Med. J.* **2022**, *8*, 121–126. [CrossRef]
42. Fukuchi, C.A.; Fukuchi, R.K.; Duarte, M. Effects of Walking Speed on Gait Biomechanics in Healthy Participants: A Systematic Review and Meta-Analysis. *Syst. Rev.* **2019**, *8*, 153. [CrossRef] [PubMed]
43. Hesse, S.; Waldner, A.; Tomelleri, C. Innovative Gait Robot for the Repetitive Practice of Floor Walking and Stair Climbing up and down in Stroke Patients. *J. Neuroeng. Rehabil.* **2010**, *7*, 30. [CrossRef]
44. Nascimento, L.R.; de Oliveira, C.Q.; Ada, L.; Michaelsen, S.M.; Teixeira-Salmela, L.F. Walking Training with Cueing of Cadence Improves Walking Speed and Stride Length after Stroke More than Walking Training Alone: A Systematic Review. *J. Physiother.* **2015**, *61*, 10–15. [CrossRef]
45. Goffredo, M.; Iacovelli, C.; Russo, E.; Pournajaf, S.; Di Blasi, C.; Galafate, D.; Pellicciari, L.; Agosti, M.; Filoni, S.; Aprile, I.; et al. Stroke Gait Rehabilitation: A Comparison of End-Effector, Overground Exoskeleton, and Conventional Gait Training. *Appl. Sci.* **2019**, *9*, 2627. [CrossRef]
46. Hollman, J.H.; McDade, E.M.; Petersen, R.C. Normative Spatiotemporal Gait Parameters in Older Adults. *Gait Posture* **2011**, *34*, 111–118. [CrossRef]
47. Ardestani, M.M.; Ferrigno, C.; Moazen, M.; Wimmer, M.A. From Normal to Fast Walking: Impact of Cadence and Stride Length on Lower Extremity Joint Moments. *Gait Posture* **2016**, *46*, 118–125. [CrossRef] [PubMed]
48. Eng, J.J.; Tang, P.F. Gait Training Strategies to Optimize Walking Ability in People with Stroke: A Synthesis of the Evidence. *Expert. Rev. Neurother.* **2007**, *7*, 1417–1436. [CrossRef] [PubMed]
49. Teodoro, J.; Fernandes, S.; Castro, C.; Fernandes, J.B. Current Trends in Gait Rehabilitation for Stroke Survivors: A Scoping Review of Randomized Controlled Trials. *J. Clin. Med.* **2024**, *13*, 1358. [CrossRef] [PubMed]
50. Katz, R.T.; Rymer, W.Z. Spastic Hypertonia: Mechanisms and Measurement. *Arch. Phys. Med. Rehabil.* **1989**, *70*, 144–155.

Journal of
Functional Morphology and Kinesiology

MDPI

Article

Surf's Up for Postural Stability: A Descriptive Study of Physical Activity, Balance, Flexibility, and Self-Esteem in Healthy Adults

Guillermo De Castro-Maqueda [1,*], Miguel Ángel Rosety-Rodríguez [1], Macarena Rivero-Vila [1], Jorge Del Rosario Fernández-Santos [1] and Teppei Abiko [2]

1 Department of Physical Education, School of Education Science, University of Cádiz, Puerto Real, 11407 Cádiz, Spain; miguelangel.rosety@uca.es (M.Á.R.-R.); macarenariverovila@hotmail.com (M.R.-V.); jorgedelrosario.fernandez@uca.es (J.D.R.F.-S.)

2 Department of Physical Therapy, Faculty of Health Sciences, Kyoto Tachibana University, Kyoto 567-0031, Japan; abiko@tachibana-u.ac.jp

* Correspondence: guillermoramon.decastro@uca.es

Abstract

Background: This study examines balance, flexibility and self-esteem among healthy individuals who engage in surfing compared to those who do not surf. **Methods:** A cross-sectional study design was conducted with 124 participants divided into the following groups: Group 1: Surfers $n = 42$; Group 2: individuals performing over 3 h of physical activity per week $n = 43$; and Group 3: individuals performing fewer than 3 h of physical activity per week $n = 39$. To assess balance, the Star Excursion Balance Test (SEBT) and the Flamenco Test (FBT) were used, the sit-and-reach test (SRT) was used to measure hamstring extensibility, the Rosenberg Scale was used to measure self-esteem, and the International Physical Activity Questionnaire (IPAQ) was used to measure physical activity levels. **Results:** Regarding descriptive characteristics, G1 participants were significant older than those of G2 and G3 ($p < 0.05$ and $p < 0.001$, respectively). Moreover, there was a higher proportion of females in G3 than in G1 and G2 ($p < 0.05$). The results revealed significant differences in balance between the surfers and those engaging in fewer than 3 h of activity per week ($p < 0.05$). G1 obtained significantly higher results in SEBT-left leg than G2 and G3 ($p < 0.001$) and higher result in SEBT-right leg and FBT than G3 ($p < 0.05$) but no significant differences in self-esteem were found. Significant differences in flexibility were observed between males and females ($p < 0.001$). **Conclusions:** This result suggests that surfing could have a positive effect on balance.

Keywords: aquatic sports; stability; flexibility; extensibility; self-esteem

1. Introduction

Surfing is an aquatic sliding sport that demands muscular strength, balance, and flexibility, enabling the surfer to stay on the board and make the necessary adjustments according to the manoeuvres being performed and the behaviour of the wave [1].

As an outdoor sport, it not only benefits physical health but also mental health, promoting concentration, coordination, and stress reduction [2]. Exercising outdoors is associated with improvements in mental health [3], and the complex aquatic environment requires the development of postural control strategies involving visual, vestibular, and proprioceptive systems [4].

These capacities are essential for adapting the body to the anterior–posterior and lateral demands generated when manoeuvring on a surfboard in an unstable, slippery environment [1,4,5].

Postural control is an essential component of performing daily living activities. It relies on the central nervous system's ability to integrate sensory inputs—including visual, vestibular, and somatosensory information—to generate a coordinated motor response [6].

This process involves complex biomechanical strategies and neuromuscular adaptations that stabilize body segments against gravity and maintain stability during upright stance. The vestibular system, in particular, provides information on the body's orientation relative to the environment, influencing athletic performance and safety during both training and competition. It plays a key role in both static and dynamic balance [5,7].

Building on this, recent studies in healthy subjects have begun to assess how sport practice, in particular, repetitive balance training of competitive athletes for long periods, helps develop the plasticity of postural function by improving the proprioceptive, improving balance control [8].

Sports requiring constant balance also improve postural control, which is a limiting factor in performance, since no technical sports movement whether at an amateur or professional level can be efficiently executed without effective postural balance control [9].

Surfing additionally involves the dynamic nature of waves, requiring continuous adjustment, and demands prior experience and situational awareness for adequate balance strategies [1,4,5].

Moreover, the psychological benefits of physical activity suggest that sports such as surfing can positively influence self-esteem and overall wellbeing in children and adolescents [10–12]. In the context of rehabilitation, incorporating activities that concurrently provide both physical and psychological benefits may optimise treatment outcomes by fostering a more enjoyable exercise environment in natural settings, thereby reducing stress and improving self-perception [10–13].

Surfing may also play a pivotal role in preventing musculoskeletal injuries due to the physical demands of the sport, including significant strengthening of the core and stabilising muscles. These adaptations, combined with the inherent balance challenge in surfing encompassing both static and dynamic balance, may be beneficial for patients recovering from physical or psychological injuries [14,15].

The benefits of surfing are not limited to the physical realm; the marine environment in which it is practiced also contributes to improved mood and reduced anxiety levels, as confirmed by recent research into water sports [16–18]. Aquatic-based rehabilitation techniques have also been shown to improve both static and dynamic balance in adults [19].

This study aims to evaluate and compare the levels of balance among individuals who practise surfing and people with varying levels of physical activity. It also seeks to determine whether there is a direct relationship between sports practice and self-esteem, thereby assessing the potential role of surfing as a therapeutic tool in clinical contexts.

2. Materials and Methods

2.1. Participants

In this cross-sectional study, 138 healthy white individuals aged 18 to 55 were recruited. A total of 13 participants were excluded for not meeting the inclusion/exclusion criteria, resulting in a final total of 124 participants. Exclusion criteria for the total sample included the following: having any balance disorder, not fitting the established age range (2 participants), experiencing lower-limb musculoskeletal injuries in the past two years (3 participants), suffering from any major visual or auditory impairment (such as blindness, vertigo, or deafness), having an oncological or neurological illness, or taking medication that could affect balance (3 participants). Pregnancy was also an exclusion criterion, along with failing to complete the requested questionnaires fully (5 participants).

All participants were instructed not to perform any physical exercise within 24 h prior to the assessments to eliminate any potential influence on the results. They were informed of the study protocol and the associated risks/benefits, and they signed informed consent forms. They also retained the right to withdraw from the study at any time, although none chose to do so. All procedures were approved by an Institutional Ethics Review Committee, Ref. UCAGM 3/23 (University of Cádiz, Spain) in accordance with current national and international laws and regulations for human subjects (Declaration of Helsinki, Fortaleza, Brazil, 2013). All data were recorded anonymously and handled in strict compliance with Spanish data protection laws (Law 41/2002 of 14 November and Law 15/1999 of 13 December).

The participants were divided into three groups: Group 1 (G1): 42 surfers (31 men, 11 women; mean age = 29.7 ± 8.8 years; surfing experience = 11.05 ± 10.12 years). Inclusion/exclusion criteria for G1 required at least two years of surfing experience and at least 3 h of physical activity included surfing; the participants were permitted to practise other sports. Individuals with visual and/or auditory impairments (myopia or hypoacusis) were included in all the groups as long as those conditions were well managed.

Group 2 (G2): 43 individuals performing more than 3 h of weekly physical activity (28 men, 15 women; mean age = 25.0 ± 8.42 years). Inclusion criterion: practising a minimum of 3 h of physical activity per week, excluding surfing.

Group 3 (G3): 39 individuals performing fewer than 3 h of weekly physical activity (18 men, 21 women; mean age = 23.3 ± 5.6 years). Inclusion/exclusion criteria for G3 required that participants practise 3 or fewer hours of physical activity per week and not engage in surfing.

2.2. Measures

All measurements were taken in April 2024. Each participant attended one assessment session. They were contacted through emails sent to surf centres and schools, and via posters placed in universities, university schools, surf clubs, and various sports facilities. These emails provided detailed information about the tests and questionnaires. All instruments employed in this study have scientific validation.

Body Mass Index (BMI): Height and body mass were measured while the participants were barefoot, wearing shorts and a t-shirt. Height was measured to the nearest 0.1 cm using a stadiometer (Holtain Ltd., Crymych, Pembrokeshire, UK), and body mass was measured to the nearest 0.1 kg using a Seca scale (SECA 861, Leicester, UK). Instruments were calibrated for accuracy. BMI was calculated as body mass (kg) divided by stature squared (m^2).

Star Excursion Balance Test (SEBT): This test is widely used to assess dynamic stability and proprioception, having been validated for various populations with high reliability [20–23]. Eight metric lines were placed on the floor, arranged like a star with 45° angles between them, each line ranging from 200 to 250 cm in length. Two calibrated lines were first placed in vertical and horizontal orientations (forming a symmetrical cross), followed by two diagonal lines in the shape of an "X", all intersecting at the same central point. Each arm was labelled according to the direction in which the leg should move. Before starting the test, the length of both lower limbs was measured from the highest point of the anterior superior iliac spine to the centre of the fibular malleolus (Figure 1).

During the test, the participants stood at the intersection point of all lines on one leg (single-leg stance), keeping the supporting foot oriented towards the anterior direction of the star (1-A). The supporting foot remained in full contact with the floor without shifting or lifting the heel. With the other foot, the participants reached as far as possible, touching the floor lightly with the tip of the big toe in each of the eight directions, returning to the starting point before moving on to the next direction. When the tested foot was the left foot, the sequence began in the anterior direction and proceeded clockwise; with the right foot, it progressed anticlockwise. The farthest point reached was recorded, and this test was performed twice per leg, with a 2 min rest between trials.

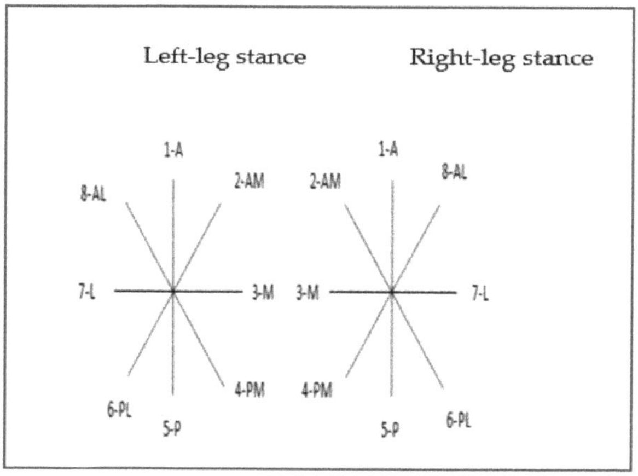

Figure 1. Note: 1-A. Anterior, 2-Am. Anteromedial, 3-M. Medial, 4-PM, Posteromedial, 5-P Posterior, 6-PL. Posterolateral, 7-L. Lateral, 8-AL. Anterolateral.

To determine the final score, the mean of all measurement results was divided by 8 times the total leg length and then multiplied by 100 to obtain a percentage. Two quantitative variables thus emerged: the result for the left leg (SEBT left) and the result for the right leg (SEBT right)

$$\text{SEBT} = \frac{\text{Mean of total reach distance}}{(\text{Total leg length} \times 8)} \times 100$$

ref. [24] (Plisky et al., 2006).

Flamenco Test: This simple, reliable test assesses static balance and is used in both clinical and sports contexts [25]. The starting position involved placing one foot on the floor and the other on a 4 × 2 × 45 cm metallic board, secured at both ends by wooden supports, elevating it 8.5 cm above the floor. On a given signal, the participants adopted a single-leg stance on the board, bending the free leg and holding it with the hand on the same side. The stopwatch began running when the participant was balanced on the board and was stopped whenever they lost balance (with either foot contacting the ground). Each time balance was lost, the participant resumed the starting position, and timing continued until a total of 1 min on the board was reached. The number of falls from the board in that minute was recorded. If the participants fell more than 15 times in the first 30 s, the test was terminated. The test was performed twice with a 1 min rest between attempts.

Rosenberg Scale: Originally developed to assess self-esteem, this scale has shown utility in evaluating psychological factors and emotional wellbeing [26–28]. Each participant completed a validated questionnaire (10 items) prior to the balance tests. Of these 10 items, 5 are worded positively and 5 negatively, measuring the individual's feeling of satisfaction with themselves.

For items 1 to 5, the responses from A to D were scored 4 to 1, respectively, while for items 6 to 10, the responses from A to D were scored 1 to 4. The results were interpreted as follows: 30–40 points indicates high self-esteem, 26–29 indicates average self-esteem, and below 25 indicates low self-esteem.

Physical activity and sports history: The level of physical activity was measured using the International Physical Activity Questionnaire (IPAQ, 2011) [29], which, among other items, queries the frequency and duration (at least 10 min per episode) of physical activity over the last seven days. The participants were also asked if they were members of any sports federation or had engaged in regular sports practice in the past two years. This questionnaire was supplemented with questions about surfing experience and weekly surfing frequency. Based on the information provided, each participant was classified as physically active or inactive.

Hamstring flexibility: This component was evaluated using the sit-and-reach test (SRT) following the established protocol [30]. This test has high validity and reliability [31,32] and is one of the most commonly used linear methods [33]. In the SRT, initially described by Wells & Dillon [34], the participants sat on the floor with their legs together and extended, and their feet flexed at 90° against a measurement box marked with a ruler, Fabrication Enterprises Inc., White Plains, NY, USA). The participants wore sports clothing (top and shorts) without shoes. With their palms facing downwards and fingers extended, they were instructed to reach forward as far as possible, sliding their hands along the ruler, holding the position for at least two seconds. The SRT score (in cm) was recorded as the final position reached by the fingertips on the ruler, with higher scores indicating better performance. The test was performed twice and the higher score was recorded [32–34].

2.3. Procedure

Upon arriving at the assessment area and prior to the balance and flexibility tests, the participants completed questionnaires on health habits, physical activity (IPAQ), and self-esteem (Rosenberg Scale). They also signed an informed consent form regarding their participation and permission to be recorded during the tests. All tests were conducted indoors under stable climatic conditions, with the ambient temperature between 22° and 24°. Each participant performed a short warm-up consisting of 5–10 min on a stationary bicycle or jogging.

Additionally, the participants completed a questionnaire on their age, sex, occupation, sports activities (type and duration), surfing experience, history of trauma or pathologies, unhealthy habits, medications taken, and any relevant personal history.

2.4. Data Analysis

Descriptive characteristics were reported as mean and standard deviation for quantitative variables and frequencies and percentage for qualitative variables. Data normality was assessed using the Shapiro–Wilk test for all quantitative variables. One-way ANOVA and chi-squared tests were conducted to examine differences in the descriptive characteristics between groups for quantitative and qualitative variables, respectively. ANCOVA was performed with age and sex as covariates to assess differences between groups in test results. RSES differences were modelled using a multinomial logistic regression with group category as the main predictor and age and sex as covariates.

All model assumptions were verified prior to analysis. When significant main effects were found, post hoc pairwise comparisons were performed using Bonferroni's correction. A significance level of $\alpha = 0.05$ was set for all hypothesis testing. All analyses were conducted using the R programming language for statistical computing (version 4.2.2).

3. Results

3.1. Participant Characteristics

A total of 124 healthy male and female aged 18 to 55 took part in this study (77 males). Participant characteristics in each category were classified as G1 (29.7 ± 8.8 years), with a mean of 11.05 ± 10.12 years of surfing experience; G2 (25.0 ± 8.42 years); and G3 (23.3 ± 5.6 years). The G1 participants were significantly older than those of G2 and G3 ($p < 0.05$ and $p < 0.001$, respectively). Moreover, there was a higher proportion of females in G3 than in G1 and G2 ($p < 0.05$).

Table 1 summarises the characteristics for the overall group. The mean (±SD) BMI values recorded were 24.0 ± 4.5 for the whole group, 24.1 ± 3.4 for female, and 23.8 ± 3.2 for male.

Table 1. Descriptive characteristics of the sample.

Variables		All (n = 124)	G1 (n = 42)	G2 (n = 43)	G3 (n = 39)
Age (years)		26.1 ± 8.2	29.7 ± 8.8 ^{a}	25.0 ± 8.4 ^{b*}	23.3 ± 5.6 ^{b***}
Sex	Male	77 (62)	31 ^{a}	28 ^{a}	18 ^{b*}
(n (%))	Female	47 (38)	11	15	21
Height (cm)		170.3 ± 11.7	174.3 ± 11.7	169.5 ± 10.8	170.2 ± 11.8
Weight (kg)		69.0 ± 8.8	69.8 ± 9.0	66.5 ± 9.8	71.1 ± 6.8
BMI (kg/m^2)		24.0 ± 4.5	23.2 ± 4.3	27.6 ± 4.7	24.9 ± 4.4

Different superscript letters indicate significant differences between groups. BMI = Body Mass Index. * $p < 0.05$; *** $p < 0.001$.

3.2. Balance Tests

For the test variables, G1 obtained significantly higher results in SEBT-left leg than G2 and G3 ($p < 0.001$) and higher results in SEBT-right leg and FBT than G3 ($p < 0.05$).

Regarding the Star Excursion Balance Test, the greatest reach distances and highest averages for each leg were recorded in the surfer group compared to the other two groups. In the Flamenco Test, higher scores correspond to more falls, which implies poorer performance. The G3 members exhibited the highest number of falls. Table 2 displays the descriptive results for each group and the different balance tests.

Table 2. Test results by experimental group.

Test		G1 (n = 42)	G2 (n = 43)	G3 (n = 39)
Sit-and-Reach Test (cm)		2.7 ± 6.2	3.7 ± 6.4	4.6 ± 5.6
SEBT—left leg		15.1 ± 2.2 ^{a}	13.4 ± 1.5 ^{b***}	12.6 ± 2.3 ^{b***}
SEBT—right leg		14.2 ± 1.9 ^{a}	13.3 ± 1.7 ^{ab}	13.0 ± 1.8 ^{b*}
Flamenco Balance Test (falls)		3.4 ± 3.1 ^{a}	8.4 ± 5.5 ^{ab}	12.4 ± 5.8 ^{b*}
	High	37 (88)	36 (84)	33 (85)
RSES (n (%))	Moderate	5 (12)	7 (16)	4 (10)
	Low	0 (0)	0 (0)	2 (5)

SEBT indicates Star Excursion Balance Test; RSES, Rosenberg Self-Esteem Scale. Different superscript letters indicate significant differences between groups. * $p < 0.05$; *** $p < 0.001$.

As regards the SEBT for the left leg, when comparing the three groups, no significant differences were found between G1 and G2, though differences did exist between G1 and G3. In comparing all three groups in the Flamenco Test, a significant difference emerged between surfers and both other groups ($p < 0.05$). The difference between G2 and G3 was not significant.

In addition, the relationship between the balance tests and age was examined to see if older or younger participants performed better or worse. The results showed no relationship between age and performance in both balance tests.

3.3. Hamstring Flexibility

G1 obtained the lowest performance in the flexibility test compared to the other groups, which may be attributed to the lower proportion of women in this group. When analysed by sex, women significantly outperformed men in the flexibility test ($p < 0.001$), despite men reporting higher levels of physical activity ($p < 0.05$). In the sit-and-reach test (SRT), women achieved a mean score of 5.3 ± 5.1 cm, while men scored 2.1 ± 5.3 cm. These differences may be explained by biological or hormonal factors associated with sex. No significant positive correlations were found with other measured variables.

3.4. Self-Esteem

With regard to the Rosenberg Self-Esteem Scale, 88.0% of participants in Group 1 exhibited high self-esteem, 10.5% demonstrated average self-esteem, and none presented with low self-esteem. In G2, 84.2% had high self-esteem, 15.7% had average self-esteem, and none had low self-esteem. In G3, 84.21% had high self-esteem, 10.5% had average self-esteem, and 5.2% had low self-esteem. No differences were found across groups, nor was any association detected between sports practice and self-esteem.

4. Discussion

The present study links the practice of surfing to a significant improvement in both dynamic and static balance, compared to other populations and different sports disciplines. The findings indicate that sports requiring continuous adaptation to unstable environments strengthen postural control, as is the case in surfing, snowboarding, and ice hockey [1,4,35–37]. These observations are supported by studies describing the physiological demands of surfing, emphasising not only the aerobic and anaerobic capacity required but also the importance of effective postural control to maintain balance on the board in constantly changing aquatic conditions [38].

Constant exposure to unstable surfaces promotes proprioception and intermuscular coordination, encouraging more advanced postural strategies that could be harnessed in therapeutic contexts. The results demonstrate a significant difference in the SEBT (dynamic balance) between people who surf and those engaging in fewer than three hours of physical activity weekly. Notably, within the group performing under three hours of exercise per week, 12 participants did not perform any physical activity. Meanwhile, all participants in the surfer group also practised another sport, supporting the idea that better balance in this group is due to both surfing and regular physical activity. This aligns with a published study indicating that physical activity improves both static and dynamic balance compared to inactivity [39].

No significant differences in dynamic balance were found between the group performing more than three hours of physical activity per week and the group performing fewer than three hours. This suggests that if practising any sport were the sole contributor to better balance, one would expect significant differences between these two groups. Hence, it is likely that the practice of surfing leads to improved dynamic balance.

Research has shown that proprioception, strength, and power are key components in aquatic sports like surfing, where ongoing exposure to unstable surfaces enhances intermuscular coordination and reflex responses [1,4,5,40]. Surfing also exerts a positive impact on specific populations, with its physical, psychological, and social benefits demonstrated by extensive intervention programmes [8,9,41]. Additionally, aquatic physiotherapy research has documented similar improvements albeit in a less challenging setting for rehabilitation, achieving significant advances in postural control and general mobility of the treated area [42–44].

With respect to balance, studies have compared dynamic balance, measured by the Star Excursion Balance Test, among hockey and football players. For instance, Bhat and Ali-Moiz [45] found no significant differences between the two groups, suggesting that better balance may be linked to sports participation in general rather than the specific type of sport. This was also observed in our study, where the surfing group reported engaging in another sport as well.

However, focusing on the development of dynamic lower-limb strength, the SEBT appears to be a solid adjunct for detecting bilateral performance differences, possibly indicating the efficacy of surfing training in reducing lower-limb asymmetry and improving postural control [46].

Furthermore, Reed et al. suggested that regular outdoor sports practice may help alleviate stress [12,47], a benefit that also appears in surfing through its combination of physical exercise and contact with nature. This highlights the potential of surfing not just as a recreational pursuit but also as a therapeutic tool. It not only aids balance and coordination but also provides a relaxing environment that may counteract chronic stress.

Regarding self-esteem, measured by the Rosenberg Scale, most participants scored in the high range; so, this study did not find a relationship between sports practice and self-esteem. These findings are consistent with the work of Molina-García et al. [48], who likewise found no significant differences between physically active and inactive participants for both sexes. Compared to a study by Monteiro et al., no significant differences in self-esteem were observed between those who did and did not practise dance [49]. Nevertheless, surfing could contribute to reducing depressive symptoms, which, in turn, may be related to improvements in self-esteem [50].

As for hamstring extensibility, our study found that women surfers exhibited greater flexibility than their male counterparts. These data match other studies using the SRT [31–33], and this difference could be due to biological or hormonal factors related to sex. However, we did not observe significant differences with other variables.

Our findings indicate that longitudinal studies are warranted to assess the long-term benefits of surfing across different populations. Future studies might explore how to combine surfing with other conventional aquatic therapies to maximise proven benefits [43,44]. Investigations should also delve into the psychological mechanisms that enhance balance and self-esteem and consider designing personalised interventions for specific clinical groups.

5. Conclusions

In conclusion, this study confirms that practising surfing and physical activity improves both dynamic and static balance in healthy individuals. However, within the age ranges studied, no definitive relationship was found between age and balance performance. Regarding self-esteem, no differences were detected between surfers and other participants, though further research is needed to corroborate this finding. Moreover, the potential therapeutic applications of surfing for populations with balance disorders were highlighted.

Our results suggest that this approach could offer a solid foundation for future research and for integrating surfing into innovative rehabilitation protocols. Surfing may serve as a complementary technique in rehabilitative treatments for patients with balance disorders, and further studies should explore these benefits in clinical settings.

6. Limitations

This study has several limitations worth noting. Firstly, its observational, cross-sectional design limits the ability to establish causal relationships between surfing practice and improved balance. Longitudinal or experimental designs would provide a clearer picture of how surfing influences balance and whether this effect persists over time. Secondly, the participants were recruited from a single geographical region, which may affect the generalisability of the findings to broader or more diverse populations. Thirdly, self-reported data on physical activity (e.g., hours of exercise per week) could introduce recall bias or inaccuracies that affect the reliability of group classification.

Furthermore, the environmental variability in surfing conditions (for example, wave height, water temperature, or currents), gender differences and the balance of participants were not standardized, which could influence the magnitude of balance adaptations. Finally, although the age range was fairly broad (18–55), the sample did not include individuals with clinically diagnosed balance disorders or other relevant comorbidities, limiting the application of these results to more specialised or clinical populations. Future research addressing these limitations, such as by conducting randomised controlled trials, recruiting more diverse cohorts, and systematically monitoring environmental factors, would help confirm and extend the conclusions drawn here.

7. Practical Applications

Despite these limitations, the findings offer several practical applications. Firstly, surfing-based exercise programmes may be considered as an adjunct to traditional balance training for healthy adults, given the positive effect observed on dynamic and static balance. Health and fitness professionals could incorporate surf-specific drills or balance-related manoeuvres (e.g., simulation training on unstable surfaces) into broader exercise regimens to enhance postural control.

Secondly, sports coaches and athletic trainers can use surf-like training environments (e.g., surf simulators, balance boards) to diversify their athletes' conditioning routine, potentially improving proprioception and postural stability.

Thirdly, the data suggest that long-term participation in an activity requiring dynamic postural adjustments (such as surfing) might confer benefits in daily tasks that involve balance and coordination, which could be particularly relevant for injury prevention in other sports.

Finally, although not tested directly in clinical populations, the results hint that surf-related activities may hold therapeutic potential for individuals undergoing rehabilitation for mild balance disorders. Engaging in enjoyable physical activities could facilitate greater adherence to rehabilitation protocols and potentially accelerate improvements in postural control.

Author Contributions: Conceptualization; G.D.C.-M., M.Á.R.-R. and M.R.-V.; Methodology, G.D.C.-M. and J.D.R.F.-S.; Writing, G.D.C.-M. and J.D.R.F.-S.; Original Draft Preparation, G.D.C.-M., M.Á.R.-R. and T.A.; Visualization and Investigation, M.Á.R.-R., T.A., G.D.C.-M. and M.R.-V.; Data Curation and Supervision, J.D.R.F.-S.; Writing—Reviewing and Edition, G.D.C.-M., T.A., M.R.-V. and J.D.R.F.-S. All authors have read and agreed to the published version of the manuscript.

Funding: This research received no external funding.

Institutional Review Board Statement: All procedures were approved by an Institutional Ethics Review Committee, Ref. UCAGM 3/23 (University of Cádiz, Spain, 12 March 2023) in accordance with current national and international laws and regulations for human subjects (Declaration of Helsinki, Fortaleza, Brazil, 2013). All data were recorded anonymously and handled in strict compliance with Spanish data protection laws (Law 41/2002 of 14 November and Law 15/1999 of 13 December).

Informed Consent Statement: Informed consent was obtained from all subjects involved in the study and Written informed consent has been obtained from the patient(s) to publish this paper.

Data Availability Statement: The raw data supporting the conclusions of this article will be made available by the authors on request.

Acknowledgments: The authors would like to thank all the participants in this study, including university students and surf schools, as well as the technical coaches of surf clubs, for their generous time and effort.

Conflicts of Interest: The authors declare no conflicts of interest.

References

1. Secomb, J.L.; Farley, O.R.L.; Lundgren, L.; Tran, T.T.; King, A.; Nimphius, S.; Sheppard, J.M. Associations between the Performance of Scoring Manoeuvres and Lower-Body Strength and Power in Elite Surfers. *Int. J. Sports Sci. Coach.* **2015**, *10*, 911–918. [CrossRef]
2. Buckley, R.C.; Cooper, M.A. Mental health contribution to economic value of surfing ecosystem services. *npj Ocean. Sustain.* **2023**, *2*, 20. [CrossRef]
3. Mahindru, A.; Patil, P.; Agrawal, V. Role of Physical Activity on Mental Health and Well-Being: A Review. *Cureus* **2023**, *15*, e33475. [CrossRef] [PubMed] [PubMed Central]
4. Chapman, D.W.; Needham, K.J.; Allison, G.T.; Lay, B.; Edwards, D.J. Effects of experience in a dynamic environment on postural control. *Br. J. Sports Med.* **2008**, *42*, 16–21. [CrossRef] [PubMed]
5. Marigold, D.S.; Patla, A.E. Strategies for dynamic stability during locomotion on a slippery surface: Effects of prior experience and knowledge. *J. Neurophysiol.* **2002**, *88*, 339–353. [CrossRef] [PubMed]
6. De Blasiis, P.; Fullin, A.; De Girolamo, C.I.; Amata, O.; Caravaggi, P.; Caravelli, S.; Mosca, M.; Lucariello, A. Posture and vision: How different distances of viewing target affect postural stability and plantar pressure parameters in healthy population. *Heliyon* **2024**, *10*, e39257. [CrossRef] [PubMed] [PubMed Central]
7. Hrysomallis, C. Balance ability and athletic performance. *Sports Med.* **2011**, *41*, 221–232. [CrossRef] [PubMed]
8. De Blasiis, P.; Fullin, A.; Caravaggi, P.; Lus, G.; Melone, M.A.; Sampaolo, S.; DELuca, A.; Lucariello, A. Long-term effects of asymmetrical posture in boxing assessed by baropodometry. *J. Sports Med. Phys. Fit.* **2022**, *62*, 350–355. [CrossRef] [PubMed]
9. Marcolin, G.; Supej, M.; Paillard, T. Editorial: Postural Balance Control in Sport and Exercise. *Front. Physiol.* **2022**, *13*, 961442. [CrossRef] [PubMed] [PubMed Central]
10. Olive, L.; Dober, M.; Mazza, C.; Turner, A.; Mohebbi, M.; Berk, M.; Telford, R. Surf therapy for improving child and adolescent mental health: A pilot randomised control trial. *Psychol. Sport Exerc.* **2023**, *65*, 102349. [CrossRef] [PubMed]
11. Carneiro, L.; Clemente, F.M.; Claudino, J.G.; Ferreira, J.; Ramirez-Campillo, R.; Afonso, J. Surf therapy for people with mental health disorders: A systematic review of randomized and non-randomized controlled trials. *BMC Complement. Med. Ther.* **2024**, *24*, 376. [CrossRef] [PubMed] [PubMed Central]
12. Reed, K.; Wood, C.; Barton, J.; Pretty, J.N.; Cohen, D.; Sandercock, G.R. A repeated measures experiment of green exercise to improve self-esteem in UK school children. *PLoS ONE* **2013**, *8*, e69176. [CrossRef] [PubMed] [PubMed Central]
13. Moreira, M.; Peixoto, C. Qualitative task analysis to enhance sports characterization: A surfing case study. *J. Hum. Kinet.* **2014**, *42*, 245–257. [CrossRef] [PubMed] [PubMed Central]
14. Becker, B.E. Aquatic therapy: Scientific foundations and clinical rehabilitation applications. *PMR* **2009**, *1*, 859–872. [CrossRef] [PubMed]
15. Melo, R.S.; Cardeira, C.S.F.; Rezende, D.S.A.; Guimarães-do-Carmo, V.J.; Lemos, A.; de Moura-Filho, A.G. Effectiveness of the aquatic physical therapy exercises to improve balance, gait, quality of life and reduce fall-related outcomes in healthy community-dwelling older adults: A systematic review and meta-analysis. *PLoS ONE* **2023**, *18*, e0291193. [CrossRef] [PubMed] [PubMed Central]
16. González-Devesa, D.; Vilanova-Pereira, M.; Araújo-Solou, B.; Ayán-Pérez, C. Effectiveness of surfing on psychological health in military members: A systematic review. *BMJ Mil. Health* **2024**, military-2024-002856. [CrossRef] [PubMed]
17. Rocher, M.; Silva, B.; Cruz, G.; Bentes, R.; Lloret, J.; Inglés, E. Benefits of Outdoor Sports in Blue Spaces. The Case of School Nautical Activities in Viana do Castelo. *Int. J. Env. Res. Public Health* **2020**, *17*, 8470. [CrossRef] [PubMed] [PubMed Central]
18. Godfrey, C.; Devine-Wright, H.; Taylor, J. The positive impact of structured surfing courses on the wellbeing of vulnerable young people. *Community Pract.* **2015**, *88*, 26–29. [PubMed]
19. Roth, A.E.; Miller, M.G.; Ricard, M.; Ritenour, D.; Chapman, B.L. Comparisons of static and dynamic balance following training in aquatic and land environments. *J. Sport Rehabil.* **2006**, *15*, 299–311. [CrossRef]
20. Powden, C.J.; Dodds, T.K.; Gabriel, E.H. The reliability of the star excursion balance test and lower quarter y-balance test in healthy adults: A systematic review. *Int. J. Sports Phys. Ther.* **2019**, *14*, 683–694. [CrossRef] [PubMed] [PubMed Central]
21. Hyong, I.H.; Kim, J.H. Test of intrarater and interrater reliability for the star excursion balance test. *J. Phys. Ther. Sci.* **2014**, *26*, 1139–1141. [CrossRef] [PubMed] [PubMed Central]

22. Gribble, P.; Hertel, J. Considerations for normalizing measures of the Star Excursion Balance Test. *Meas. Phys. Educ. Exerc. Sci.* **2003**, *7*, 89–100. [CrossRef]
23. Gribble, P.A.; Hertel, J.; Plisky, P. Using the Star Excursion Balance Test to assess dynamic postural-control deficits and outcomes in lower extremity injury: A literature and systematic review. *J. Athl. Train.* **2012**, *47*, 339–357. [CrossRef] [PubMed] [PubMed Central]
24. Plisky, P.J.; Rauh, M.J.; Kaminski, T.W.; Underwood, F.B. Star Excursion Balance Test as a predictor of lower extremity injury in high school basketball players. *J. Orthop. Sports Phys. Ther.* **2006**, *36*, 911–919. [CrossRef] [PubMed]
25. Gergüz, Ç.; Aras Bayram, G. Effects of Yoga Training Applied with Telerehabilitation on Core Stabilization and Physical Fitness in Junior Tennis Players: A Randomized Controlled Trial. *Complement Med. Res.* **2023**, *30*, 431–439. [CrossRef] [PubMed]
26. Schmitt, D.P.; Allik, J. Simultaneous administration of the Rosenberg Self-Esteem Scale in 53 nations: Exploring the universal and culture-specific features of global self-esteem. *J. Pers. Soc. Psychol.* **2005**, *89*, 623–642. [CrossRef] [PubMed]
27. Frieiro, P.; González-Rodríguez, R.; Domínguez-Alonso, J. Self-esteem and socialisation in social networks as determinants in adolescents' eating disorders. *Health Soc. Care Community* **2022**, *30*, e4416–e4424. [CrossRef] [PubMed] [PubMed Central]
28. Zurita-Ortega, F.; Castro-Sánchez, M.; Rodríguez-Fernández, S.; Cofré-Boladós, C.; Chacón-Cuberos, R.; Martínez-Martínez, A.; Muros-Molina, J.J. Actividad física, obesidad y autoestima en escolares chilenos: Análisis mediante ecuaciones estructurales [Physical activity, obesity and self-esteem in chilean schoolchildren]. *Rev. Med. Chil.* **2017**, *145*, 299–308. [CrossRef] [PubMed]
29. Hallal, P.C.; Victora, C.G. Reliability and validity of the International Physical Activity Questionnaire (IPAQ). *Med. Sci. Sports Exerc.* **2004**, *36*, 556. [CrossRef] [PubMed]
30. Wells, K.F.; Dillon, E.K. The sit and reach—A test of back and leg flexibility. *Res. Q* **1952**, *23*, 115–118. [CrossRef]
31. Chillón, P.; Castro-Piñero, J.; Ruiz, J.R.; Soto, V.M.; Carbonell-Baeza, A.; Dafos, J.; Vicente-Rodríguez, G.; Castillo, M.J.; Ortega, F.B. Hip flexibility is the main determinant of the back-saver sit-and-reach test in adolescents. *J. Sports Sci.* **2010**, *28*, 641–648. [CrossRef] [PubMed]
32. Ponce-González, J.G.; Gutiérrez-Manzanedo, J.V.; De Castro-Maqueda, G.; Fernández-Torres, V.J.; Fernández-Santos, J.R. The federated practice of soccer influences hamstring flexibility in healthy adolescents: Role of age and weight status. *Sports* **2020**, *8*, 49. [CrossRef] [PubMed]
33. Gutiérrez-Manzanedo, J.V.; Fernández-Santos, J.R.; Ponce-González, J.G.; Lagares-Franco, C.; De Castro-Maqueda, G. Hamstring extensibility in female elite soccer players. *Retos. Nuevas Tend. Educ. Fís. Deportes Recreac.* **2018**, *33*, 175–178.
34. Ruiz, J.R.; Castro-Piñero, J.; Artero, E.G.; Ortega, F.B.; Sjöström, M.; Suni, J.; Castillo, M.J. Predictive validity of health-related fitness in youth: A systematic review. *Br. J. Sports Med.* **2009**, *43*, 909–923. [CrossRef] [PubMed]
35. Zemková, E.; Kováčiková, Z. Sport-specific training induced adaptations in postural control and their relationship with athletic performance. *Front. Hum. Neurosci.* **2023**, *16*, 1007804. [CrossRef] [PubMed] [PubMed Central]
36. Behm, D.G.; Wahl, M.J.; Button, D.C.; Power, K.E.; Anderson, K.G. Relationship between hockey skating speed and selected performance measures. *J. Strength Cond. Res.* **2005**, *19*, 326–331. [CrossRef] [PubMed]
37. Paillard, T.; Margnes, E.; Portet, M.; Breucq, A. Postural ability reflects the athletic skill level of surfers. *Eur. J. Appl. Physiol.* **2011**, *111*, 1619–1623. [CrossRef] [PubMed]
38. Mendez-Villanueva, A.; Bishop, D. Physiological aspects of surfboard riding performance. *Sports Med.* **2005**, *35*, 55–70. [CrossRef]
39. Igual Camacho, C.; Serra Añó, P.; Alakdar, Y.; Cebriá, M.A.; López Bueno, L. Estudio comparativo del efecto de la actividad física en el equilibrio en personas mayores sanas. *Fisioterapia* **2008**, *30*, 137–141. [CrossRef]
40. Farley, O.; Harris, N.K.; Kilding, A.E. Anaerobic and aerobic fitness profiling of competitive surfers. *J. Strength Cond. Res.* **2012**, *26*, 2243–22488. [CrossRef] [PubMed]
41. Benninger, E.; Curtis, C.; Sarkisian, G.V.; Rogers, C.M.; Bender, K.; Comer, M. Surf Therapy: A Scoping Review of the Qualitative and Quantitative Research Evidence. *Glob. J. Community Psychol. Pract.* **2020**, *11*, 1–26. [CrossRef]
42. Veldema, J.; Jansen, P. Aquatic therapy in stroke rehabilitation: Systematic review and meta-analysis. *Acta Neurol. Scand.* **2021**, *143*, 221–241. [CrossRef] [PubMed]
43. Bartels, E.M.; Juhl, C.B.; Christensen, R.; Hagen, K.B.; Danneskiold-Samsøe, B.; Dagfinrud, H.; Lund, H. Aquatic exercise for the treatment of knee and hip osteoarthritis. *Cochrane Database Syst Rev.* **2016**, *3*, CD005523. [CrossRef] [PubMed] [PubMed Central]
44. Peretro, G.; Ballico, A.L.; Avelar, N.C.; Haupenthal, D.P.D.S.; Arcêncio, L.; Haupenthal, A. Comparison of aquatic physiotherapy and therapeutic exercise in patients with chronic low back pain. *J. Bodyw. Mov. Ther.* **2024**, *38*, 399–405. [CrossRef] [PubMed]
45. Bhat, R.; Moiz, J.A. Comparison of dynamic balance in collegiate field hockey and football players using star excursion balance test. *Asian J. Sports Med.* **2013**, *4*, 221–229. [CrossRef] [PubMed] [PubMed Central]
46. Silva, B.; Clemente, F.M. Physical performance characteristics between male and female youth surfing athletes. *J. Sports Med. Phys. Fit.* **2019**, *59*, 171–178. [CrossRef] [PubMed]
47. Barton, J.; Pretty, J. What is the best dose of nature and green exercise for improving mental health? A multi-study analysis. *Environ. Sci. Technol.* **2010**, *44*, 3947–3955. [CrossRef] [PubMed]

48. Molina García, J.; Castillo Fernández, I.; Pablos, C. Bienestar psicológico y práctica deportiva en universitarios. *Eur. J. Hum. Mov.* **2007**, *18*, 79–91.
49. Monteiro, L.A.; Novaes, J.S.; Santos, M.L.; Fernandes, H.M. Body dissatisfaction and self-esteem in female students aged 9–15: The effects of age, family income, body mass index levels and dance practice. *J. Hum. Kinet.* **2014**, *43*, 25–32. [CrossRef] [PubMed] [PubMed Central]
50. Hearn, B.; Biscaldi, M.; Rauh, R.; Fleischhaker, C. Feasibility and effectiveness of a group therapy combining physical activity, surf therapy and cognitive behavioural therapy to treat adolescents with depressive disorders: A pilot study. *Front. Psychol.* **2025**, *16*, 1426844. [CrossRef] [PubMed] [PubMed Central]

MDPI AG
Grosspeteranlage 5
4052 Basel
Switzerland
Tel.: +41 61 683 77 34

Journal of Functional Morphology and Kinesiology Editorial Office
E-mail: jfmk@mdpi.com
www.mdpi.com/journal/jfmk

www.ingramcontent.com/pod-product-compliance
Lightning Source LLC
Chambersburg PA
CBHW061608210926
51850CB00009B/2252
9783725864140